The Veterinary General Practice Casebook

A harmless-looking papilloma on Monday morning, a fitting Bulldog on Wednesday afternoon, a pyometra last thing on Friday – *The Veterinary General Practice Casebook* echoes life at the coalface of companion animal practice. Organised into 'clinics', each chapter feels like a day in the life of a busy general practitioner, where emergencies are juggled with routine consultations and every so often something unexpected pops up.

Ideal for senior veterinary students, new graduates, those returning to practice, and those seeking a general practice workout, this book presents cases as they appear in real life, often messier and less complete than textbook descriptions. The clinical content is complemented by topics on wellbeing and professional practice, as well as recipes for simple and nutritious meals to feed veterinary body and soul.

This book makes a persuasive argument for general practice as a specialty in its own right and celebrates the role of general practice veterinarians and their vital contribution to animal health and welfare in the community.

The Veterinary General Practice Casebook

Companion Animal Clinics

Edited by
ANDREW GARDINER
ANNE QUAIN

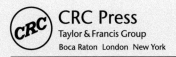

CRC Press
Taylor & Francis Group
Boca Raton London New York

CRC Press is an imprint of the
Taylor & Francis Group, an **informa** business

Cover image shows Alice Gilmour, veterinary student, examining a dog in general practice.

First edition published 2025
by CRC Press
2385 NW Executive Center Drive, Suite 320, Boca Raton, FL 33431

and by CRC Press
4 Park Square, Milton Park, Abingdon, Oxon, OX14 4RN

CRC Press is an imprint of Taylor & Francis Group, LLC

ISBN: 9781032243771 (hbk)
ISBN: 9781032243764 (pbk)
ISBN: 9781003278306 (ebk)

DOI: 10.1201/9781003278306

Typeset in Janson Text LT Pro
by Evolution Design & Digital Ltd (Kent)

To family, human & animal, passed & present
(AG)

To Stephen, with love
(AQ)

CONTENTS

Veterinary general practitioners provide comprehensive, continuing medical care to animals in the community. They work in a wide variety of places, from inner cities to remote and rural locations, and typically see a broad range of cases, drawing on knowledge from different medical disciplines. Many of these disciplines also exist as clinical specialties and general practitioners may refer cases to specialist colleagues or seek advice from them. When referral is not available or affordable, general practitioners provide care appropriate to the economic and clinical context.

In medical education, general practice (sometimes also called primary care, family medicine, or community medicine) is a fully-formed specialty. Medical GPs provide long-term continuity of care for their patients. They build relationships over time, learning not only what is normal for individuals, but gaining insights into their patients' lifestyles, relationships, and preferences. Like veterinarians, they work in a wide variety of locations, and their work is informed by knowledge of the particular community in which they practice. Dedicated postgraduate training helps doctors develop the multifaceted biomedical and social competences that are the hallmark of good general practice.

While veterinary general practice has much in common with its medical counterpart, it is not currently seen as a specialism that requires specific postgraduate training. When one of the authors asked a group of final-year veterinary students what they understood by the term general practice, the answer was, 'what is not covered by our clinical rotations'. The students found it difficult to define general practice except as a negative in this way. This could make general practice seem less desirable as a field in which to pursue a whole career. New graduates are deemed competent to enter general practice on day 1 after graduation, but if they choose to work as a specialist vet, they must undertake extensive additional training and examinations. In terms of net contribution and impact on animal care and welfare, however, general practice dwarfs all other fields. There is therefore a compelling argument for general practice to be further developed as a subject in veterinary education.

The boundaries between general and specialty practice in veterinary medicine are not always clear (Gardiner et al. 2011, McKenzie 2024). Most clinical teaching in traditional veterinary schools (i.e. those with teaching hospitals) is currently provided by specialists.* This ensures that students are exposed to high standards and the latest developments in individual specialisms. An unintended consequence could be that students graduate with knowledge of 'gold standard' treatments without being equipped to provide the spectrum of care required in general practice (Fingland et al. 2021, Quain et al. 2021, Skipper et al. 2021). It may also mean

---

* Distributed model veterinary schools do not have in-house clinics and hospitals, relying on external partners as providers. This may offer more potential for clinical teaching grounded in general practice, but may also make it more challenging to provide a consistent approach in this teaching. Each model has advantages and disadvantages.

that students gain less experience of work that features prominently in general practice but has never been a major part of the taught curriculum. A good example, at least until fairly recently, was companion animal dentistry (Anderson et al. 2017).

Fortunately, veterinary general practice is experiencing something of a renaissance. Practitioners in the UK can apply for Advanced Practitioner status in small animal practice.* The Australian and New Zealand College of Veterinary Scientists (ANZCVS) has offered membership in small animal practice by examination since 2019.† Veterinary school accrediting bodies, including the Royal College of Veterinary Surgeons (RCVS), the American Veterinary Medical Association (AVMA), and the Australasian Veterinary Boards Council (AVBC), now emphasise the importance of equipping veterinary graduates with general practice competences. And the RCVS stipulates that 70% of students' experience of cases should reflect general practice.

RATIONALE FOR THIS BOOK

The self-assessment colour review format was originally developed within medical education, but soon found its way into veterinary publishing. Currently available books tend to focus on specific companion animal disciplines and are invaluable for experienced practitioners in pursuit of extra information and those working towards further qualifications. This book uses the same engaging format, but addresses the interests of those who seek an overview of the whole field of companion animal practice, whether they are clinical veterinary students, recent graduates, returning to practice after a break, or moving from another field. It presents a variety of cases in a way that reflects the unpredictable real world of the clinic, which calls for ophthalmology at one moment and orthopaedics the next. Each chapter represents a day of the week and the case headers present information in the – occasionally misleading – way that this appears on consulting room screens. The answers are comprehensive and include a few references.

Of course, there is a limit to what can be done in *c.* 300 pages. But even if it were possible to cover every condition likely to be seen in general companion animal practice, we would not wish to do so. The joy and intellectual challenge of general practice lie in the unpredictability and variety of presentations, diagnoses, contexts, and constraints encountered on a daily basis. In working through this book, the reader will develop an approach that can be applied to all cases, including those in which a definitive diagnosis is not possible – a not uncommon situation.

Taking time to rest, refuel, and reflect is vital but easy to ignore in practice. We know from experience that team members – like our patients – are embodied beings who cannot function well when energy runs low. As a reminder – and it is a serious one – we have included several wellbeing items and a few quick recipes in the text (all recipes have been tested multiple times).

Both editors work as small animal general practitioners and academics. We have 45 years of clinical experience between us. Our contributors have extensive experience of general practice, whether they currently work in this field or remain active in it through teaching and/or research. Some have gained advanced practitioner status on the basis of the diverse caseloads typical of primary care; others have acquired clinical or non-clinical specialisms but still maintain strong connections with general practice. They work in a range of countries and jurisdictions, so the cases reflect a variety of practice contexts, including in terms of legislation and prescribing practices.

---

*   See *www.rcvs.org.uk/lifelong-learning/professional-accreditation/advanced-practitioner-status/*.

†   See *www.anzcvs.org.au/chapters/veterinary+practice+small+animal*.

In writing this book, we had the luxury of space to reflect on and read about cases, and to seek the opinions of multiple colleagues. In several instances, their views on patient assessment and management differed, but were supported by equally compelling justifications – even in this era of evidence-based veterinary medicine. We acknowledge that, for valid reasons, readers may sometimes disagree with the answers in this book. The ability to make a decision in the face of conflicting information and/or interests is part of the art of veterinary practice.

This book provides an overview of veterinary practice at a time of increasing debate about what should come into the remit of general practice and what requires specialist care (McKenzie 2024). We believe it is important that this debate continues, and that it should begin to feature in veterinary education. We were interested by how many of the general practitioners we invited to contribute to this book hesitated because they were 'just a GP' or 'might not know enough' or believed themselves 'not qualified enough to write for publication' – sometimes after decades of relevant experience. Do general practitioners have a higher incidence of impostor syndrome than specialist colleagues (Kogan et al. 2020)? The profession needs more initiatives that enable general practitioners to contribute to veterinary education, ones that recognise their expertise in managing complexity and understanding contexts when dealing with the many multifactorial human–animal issues encountered on a daily basis.

HOW TO USE THIS BOOK

If you are moved to discuss cases with a colleague or mentor, if you find yourself sourcing veterinary and medical textbooks, if the questions (signified by blue banners) raise additional questions you feel compelled to answer, if you download articles onto your device to dive deeper, go to a library, or start a conversation with a colleague, then we will have achieved what we set out to do.

The model answers in this book (signified by red banners) reflect the particular approaches of our contributors. There are, however, often several different ways to address the questions posed. The answers are not intended to provide definitive solutions, nor could they hope to do so; veterinary practice is a rapidly evolving field, with new products, techniques, research, and guidelines emerging at pace. Similarly, when we ask readers to make lists, we do not expect them to nail every item that appears in the answer.

Questions and answers with a wellbeing theme are signified by green banners, while recipes are signified by orange banners. Most of the references cited appear in the answers section, with the publications listed at the end of each case discussion. Where a reference is occasionally mentioned in the questions section, the relevant publication details will be found in the answers.

While factual information is undoubtedly empowering, it is more important to know where to find information than to be able to regurgitate it, and even more vital not to overlook the evidence that is presented to the clinician's senses in the consulting room and operating theatre. To repurpose an old clinical pearl that seems especially relevant to general practice: *More is missed by not looking than not knowing.*

We hope you enjoy this book.

Andrew Gardiner, Edinburgh
Anne Quain, Sydney

This book has been produced for the purposes of self-testing, and not as a textbook, handbook, or comprehensive guide to case management. Readers should be aware that information provided may not apply in the contexts in which they practise. For example, legislation and access to pharmaceuticals vary across jurisdictions. Dose rates included are a guide only and should be checked carefully before administration. Use of medications mentioned may be off-label in some cases.

REFERENCES

Anderson, J. G., Goldstein, G. S., Boudreaux, K. A. & Ilkiw, J. E. (2017) The state of veterinary dental education in North America, Canada, and the Caribbean: a descriptive study. *Journal of Veterinary Medical Education* **44**(2):358–363. doi: 10.3138/jvme.1215-204R.

Australasian Veterinary Boards Council (2023) *AVBC Day One Competencies 2024 – International Day One Competencies Map*. Available at: https://avbc.asn.au/veterinary-education/day-one-competencies/.

Fingland, R. B., Stone, L. R., Read, E. K. & Moore, R. M. (2021) Preparing veterinary students for excellence in general practice: building confidence and competence by focusing on spectrum of care. *Journal of the American Veterinary Medical Association* **259**(5):463–470. doi: 10.2460/javma.259.5.463.

Gardiner, A., Lowe, P. & Armstrong, J. (2011) Who or what is a veterinary specialist? *Veterinary Record* **169**(14):354–356. doi: 10.1136/vr.d5385.

Kogan, L. R., Schoenfeld-Tacher, R., Hellyer, P., Grigg, E. K. & Kramer, E. (2020) Veterinarians and impostor syndrome: an exploratory study. *Veterinary Record* **187**(7):271. doi: 10.1136/vr.105914.

McKenzie, B. (2024) Do it yourself or send for help? Considering specialty referral from a general practitioner perspective. *Journal of the American Veterinary Medical Association* **262**(5):1–6. doi: 10.2460/javma.23.11.0612.

Quain, A., Ward, M. P. & Mullan, S. (2021) Ethical challenges posed by advanced veterinary care in companion animal veterinary practice. *Animals* **11**(11):3010. doi: 10.3390/ani11113010.

Skipper, A., Gray, C., Serlin, R. et al. (2021) 'Gold standard care' is an unhelpful term. *Veterinary Record* **189**(8):331. doi: 10.1002/vetr.1113.

Clinical information can be found in standard texts. The following books are particularly suited to the general practice context. The older titles are still relevant and available. Books covering animal welfare and ethics are included since these disciplines can aid clinical decision-making in different contexts.

Adams, C. L. & Kurtz, S. (2017) *Skills for Communicating in Veterinary Medicine.* Parsippany, NJ: Dewpoint Publishing.

BSAVA Foundation Manuals, published by the British Small Animal Veterinary Association (Gloucester):

- Baines, S. J., Lipscomb, V. & Hitchinson, T. (eds) (2012) *Manual of Canine and Feline Surgical Principles*
- Harvey, A. & Tasker, S. (eds) (2013) *Manual of Feline Practice*
- Hitchinson, T. & Robinson, K. (eds) (2015) *Manual of Canine Practice*
- Holloway, A. & McConnell, J. F. (eds) (2013) *Manual of Canine and Feline Radiography and Radiology*
- Meredith, A. & Johnson-Delaney, C. (eds) (2010) *Manual of Exotic Pets*

Englar, R. E. & Dial, S. M. (2023) *Low-Cost Veterinary Diagnostics.* Hoboken, NJ: Wiley Blackwell.

Gorrel, C. (2013) *Veterinary Dentistry for the General Practitioner*, 2nd edition. London: Elsevier.

Gough, A. & Murphy, K. F. (2015) *Differential Diagnosis in Small Animal Medicine*, 2nd edition. Oxford: Wiley Blackwell.

Hill, P., Warman, S. & Shawcross, G. (2011) *100 Top Consultations in Small Animal General Practice.* Oxford: Wiley Blackwell.

Hunt, G. B. (ed.) (2017) *Pitfalls in Veterinary Surgery.* Oxford: Wiley Blackwell.

Maddison, J. E., Volk, H. A. & Church, D. B. (2022) *Clinical Reasoning in Small Animal* Practice, 2nd edition. Oxford: Wiley Blackwell.

Mullan, S. & Fawcett, A. (2017) *Veterinary Ethics: Navigating Tough Cases.* Sheffield: 5m Publishing Limited.

Shepherd, K. (2021) *Demystifying Dog Behaviour for the Veterinarian.* Abingdon: CRC Press.

Yeates, J. (2013) *Animal Welfare in Veterinary Practice.* Wheathampstead: UFAW/Wiley Blackwell Animal Welfare Series.

The editors would like to thank the following individuals who have freely given time, ideas, and expertise to help in the development of this project at different stages in its gestation. Their generosity, insights, image libraries, subject matter expertise, moral support, and practical assistance have been invaluable.

Dr Graeme Allan, Professor Sarah Baillie, Sue Bradley, Emeritus Professor Paul Canfield, Dr Georgina Child, Dr Megan Clisby, Dr Sarah Davies, Tracy Duffy, Dr Timothy Foo, Dr Allan Gunn, Dr Norman Johnston, Professor Tiziana Liuti, Dr Josephine Lusk, Frances MacAllister, Dr Erin Mooney, Professor John Munday, Professor Jacqueline Norris, Dr Stephen Page, Cheryl Palmer, Professor Susan Rhind, Antoinette, John, and Ron Riley, Professor Tobias Schwarz, Dr Glenn Shea, Amy Shi, Professor Jan Šlapeta, Dr Robin Stanley, The Unusual Pet Vets, Professor Denis Verwilghen, Kristina Vesk OAM, Veterinary Medical Education Division (VMED) at the Royal (Dick) School of Veterinary Studies, Dr Jeremy Watson and Brimbank Veterinary Clinic, Holly Webb, Dr Jane Whitley, and 10 anonymous international reviewers.

Thank you to Alice Gilmour and rescue puppy Neville for allowing us to feature you both on the cover. We would also like to thank the team at Potts Point Veterinary Hospital, the Sydney School of Veterinary Science, and the Society of Authors for their support.

We are very grateful to the guardians of animals who allowed photographs to be taken specifically for inclusion in this book. Veterinary education depends on exposure to clinical cases, and these images are invaluable. There are some concepts that, for ethical or practical reasons, we were not able to capture using photos. Sally Pope (*www.spediting.com.au*) worked with us to create beautiful bespoke illustrations to support the text.

Bringing this book to life would not have been possible without the support of Alice Oven, Shikha Garg, Alison Nick, Linda Leggio (Taylor & Francis/CRC Press), and Claire Furey (*www.editingfurey.com*). We sought to create a book that reflected the reality of veterinary general practice, and the publishing professionals got behind it enthusiastically.

Sam Abraham A5.21; **Lucinda Alderton-Sell** 5.8; **Graeme Allan** 1.12ab, A2.19ab, A3.10ab, 5.12; **Annie Basile** 4.1a; **Jude Bradbury** 2.13ab, A2.13a–g, 4.4, 4.15, 5.1a–c, 'Cheesecake' 1–16; **Nichola Calvani** A4.9, 5.14, A5.14; **Chantal Celindano** A4.8; **Wesley Cheung** 4.6; **Stephen Cutter** 1.21a, 3.14, 4.14ab; **Sarah Davies** A1.8ab, A4.16ab, 4.19b, A4.19a–d; **Louise Dingley** 3.9ab, A3.9; **Kiterie Faller** 5.17; **Timothy Foo** 4.18bc; **Andrew Gardiner** 1.7b, A1.9, 1.13ab, 1.14ab, 1.16, A1.16ab, 1.17, A2.4, 2.7, 2.8, 2.11, 2.15, 3.2, 3.17a–c, A3.3a, 4.1b, 4.3, A4.3; **Mike Guilliard** 1.15, A1.15ab, 4.10, A4.10ab; **Christine Hawke** A1.3, 5.16, A5.16; **Robert Johnson** 3.16a–c, A3.16ab; **Norman Johnston** 1.11a–c; **Katherine Littlewood** 5.4b; **Tiziana Liuti** 1.17, 3.3, 4.7a; **Fabrizio Montarsi** A4.12; **Tanya Moroney** 1.6; **Sonja Olson** 5.23a; **Sally Pope** A1.20, A2.8, A3.3b, A3.20, A4.10c, A5.15ab, A5.19bc; **Anne Quain** 1.1, 1.2, 1.3a–d, 1.4, 1.5, 1.7a, 1.8ab, 1.9, 1.10, A1.4a–d, A1.10ab, 1.21b, A1.21, 1.22, 2.1, 2.2, 2.3, 2.9a–c, 2.10, A2.11, 2.12, 2.14, 2.16, 2.18, 2.19, A2.20, 2.21ab, 3.1, A3.1, A3.3c, 3.5ab, 3.7, 3.8ab, A3.8, 3.10, 3.13, A3.14ab, 3.15, 3.18, 3.20, 3.21ab, 3.22ab, 4.2ab, 4.5ab, 4.8ab, 4.9, 4.16, 4.18a, 4.20, A4.20, 4.21ab, 5.2, 5.4a, 5.6, A5.8, 5.10ab, 5.11ab, 5.13ab, 5.15, 5.18ab, 5.19ab, A5.19a, 5.21, 5.22, A5.22ab, 5.23b; **Andrea Roe** 1.19; **Kendal Shepherd** A2.2; **Shutterstock** 4.13, 5.7; **Jan Šlapeta** 3.19; **Anna Sri** 1.18ab, A1.18; **Robin Stanley** 2.4, 4.11b; **Jenny Stavisky** 4.11a, 4.11c; **Kate Toyer** 2.20, 3.4ab, A3.4; **Unusual Pet Vets** 2.5, A2.5, 2.17, A3.13ab; **Rob Ward** 3.12, 4.7b, 4.17, 5.5; **Jeremy Watson** 4.12ab; **Heather Woodke** 5.3ab, 5.20ab; **Kate Worthing** 4.19a; **Holly Yang** A1.1ab.

2.6ab, A2.6a: Reproduced with permission from Verstraete, F. J. M. & Tsugawa, A. J. (eds) (2016) *Self-Assessment Color Review of Veterinary Dentistry*, 2nd edition. Boca Raton, FL: CRC Press.

A2.6b: Reproduced with permission from Niemiec, B. A. (2012) *A Colour Handbook of Small Animal Dental, Oral and Maxillofacial Disease*. Boca Raton, FL: CRC Press.

Andrew Gardiner *BVM&S Cert SAS MSc PhD DipECAWBM (AWSEL) MRCVS* spent 16 years in general practice, during which time he obtained the Royal College of Veterinary Surgeons (RCVS) Certificate in Small Animal Surgery. He was awarded a doctoral scholarship in medical humanities to research 20th-century British veterinary education and practice at the Wellcome Unit for the History of Medicine, University of Manchester, after which he joined the staff of the Royal (Dick) School of Veterinary Studies (R(D)SVS), University of Edinburgh, as a veterinary clinical lecturer focusing on general practice. Since 2009, working with students and volunteer veterinarians, he has run All4Paws, an accessible veterinary care practice for homeless and vulnerably-housed animal owners in Edinburgh. He is a Diplomate of the European College of Animal Welfare and Behavioural Medicine in Animal Welfare Science, Ethics and Law, and Professor of Veterinary Medical Humanities at the R(D)SVS.

Anne Quain *BA BScVet BVSc MVetStud GradCertEdStud(HigherEd) MANZCVS (Animal Welfare) DipECAWBM (AWSEL) PhD* graduated with her BVSc from the University of Sydney in 2005. She is a senior lecturer in the Sydney School of Veterinary Science and also works in private practice. She is a member of the Australian and New Zealand College of Veterinary Scientists (ANZCVS) in Animal Welfare Science, Ethics and Law; a Diplomate of the European College of Animal Welfare and Behavioural Medicine in Animal Welfare Science, Ethics and Law; and has a PhD in veterinary ethics. Together with Siobhan Mullan, she co-wrote *Veterinary Ethics: Navigating Tough Cases*. She also co-edited *The Vet Cookbook: A Collegial Collaboration* and is working on the second edition. She is passionate about general practice, clinical and ethical decision-making, and animal welfare. In 2023, she received a Fear Free Research Award in recognition of her commitment to alleviating fear, anxiety, and stress in animals through research, and in 2024, a Centenary Medal from the NSW Veterinary Practitioner's Board for Animal Welfare Leadership in Veterinary Ethics and Animal Welfare.

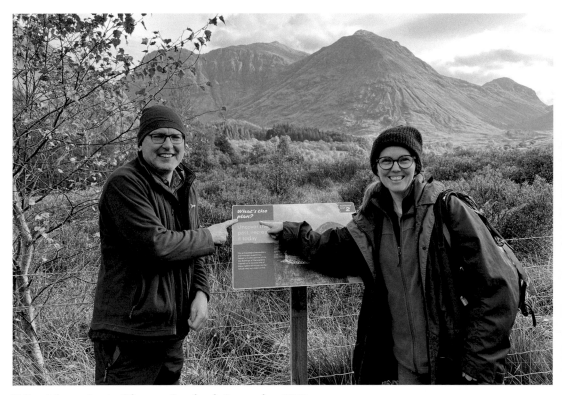

Editorial meeting in Glencoe, Scotland, September 2023.

Lucinda Alderton-Sell *BVetMed GPCert(SAM) MANZCVS (Medicine of Cats) MRCVS* graduated from the Royal Veterinary College, London. She had always wanted to work in the charitable sector, and so joined the People's Dispensary for Sick Animals (PDSA) after qualification. In 2013, Lucinda completed her General Practitioner Certificate in Small Animal Medicine, which helped cement her interest in everything feline. She then moved to Cats Protection, where she combines her love of feline medicine and welfare with pragmatic charity medicine. Lucinda has a particular interest in contextualised care and its application in general practice. She gained membership of the ANZCVS in Medicine of Cats in 2021. (Case 5.8)

Jude Bradbury *BVSc CertAVP(SAM) PGDipVetEd FHEA MRCVS* graduated from Liverpool University in 2010 and worked in general, referral, and emergency practice. She has built her career promoting evidence-based veterinary general practice, with numerous peer-reviewed publications spanning internal medicine and emergency and critical care. She left clinical practice to move into education, teaching veterinary nurses, then managing the RCVS Statutory Membership Examination for overseas veterinarians wishing to work in the UK. Jude continues to educate both veterinary and veterinary nurse students and graduates in general practice in her current role as Senior Teaching Fellow at the Royal Veterinary College, London. (Cases 2.13, 4.4, 4.15, 5.1)

Victoria Brookes *BVM&S GCLTHE MANZCVS (Avian Health) MPH&TM PhD FHEA FANZCVS (Epidemiology) FRCVS* spent 15 years in general practice in the UK and Australia, where she had diverse interests including avian health, orthopaedics, and production animal medicine. Since completing her PhD in 2014, she has focused on epidemiology and combining her broad experience and expertise across animal and human health to promote One Health (integrated animal, human, and ecosystem health). As well as teaching, she researches emerging infectious diseases in the Asia-Pacific region, contributing to national and international policy and practice for emerging infectious disease response and pandemic preparedness. (Case 5.9)

Nichola Calvani *AVBS PhD* is a lecturer in parasitology and an Australian Research Council Discovery Early Career Researcher Award Fellow at the University of Sydney, Australia. She completed a PhD on the molecular diagnosis and distribution of *Fasciola* spp. in Southeast Asia, before embarking on a postdoctoral research position at the University of Galway, Ireland. There she worked on immunology, cell biology, and immunodiagnosis of helminths under the supervision of Professor John Dalton. Alongside her academic pursuits, she is an advocate for gender equity in the discipline of parasitology, as evidenced by her initiative 'Herminthology'. She also has extensive experience working in commercial and government diagnostic laboratories. (Cases 4.9, 5.14)

Chantal Celindano *BVSc MANZCVS (Medicine of Cats) ISFM AdvCert FB* has dedicated her 20 years in practice to feline medicine, working in cat hospitals in Melbourne, Sydney, Brisbane, and London. She has obtained postgraduate qualifications in feline medicine and is an International Society for Feline Medicine (ISFM) Advanced Practitioner and an ANZCVS mentor. Chantal also runs a house-call clinic exclusively for cats called Feline Fine Mobile Vet in Brisbane, Australia. Her passion is addressing the cat as a whole, within their environment, as well as preventive medicine to give cats the highest quality of life possible, as every cat deserves. (Cases 4.8, 5.6)

Wesley Cheung *BVSc* graduated from the University of Sydney and started his career in small animal general practice. He later undertook an internship in emergency and critical care and worked as an emergency veterinarian. During this time, he also volunteered with animal shelters and community programmes. Following this passion for shelter medicine, he pursued a shelter medicine internship at Cornell University, and served as a shelter veterinarian at Toronto Humane Society. He is currently the first clinical resident in shelter medicine in Canada, based at the Ontario Veterinary College, and is involved in teaching, shelter consultative work, and community medicine clinics. (Case 4.6)

Stephen Cutter *BVSc* has spent 29 years in diverse general practice, mostly in the Northern Territory of Australia. During that time, he has regularly provided veterinary services to remote indigenous communities across the northern west quarter of Australia. He helped establish Animal Management in Rural and Remote Indigenous Communities (AMRRIC), a registered charity that helps provide remote veterinary services sustainably.

Stephen also runs The Ark Animal Hospital, a busy general practice in Palmerston, out of Darwin, and provides veterinary services to several wildlife parks. (Case 4.14)

Louise Dingley *BVMS PGCert FHEA MRCVS* graduated from the University of Glasgow in 2012 and worked in general practice for 2 years in her home county of Lancashire. She then moved to Edinburgh to complete a small animal rotating internship at the R(D)SVS, followed by locum GP work throughout the UK, while developing interests in soft tissue and laparoscopic surgery. She returned to the R(D)SVS and its Dick Vet General Practice, where she introduced laparoscopic spays to the service. A developing love of teaching in the general practice context led to a move to academia in 2024: she took up a lectureship in Veterinary Primary Care and Leadership at the University of Central Lancashire (UCLan). She is currently responsible for a part-time, online postgraduate certificate and Master's programme in Veterinary Primary Care and Leadership at UCLan. (Case 3.9)

Kiterie Faller *DVM DPhil DipECVN MRCVS* is Professor of Comparative Neurology at the R(D)SVS, University of Edinburgh. After graduating from the École Nationale Vétérinaire de Toulouse, she underwent residency training at the University of Glasgow and obtained a PhD from the University of Oxford. As a specialist in neurology with a strong research background, her work combines her interests in clinical neurology, research, and teaching. (Case 5.17)

Mike Guilliard *MA VetMB Cert SAO FRCVS* has been in general practice for over 50 years, during which he has maintained a professional interest in Greyhound injuries, resulting in numerous peer-reviewed publications, book chapters, and lecture invitations. In 2012, he was made a Fellow of the RCVS for his thesis entitled 'The nature, incidence and response to treatment of injuries to the distal limbs in the racing Greyhound'. In 2014, he was awarded the British Small Animal Veterinary Association (BSAVA) Simon Award for outstanding contributions in the field of veterinary surgery. (Cases 1.15, 4.10)

Christine Hawke *BSc(Vet) BVSc PhD MANZCVS (Veterinary Dentistry)* spent several years in general practice in Australia and the UK before completing her PhD studies in immunogenetics. Following this, she worked at the University of Sydney, teaching general practice and professional practice skills to undergraduate veterinary students. This is where she became addicted to small animal dentistry. She became a member (by examination) of the ANZCVS in the field of veterinary dentistry in 2006, and has worked exclusively in this field ever since. She is currently in private referral practice in Sydney. (Case 5.16)

James Hunt *BVetMed MSc PhD CertVA DipECAWBM(AWSEL) MRCVS* spent 15 years working in general practice prior to undertaking research in canine and feline analgesia. He currently divides his time between operating a chronic pain management service and working as a clinical anaesthetist in a referral hospital. (Case 2.14)

Louisa Johnson *BVSc MOccHlthSfty MANZCVS (Small Animal Medicine) Cert IV TAE* has a keen interest in veterinary team welfare, and works to improve the health and safety outcomes for veterinarians, veterinary nurses, and veterinary students through research, evidence-based health and safety training, and support. Her Master's thesis was on the health and safety of Australian veterinarians, veterinary nurses, and veterinary students. (Case 3.21)

Robert Johnson *AM BVSc BA MANZCVS FAVA* graduated from the University of Sydney in 1977. He is a Fellow and Past President of the Australian Veterinary Association and a Life Member of ANZCVS, and he holds a Certificate in Zoological Medicine from the RCVS (UK). Robert taught reptile and wildlife medicine at James Cook University and is currently a tutor at the University of Sydney. In 2022, he was appointed a Member of the Order of Australia for distinguished service to veterinary science. During his final year in clinical practice, Robert was bitten by an eastern brown snake; he recovered, and so did the snake. (Case 3.16)

Corinna Klupiec *BVSc PhD GradCertEdStud(HigherEd)* is a graduate of the University of Sydney. Her professional experience spans clinical practice, research, veterinary education, digital/audiovisual communication, and industry. Corinna's special interests include education and environmental sustainability, with a particular emphasis on the urgent need for climate action. (Cases 2.4 [with AQ], 4.12)

Margaret (Peggy) Root Kustritz *DVM, PhD, DACT, MMedEd* is a 1987 graduate of the University of Minnesota College of Veterinary Medicine, where she earned her DVM and PhD and completed a residency in theriogenology. Her PhD thesis was entitled 'The effect of prepuberal and postpuberal gonadectomy on the general health and development of obesity in the male and female domestic cat'. She completed a Master's in Medical Education and Leadership in 2015. She is currently employed as a Professor in Small Animal Reproduction at the University of Minnesota College of Veterinary Medicine, where she also serves as Associate Dean of Education. (Cases 3.15, 4.16)

Kat Littlewood *BVSc PGDipVCS AFHEA PhD FANZCVS(AWSEL)* is a Senior Lecturer at Massey University in New Zealand. She is a registered veterinary specialist in Animal Welfare Science, Ethics and Law. Kat is passionate about enhancing veterinarians' understanding of their role as animal welfare experts. She also works to operationalise the Five Domains Model for animal welfare assessment and training. Kat's research employs social science approaches to improve our understanding of complex human–animal interactions and ethically challenging situations. She aims to develop a nuanced understanding of why and how people manage animals. (Case 5.4)

Laura McGuffog *DVM CHPV, CPEV* completed her veterinary studies at the University of Sydney in 2019. Prior to this she attended the Australian National University where she majored in zoology and immunology/microbiology. Laura is the lead veterinarian for Rest Your Paws in the Australian state of Victoria. Rest Your Paws provides end-of-life care for animals in the comfort of their own home. Laura is accredited with both the International Association for Animal Hospice and Palliative Care and the Companion Animal Euthanasia Training Academy. Working with Rest Your Paws allows her to celebrate the human–animal bond and provide pets with an ending that honours the lives they have lived. (Cases 1.20, 2.11, 3.18, 4.13)

Amy Miele *BVM&S Cert Anim Behav PhD MRCVS* graduated from the R(D)SVS in 2006 and spent 5 years in mixed and small animal general practice before returning to complete her PhD. Amy is currently undertaking a part-time residency in Behavioural Medicine and is the Programme Director for the University of Edinburgh MSc in Clinical Animal Behaviour. (Cases 1.19, 3.6)

Sonja Olson *DVM* grew up in Maryland, USA. She graduated from the Virginia–Maryland Regional College of Veterinary Medicine with a focus on exotic animal and conservation medicine. She has over 25 years experience in small animal and exotic emergency medicine. Dr Olson is currently Veterinary Wellness Educator for her own business, Heartstorming Wellness LLC, based in Vancouver, Washington State. She is an advisory board member for MentorVet and the Washington State Veterinary Medical Association (WSVMA) Board of Directors Committee Lead for Veterinary Wellbeing on the Diversity Equality Inclusion Wellbeing (DEIW) Committee. She is a Certified Instructor in Mental Health First Aid, Mindful Meditation, Emotional Intelligence and Psychological Safety for Leaders and AVMA Train-the-Trainer for Wellbeing in the Workplace. She is the author of *Creating Well-being and Building Resilience in the Veterinary Profession: A Call to Life* (2022). (Case 5.23)

Ri Scarborough *BVSc* is a veterinarian with an interest in One Health. She is currently undertaking a PhD examining veterinary antimicrobial use at the Melbourne Veterinary School and the multidisciplinary National Centre for Antimicrobial Stewardship (NCAS). Her main interest is the complexity of clinical decision-making and how best to support clinicians to use antimicrobials well. (Cases 1.9, 2.16)

Sallianne Schlacks *DVM DACVIM* is an internal medicine specialist who teaches preclinical veterinary medicine at the University of Arizona. Prior to joining the university faculty, she practised for 7 years at the Veterinary Specialty Center of Tucson, a large specialty and emergency hospital in Tucson, Arizona. Sallianne completed her veterinary school training and residency training at the University of Illinois, then promptly moved to the more inviting climate of the southwestern desert in Tucson. When not teaching or practising medicine, she enjoys hiking, camping, and exploring music. (Case 4.19)

Kendal Shepherd *BVSc MRCVS* qualified from Bristol University in 1978. Alongside extensive experience in general practice, in 2005 she was the first veterinary surgeon in the UK to be accredited by the Association for the Study of Animal Behaviour as a certificated clinical animal behaviourist. She has been heavily involved in the anatomical and behavioural assessment of dogs for the English courts under both Sections 1 and 3 of the Dangerous Dogs Act 1991. Her present particular passions are routine education, particularly of children, in the understanding of canine communication and prevention of aggression and dog-bite incidents; the abolition of Breed Specific Legislation and a complete overhaul of the Dangerous Dogs Act; and the encouragement of all veterinary professionals to routinely safeguard the behaviour of their patients in all cases that they treat. (Cases 2.2, 4.2, 5.7)

Anna Sri *BVSc MPH* is a small animal general practice veterinarian and also has an interest in One Health. She is completing her PhD with NCAS and the Asia-Pacific Centre for Animal Health, focusing on antimicrobial stewardship in Australian veterinary practice. (Case 1.18)

Jenny Stavisky *BVM&S PhD PGCHE FHEA MRCVS* qualified as a vet from the University of Edinburgh in 2002. After some years in general practice, she took a PhD in epidemiology and virology at the University of Liverpool. Following another spell in general practice, she joined the University of Nottingham in 2010, initially as Research Fellow at the Centre for Evidence-Based Veterinary Medicine, and later as Assistant Professor in Shelter Medicine. She is a founder and honorary member of the Association of Charity Vets, co-editor of the *BSAVA Manual of Canine and Feline Shelter Medicine*, and founded Vets in the Community, a student-led service providing free veterinary care for homeless people. She joined VetPartners in 2021 as Clinical Research Manager. (Case 4.11)

Kate Toyer *BVSc MANZCVS(Surg)* Who am I? I'm Kate. Yes, I'm a vet, but most of you reading this are also vets and all the vetty degrees and stuff are kinda boring. So here is the interesting stuff. Wife, Father, Equality Advocate, Musician, Surfer, Dancer, Cancer Survivor, Trans Woman. Founder of Australian Rainbow Vets and Allies and of The Veterinary Kaleidoscope, and the recipient of a PrideVMC 2023 Leadership Award, I was named one of 15 women to watch in 2023 according to the American Animal Hospital Association and the Women's Veterinary Leadership Development Initiative. In 2024, I received a NSW Veterinary Practitioners Board Centenary Medal for service and leadership in diversity and inclusion in the veterinary profession. Oh, I also do surgery. I'm not bad at it apparently, at least that's what people say. (Cases 2.20, 3.4)

Rob Ward *BSc BVM&S FHEA DipECVAA MRCVS* qualified from the R(D)SVS in 2010 and, after a period in general practice, has pursued a career in veterinary anaesthesia, having completed internships at the R(D)SVS and an anaesthesia residency at the University of Cambridge. He was awarded the European Diploma in Veterinary Anaesthesia and Analgesia in 2023. He teaches undergraduate and postgraduate veterinary anaesthesia and has written various peer-reviewed publications on a range of topics. A current interest is the expanding use of technology in veterinary medicine. (Cases 1.16, 2.10, 3.12, 4.7, 4.17, 5.5)

Danielle Wille *BVSc* graduated from the University of Sydney in 2016. Since then she has worked in general practice on Sydney's Northern Beaches, and she is currently studying for a Foundation Certificate in Emergency & Critical Care. She also has an interest in endocrinology, inspired by her late dog Cleo's complex medical journey, on whom her contributed case is based. Danielle was the pianist for a ballet school for many years, and on her days off can be found playing the flute in a local orchestra, practising her French, and reading. (Case 4.18)

Heather Woodke *DVM MA* has been a practising veterinarian for 22 years. Following work providing ambulatory services for small ruminants and camelids in rural Washington State, she moved to Seattle to provide relief services for companion animals. During this time, she received a Master's in Bioethics and Humanities from the University of Washington. She spends most of her spare time walking the dogs on secret paths and volunteering for the Society for Veterinary Medical Ethics, a non-profit organisation dedicated to advancing work in veterinary ethics education, research, and service. (Cases 5.3, 5.20)

Kate A. Worthing *BVSc PhD PGCert (Veterinary Epidemiology and Public Health)* is a clinical veterinary microbiologist who teaches microbiology in the Sydney School of Veterinary Science during the week and moonlights in a busy general practice at weekends. After graduation from the University of Sydney, she worked in general practice before completing an internship in medicine and emergency medicine at the Animal Referral Hospital, Homebush. She returned to general practice part-time while completing a PhD in antimicrobial resistance. She enjoys teaching and nerding out over complex infectious disease cases. Outside work, she enjoys gardening and watching the adventures of her glorious chooks. (Case 4.19)

Holly Yang *BPsych, BVB, DVM* graduated from Sydney University in 2019, initially working in small animal general practice in Perth, Western Australia, before joining the Unusual Pet Vets where she treats non-traditional companion animals. She is currently a locum veterinarian at the Royal Society for the Prevention of Cruelty to Animals (RSPCA) Western Australia, treating both traditional and non-traditional companion animals. Since 2022, she has been a member of the World Small Animal Veterinary Association (WSAVA) Professional Wellness Committee, and contributed to its global Professional Wellness Guidelines. (Cases 2.5, 2.17, 3.13)

ACE	angiotensin-converting enzyme
ACL	anterior cruciate ligament (= cranial cruciate ligament)
ACTH	adrenocorticotropic hormone
ACVIM	American College of Veterinary Internal Medicine
ALP	alkaline phosphatase
ALT	alanine aminotransferase
AMRRIC	Animal Management in Rural and Remote Indigenous Communities
ANZCVS	Australian and New Zealand College of Veterinary Scientists
Apgar	appearance, pulse, grimace, activity, respiration
APTT	activated partial thromboplastin time
ASA	American Society of Anesthesiologists
ASIT	allergen-specific immunotherapy
ASPCA	American Society for the Prevention of Cruelty to Animals
AST	aspartate aminotransferase
ASV	Association of Shelter Veterinarians
AV	atrioventricular
AVBC	Australasian Veterinary Boards Council
AVMA	American Veterinary Medical Association
BAR	bright, alert, responsive
BCS	body condition score
BID	bis in die (twice daily)
BP	blood pressure
BPH	benign prostatic hyperplasia
bpm	beats per minute
BSAVA	British Small Animal Veterinary Association
BUN	blood urea nitrogen
C&S	culture and sensitivity
CBC	complete blood count
CBD	cannabidiol
CCL	cranial cruciate ligament
CDA	colour dilution alopecia
CED	canine ectodermal dysplasia
CK	creatine kinase
CKCS	Cavalier King Charles Spaniel
CKD	chronic kidney disease
CNS	central nervous system
COX	cyclooxygenase
CPR	cardiopulmonary resuscitation
CPV1	canine papillomavirus 1
CRI	constant rate infusion
CRT	capillary refill time
CSF	cerebrospinal fluid
CT	computerised tomography
DDF	deep digital flexor
DIP	distal interphalangeal
DHPP	distemper–hepatitis–parvovirus–parainfluenza
DLH	Domestic Longhair (cat)
DOCP	desoxycorticosterone pivalate
DSH	Domestic Shorthair (cat)
DV	dorsoventral
ECG	electrocardiogram
EGC	eosinophilic granuloma complex
ELISA	enzyme-linked immunosorbent assay

FCV	feline calicivirus		**MCH**	mean cellular haemoglobin
FE	female entire		**MCHC**	mean corpuscular haemoglobin concentration
FeLV	feline leukaemia virus		**MCS**	muscle condition score
FHV	feline herpesvirus		**MCV**	mean corpuscular volume
FIP	feline infectious peritonitis		**ME**	male entire
FIV	feline immunodeficiency virus		**MM**	mucous membranes
FLUTD	feline lower urinary tract disease		**MMVD**	myxomatous mitral valve disease
FN	female neutered		**MN**	male neutered
FN	false negative		**mo**	months old (i.e. age)
FNA	fine-needle aspirate			
			NAD	no abnormality detected
GDV	gastric dilatation and volvulus		**NCAS**	National Centre for Antimicrobial Stewardship
GGT	gamma-glutamyl transferase		**NHS**	National Health Service (of UK)
GIBOR	Gender Identity Bill of Rights		*NPV*	negative predictive value
GIT	gastrointestinal tract		**NSAID**	non-steroidal anti-inflammatory drug
GP	general practitioner			
			O	owner
Hb	haemoglobin		**OD**	oculus dexter (right eye)
HCT	haematocrit		**OVH**	ovariohysterectomy
HL	hindlimb		**OOH**	out of hours
hpf	high-power field		**OS**	oculus sinister (left eye)
HR	heart rate		**OU**	oculus uterque (both eyes)
ICU	intensive care unit		*P*	probability
IE	idiopathic epilepsy		**PCR**	polymerase chain reaction
IM	intramuscular(ly)		**PCV**	packed cell volume
IMHA	immune-mediated haemolytic anaemia		**PDS**	polydioxanone
IMTP	immune-mediated thrombocytopenia		**PEG**	percutaneous endoscopic gastrostomy
IN	intranasal(ly)		**PO**	per os (by mouth)
IOP	intraocular pressure		**PPE**	personal protective equipment
IRIS	International Renal Interest Society		*PPV*	positive predictive value
ISCAID	International Society for Companion Animal Infectious Diseases		**PR**	pulse rate
			PreP	pre-test probability
ISFM	International Society for Feline Medicine		**PSA**	prostate-specific antigen
			PT	prothrombin time
IV	intravenous(ly)		**PU/PD**	polyuria/polydipsia
KCS	keratoconjunctivitis sicca		**q**	every
			QOL	quality of life
LH	luteinising hormone			
			RBC	red blood cell
MBA	multiple biochemical analysis (blood tests)		**RCVS**	Royal College of Veterinary Surgeons

R(D)SVS	Royal (Dick) School of Veterinary Studies	**TNR**	trap–neuter–return
RDW	red blood cell distribution width	**TP**	total protein
RECOVER	Reassessment Campaign on Veterinary Resuscitation	*TP*	true positive
		TPE	therapeutic plasma exchange
RR	respiratory rate	**TPP**	total plasma protein
		TT4	total thyroxine
SAMe	S-adenosyl-methionine	**UCO**	ungual crest ostectomy
SBT	Staffordshire Bull Terrier	**USG**	urine specific gravity
SC	subcutaneous(ly)	**USMI**	urethral sphincter mechanism incompetence
SCC	squamous cell carcinoma		
SDF	superficial digital flexor	**UTI**	urinary tract infection
SDMA	symmetric dimethylarginine		
Se	diagnostic sensitivity	**VD**	ventrodorsal
SID	semel in die (once daily)	**VOHC**	Veterinary Oral Health Council
SIRS	systemic inflammatory response syndrome		
		WBC	white blood cell
Sp	diagnostic specificity	**WHO**	World Health Organization
SSRI	selective serotonin reuptake inhibitor	**wo**	week(s) old (i.e. age)
		WSAVA	World Small Animal Veterinary Association
STT	Schirmer tear test		
TMS	trimethoprim sulfonamide	**yo**	year old (i.e. age)
TN	true negative		

TODAY'S CASE LIST

1.1 Tony, 1-yo ME Toy Poodle: sutures out

1.2 Caramel, 15-yo FN DSH: *fit in*, arthritis injection

1.3 Xanthe, 14-mo FE Mexican Hairless Dog: health check & vacc

1.4 Chanel, 12-mo FE Pomeranian: mated by accident

1.5 Miso, 12-yo FN DSH (inpatient): not eating

1.6 Bosca, 2-yo MN Wolfhound: *phone call*, ate choc muffins

1.7 Kenya, 6-yo FN Jack Russell Terrier: smells bad!

1.8 Charles, 5-yo MN Cocker Spaniel: licking left paw+++

1.9 Felix, 8-yo MN Sphynx: swelling on flank

1.10 Lucy, 15-mo FN DSH: vomiting

1.11 Ariel, 18-mo MN DSH: rehomed – sneezing & snorting

1.12 Lucy, 10-yo FE Lab (inpatient): pre-pyo, *review bloods*

1.13 Speed, 2-yo ME Australian Cattle Dog: hips

1.14 Paddy, 4-mo ME Cross-breed: another parvo? *in car*

1.15 Lady, 7-yo FN Greyhound: still lame

1.16 Mac, 1-yo ME Cross-breed: broken tooth, *heart murmur*

1.17 Sam, 12-yo MN Airedale Terrier: very sore

1.18 Xena, 6-yo FN SBT: skin problem getting worse

1.19 Minty, 9-mo MN Bengal: biting owners

1.20 Greyson, 4-yo MN SBT x Boxer: O considering euth

1.21 Staff meeting

Recipe: Banana and oat chocolate chip cookies

DOI: 10.1201/9781003278306-1

1.1 Tony, 1-yo ME Toy Poodle: sutures out

Tony presents for suture removal post-neutering. The surgical wound has healed beautifully, but just this morning the owners noticed a growth in Tony's mouth. Physical examination reveals a mass with a frond-like appearance on the left-hand side of Tony's oral cavity (Figure 1.1). The exophytic, vegetative mass is characteristic of a papilloma.

a) Using the modified Triadan system, the papilloma is sitting above the roots of which tooth?

b) The owners ask whether the papilloma could have been contracted as a result of surgery. Is this likely?
c) Would you recommend surgery in this case?
d) Is there a risk of malignant transformation of an oral papilloma in the dog?
e) Tony goes to doggy day care twice a week. What factors should be considered when determining the extent of his interactions with other dogs?

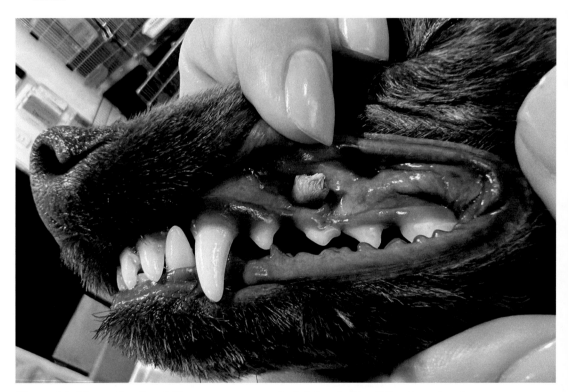

Figure 1.1 **Mass with a frond-like appearance on the left-hand side of Tony's oral cavity.**

1.2 Caramel, 15-yo FN DSH: *fit in*, arthritis injection

It is a busy Monday morning in the practice. The schedule is full, you have five surgeries to complete before afternoon consults, and one team member has just called in sick. You are asked to fit in a quick pentosan polysulfate injection for Caramel, an older 4-kg cat with degenerative joint disease. Just as you approach the pharmacy to draw up the medication

(Zydax™), a nurse asks you how she should premedicate a fractious cat prior to taking radiographs. You answer the query while drawing up the drug, return to the consultation room, give Caramel the injection, and call in your next client.

Minutes later, a receptionist rushes in to inform you that Caramel has collapsed.

On examination, Caramel is unconscious with pink mucous membranes (MMs), a capillary refill time (CRT) of <2 s and a heart rate (HR) of 184 beats per minute (bpm). You realise that you administered a sedative (Zoletil™, a combination of tiletamine and zolazepam) instead of Zydax™ (Figure 1.2).

a) What should you do first?
b) How else should you approach unintended drug administration in a patient?
c) From whom could you seek help in the case of an error that leads to patient harm?
d) How should the error be disclosed to the client?
e) Should you apologise?
f) What steps can you take to take care of yourself in the wake of such an error?

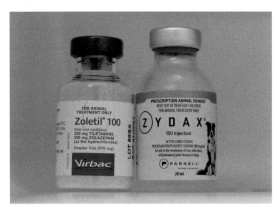

Figure 1.2 **Two drugs with similar-sounding names were stored beside each other, in alphabetical order. In this case, the incorrect medication was selected from the refrigerator and administered. A review of the way medications are stored can prevent such errors from happening in the future.**

1.3 Xanthe, 14-mo FE Mexican Hairless Dog: health check & vacc

Xanthe, a Mexican Hairless Dog (Xoloitzcuintli), presents for her annual check-up and vaccination (Figure 1.3a). Xanthe is quite nervous and head-shy during the examination, but you are able to examine her mouth briefly. After checking with her owner that she does not have any dietary intolerances and is not on an elimination diet, you offer her several large kibble pieces, which she readily chews and swallows.

The owner reports that Xanthe is in excellent health, with no concerns. She eats and drinks without any difficulty, and is fed a diet of commercial dog kibble and uncooked bones. Xanthe has never tolerated tooth-brushing. She has not had any previous dental surgery and has not incurred any trauma to the teeth.

a) From Figure 1.3b–d, what do you observe regarding Xanthe's dentition?

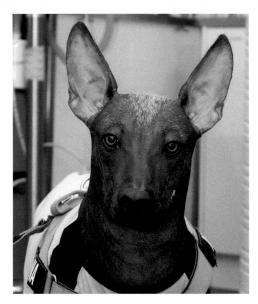

Figure 1.3a **Xanthe on presentation for her vaccination.**

b) What are the potential causes?

c) What would you do next and what might you find?

d) You take dental radiographs, which show several missing teeth. The teeth present appear normal, as do the maxilla and mandible. What is your conclusion?

e) What advice would you give Xanthe's owner regarding home dental care?

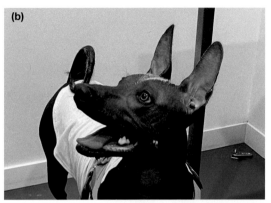

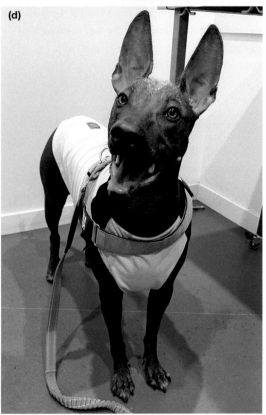

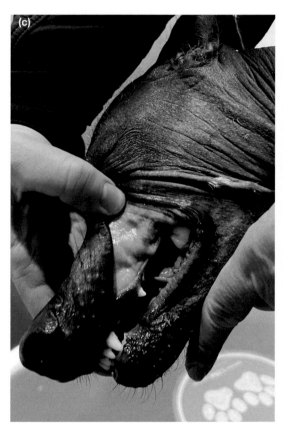

Figure 1.3b–d **Views of Xanthe's mouth at a distance.**

1.4 Chanel, 12-mo FE Pomeranian: mated by accident

The owners were planning to breed Chanel, who weighs 3 kg, with Rocco, their 18-month-old male Pomeranian, at Chanel's second heat. However, to their horror, Chanel escaped her crate approximately 18 days ago on what her owners report to be her first heat, and copulation occurred (Figure 1.4).

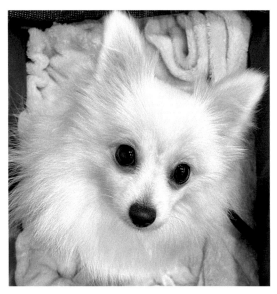

Pertinent physical findings:

- Bright, alert, responsive (BAR) +++
- Body condition score (BCS) 3/5
- Oral exam: MMs pink, CRT <1 s
- Teeth: grade 1 tartar, bilateral retained deciduous teeth
- Skin and coat: normal
- Lymph nodes: normal size
- HR = 100 = PR
- Pulmonary auscultation: no abnormalities
- Abdominal palpation: no abnormalities
- Perianal/urogenital region: normal
- Temp: 38.1 °C

Figure 1.4 Chanel escaped her crate and copulated.

a) What is the canine gestation period?
b) The owners want to know if Chanel is pregnant. How would you test pregnancy at this stage?
c) The owners ask whether, if Chanel is pregnant, they should schedule an elective caesarean section. What would you advise?
d) One of the potential complications of pregnancy in the dog is eclampsia. When is this complication most likely to occur, what signs are associated with it, and how would you confirm the diagnosis?

1.5 Miso, 12-yo FN DSH (inpatient): not eating

Miso was admitted to hospital by your colleague yesterday (Figure 1.5). She has a history of developing upper respiratory tract and ocular signs (sneezing, watery eyes) in boarding, thought to be due to recrudescence of feline herpesvirus (FHV). When she presented yesterday, Miso had a 2-day history of vomiting, and had lost approximately 400 g since her last visit (a vaccination, performed 6 months before).

Due to cost constraints, Miso's owners declined diagnostic investigations yesterday, but agreed to her admission for IV fluids. She weighs 5.4 kg and was placed on Hartmann's with an initial bolus of 5 mL/kg over 15 minutes followed by 2× maintenance (40 mL/kg/day) (Pardo et al. 2024).

Physical examination findings today are as follows:

- BCS 4/5 (body weight 5.4 kg)
- BAR
- Bilateral serous ocular discharge
- Bilateral serous nasal discharge
- MMs pink, CRT <2 s

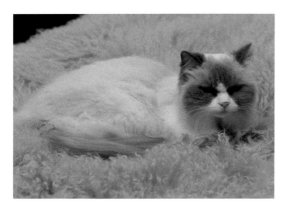

Figure 1.5 Miso shortly after admission. She was placed on fluids overnight.

- HR = 184 bpm (no murmurs)
- Lung fields clear
- Abdominal palpation: large bladder, stool in colon, no organomegaly. Difficult to palpate due to intra-abdominal fat
- Rectal temp: 39.1 °C

Overnight, Miso urinated, but has not defaecated. She has not touched her food. There is no evidence of vomitus in the cage. Her intravenous catheter is patent.

a) List as many possible causes of inappetence in Miso as you can before comparing your response to the answers.
b) You update the owners and they ask for your recommendation. What might you do next to address Miso's inappetence?
c) Miso's owners ask if you can administer something to 'get her eating'. When are appetite stimulants contraindicated?
d) What appetite stimulant(s) might be used in cats, and what potential adverse effects are possible from their use?

1.6 Bosca, 2-yo MN Wolfhound: *phone call*, ate choc muffins

Ms Drumm contacts your clinic when she discovers that Bosca has eaten some chocolate muffins that were cooling on the kitchen counter (Figure 1.6).

a) What key information do you need to manage this case?
b) Aside from chocolate, which contains the methylxanthines theobromine and caffeine, what other potentially hazardous ingredients might muffins contain, depending on the recipe used?
c) What are the potential signs of chocolate toxicity?
d) Bosca ate the muffins 60 minutes ago and is currently not showing clinical signs. Assuming the only toxic ingredient they contained was chocolate, what would you recommend?
e) The owner is reluctant to bring Bosca to you because he isn't showing clinical signs. What should you advise?

f) How would you treat Bosca if he develops clinical signs?

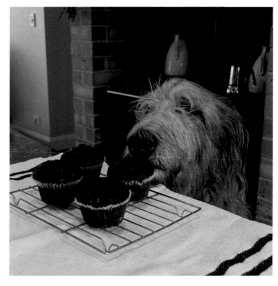

Figure 1.6 Accessible chocolate muffins are a risk to most dogs.

1.7 Kenya, 6-yo FN Jack Russell Terrier: smells bad!

Kenya's owner is worried about a bad smell she has noticed coming from her dog (Figure 1.7a). She also feels Kenya has lost weight recently. Kenya has not been seen at the practice before. There are no other problems reported by the owner. Kenya eats well, is active and energetic, and has no vomiting or polyuria/polydipsia (PU/PD).

Physical exam findings:

- HR = PR = 98 bpm, good pulse volume
- RR = 12 breaths per minute, chest sounds clear
- CRT 2 s, MMs pink and moist
- Temp: 39.3 °C
- BCS 3/5
- Abdominal palpation: no abnormality detected (NAD), perhaps a little 'squelchy' in guts
- Periodontal disease: tartar/calculus on most teeth, cementum on 204 exposed with debris entrapment caudally (especially between 205 and 206) and the furcation of 309 exposed; gingiva swollen and hyperaemic on caudal mandibular area; halitosis (Figure 1.7b)

- Both anal glands very full; expressed normal secretion
- Bilateral waxy otitis externa (tolerated otoscope)

On further questioning, the owner is insistent about weight loss and says that this happened probably within the last few months. She is unable to give any previous weight measurements, but today Kenya weighs 7.4 kg. Upon discussion of the anal glands, the owner remarks that Kenya had diarrhoea for a few days earlier in the week after scavenging the remains of an Indian takeaway.

Acting on the reported weight loss, you obtain a blood sample for your lab's 'comprehensive profile'. It gets sent to the lab the following morning, with results reported in the afternoon (Table 1.7).

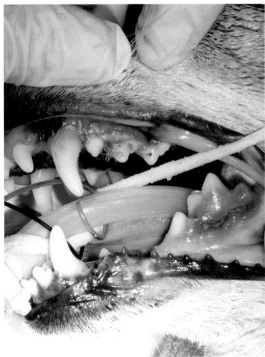

Figure 1.7b **Periodontal disease in Kenya's left upper and lower quadrants. The right side had similar changes.**

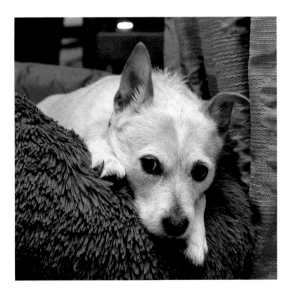

Figure 1.7a **Kenya's owner thinks her dog smells bad.**

Table 1.7 **Kenya's comprehensive profile results, with values outside normal ranges highlighted in red**

PARAMETER	KENYA'S RESULTS	LAB'S NORMAL RANGE
White blood cell (WBC) count	7.68	$6.00–15.00 \times 10^9$/L
Neutrophils (segmented)	53	40.00–80.00%
Neutrophils (segmented) %	4.070	$3.60–12.00 \times 10^9$/L
Neutrophils (non-segmented) %	0	0–1.00%
Neutrophils (non-segmented)	0	$0–0.10 \times 10^9$/L
Lymphocytes %	41.00%	10.00–36.00%
Lymphocytes (absolute number)	3.149	$0.70–4.80 \times 10^9$/L
Monocytes %	5	0.00–13.00%
Monocytes (absolute number)	0.384	$0.00–1.50 \times 10^9$/L
Eosinophils %	1.00%	2.00–10.00%
Eosinophils (absolute number)	0.077	$0.00–1.00 \times 10^9$/L
Basophils %	0.00	0.00–1.00%
Basophils (absolute number)	0.00	$0.00–0.20 \times 10^9$/L
Red blood cell (RBC) count (absolute number)	7.25	$5.5–8.5 \times 10^{12}$/L
Haematocrit	0.52	0.39–0.55%
Haemoglobin (Hb)	16.97	12.00–18.00 g/dL
Mean corpuscular volume (MCV)	71.39	60.00–77.00 fL
Mean corpuscular haemoglobin concentration (MCHC)	32.80	32.00–36.00 g/dL
Platelets (automated count)	354.00	$200.00–500.00 \times 10^9$/L
Reticulocytes (automated count)	45.98	$0.00–60.00 \times 10^9$/L
Red blood cell distribution width (RDW)	13.9	13.6–21.7%
Protein	65.33	58.00–73.00 g/L
Albumin	28.10	26.00–35.00 g/L
Globulin	37.20	18.00–37.00 g/L
Alanine aminotransferase (ALT)	19.57	21.00–102.00 U/L
Alkaline phosphatase (ALP)	143.02	20.00–60.00 U/L
Bile acids	4.90	0.00–10.50 µmol/L
Bilirubin (total)	2.70	0.00–6.80 µmol/L
Cholesterol	8.60	3.80–7.00 mmol/L
Triglycerides	1.35	0.54–1.14 mmol/L
Creatine kinase (CK)	121.00	50.00–200.00 U/L
Urea	6.30	1.70–7.40 mmol/L
Creatinine	108.00	22.00–115.00 µmol/L
Calcium (total)	1.78	2.30–3.00 mmol/L
Calcium (ionised)	0.80	1.15–1.50 mmol/L
Phosphate inorganic	0.98	0.90–2.00 mmol/L
Magnesium	0.89	0.69–1.18 mmol/L
Sodium	146.76	139.00–154.00 mmol/L
Potassium	4.94	3.50–5.60 mmol/L
Chloride	109.54	102.00–118.00 mmol/L
Canine C-reactive protein	5.55 mg/L	0.00–5.00 mg/L
Glucose	5.41 mmol/L	3.00–5.00 mmol/L

a) What are some common reasons for an owner reporting that their dog 'smells bad'?
b) Based on what you find on physical exam, how would you grade any proposed dental treatment for Kenya: simple, medium, or advanced, in terms of length and complexity of procedure?
c) The owner was sent a copy of the blood results as per practice policy and has become very worried that Kenya might have cancer due to the abnormal calcium values, and that she is becoming diabetic. Comment on the results and how you will address these concerns.
d) What is your next step with Kenya, and why?

1.8 Charles, 5-yo MN Cocker Spaniel: licking left paw+++

Charles has a long-standing history of atopic dermatitis and presents for acute licking of his left front paw over the previous 24 hours. The owner remarks that there is a red spot between Charles's toes, but Charles will not let him examine the paw. Charles has had allergies in the past, for which he often receives an injection, but this time he seems very focused on his left paw.

On examination of the dorsal aspect of the paw between digits 2 and 3, you note swelling and redness of the interdigital skin. There is a doughnut-like swelling, approximately 6 mm in diameter, surrounding what appears to be a central sinus with a small amount of serosanguinous discharge (Figure 1.8a). Charles seems painful on examination, and attempts to withdraw his paw from your grasp. His temperature is 38.3 °C.

You suspect a foreign body, syringe local anaesthetic (lignocaine, 3 mg/kg) directly into the sinus, and using micro-alligator forceps, withdraw an 8-mm grass seed (Figure 1.8b).

a) What four factors influence the presentation of grass-seed foreign-body disease?
b) How else could you approach the removal of a foreign body from a site like this?

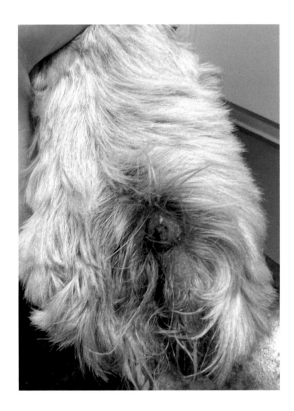

Figure 1.8a A doughnut-like swelling, approximately 6 mm in diameter, surrounding what appears to be a central sinus with a small amount of serosanguinous discharge, between digits 2 and 3.

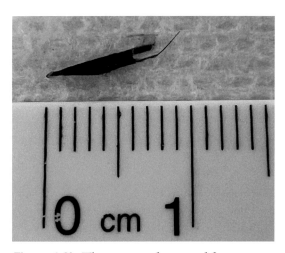

Figure 1.8b The grass seed removed from Charles's draining sinus.

c) What if you strongly suspected a foreign body, but failed to find one?
d) Is there any treatment you would recommend for Charles following the procedure?

1.9 Felix, 8-yo MN Sphynx: swelling on flank

Felix lives an indoor–outdoor lifestyle. He is up to date with all recommended vaccines. His dedicated owner, Lizzie, is a fit and sprightly retired nurse in her 60s who lives alone since her husband died a few years ago. Lizzie says she heard a cat fight three nights ago and Felix now is 'not himself' and eating slightly less than usual. On examination, Felix seems a little stressed but is bright and alert, his hydration appears normal, temperature is 39.3 °C, and he has a fluctuant swelling approximately 3 cm in diameter on his left flank, with no apparent cellulitis (Figure 1.9). Elsewhere there are no abnormal findings. Lizzie agrees to you sedating Felix and then lancing and flushing the abscess.

a) What do you understand by the term cellulitis?

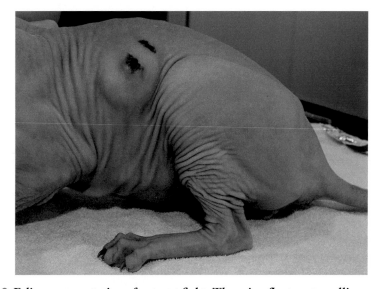

Figure 1.9 Felix on presentation after a cat fight. There is a fluctuant swelling on his flank.

b) What are the principles of achieving good drainage when lancing an abscess?
c) What solutions could you use to flush Felix's abscess?
d) What other treatment is indicated for Felix today?
e) Lizzie says that last time this happened, a few years ago, your boss gave Felix an antibiotic injection that 'worked really well'. You note in the records for the previous visit that your boss had administered cefovecin, a long-acting third-generation cephalosporin. She asks if she can have the same treatment again. How might you respond?

1.10 Lucy, 15-mo FN DSH: vomiting

Lucy presents with a history of acute vomiting (approximately five times over the previous 24 hours) and inappetence. She lives entirely indoors, and has up-to-date vaccinations and worming. She is fractious and difficult to restrain for physical examination.

a) What are the most likely causes of acute vomiting in a young, otherwise healthy cat?
b) Are there specific questions you wish to ask the owners?
c) What diagnostic tests would you recommend?
d) If the owner declines diagnostic tests, what empirical treatment might you offer?
e) What aspects of the physical examination are particularly important where you suspect a gastrointestinal tract (GIT) foreign body?
f) Radiographs (Figure 1.10) reveal a moderately radiopaque coiled linear foreign body in the region of the small intestine. How would you treat this patient?

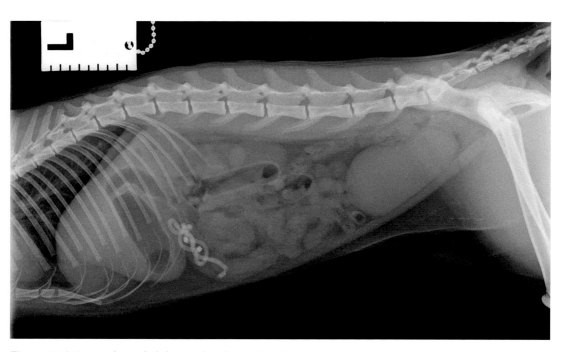

Figure 1.10 Lucy's lateral abdominal radiograph (taken under anaesthetic) showing a radiopaque coiled linear structure in the proximal small intestine. There is air in the stomach. No other radiopaque foreign bodies are present.

1.11 Ariel, 18-mo MN DSH: rehomed – sneezing & snorting

Ariel's new owners acquired him from an internet pet sales site 5 days ago, and travelled to collect him from a town 2 hours away. He's a charming, active and affectionate young adult cat, already established in his new home. The owners know there is something odd about his upper lip (Figure 1.11a). In fact, it was this that endeared him to them. Ariel eats normally but occasionally snorts and sneezes. He has come in today for a health check and vaccines.

a) What are your clinical observations from a distance?
b) You take a closer look at Ariel's oral cavity. Describe the anatomical and functional problem in Figure 1.11b,c.
c) Ariel's owners do not have a lot of money. Referral is out of the question. Outline some options for discussion with his owners at this stage.
d) If surgery was undertaken within general practice, what are some key principles and challenges to keep in mind for this type of procedure?

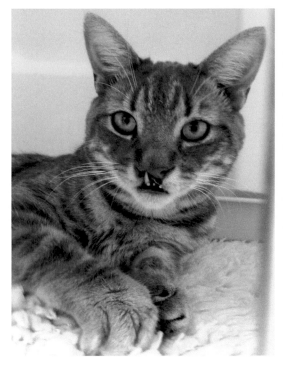

Figure 1.11a Ariel on presentation for his check-up.

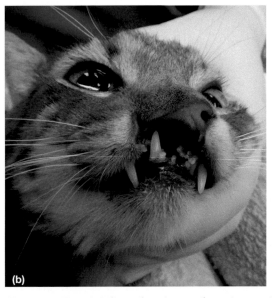

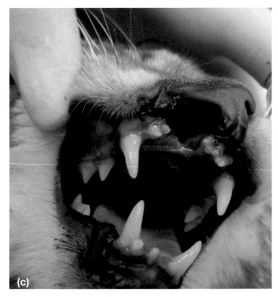

Figure 1.11b,c Ariel's oral cavity on closer inspection.

1.12 Lucy, 10-yo FE Lab (inpatient): pre-pyo, *review bloods*

Lucy presented semi-collapsed with suspected closed pyometra and was admitted by a colleague earlier today. The owner reported that Lucy had been unwell for 5 days; her last oestrus was 6 weeks ago. A lateral radiograph was taken (Figure 1.12a). The pyometra was confirmed by ultrasound (Figure 1.12b).

Lucy is currently receiving fluid resuscitation with normal saline prior to surgery and has also been given IV co-amoxiclav. An emergency point-of-care venous blood test has just been carried out (Table 1.12).

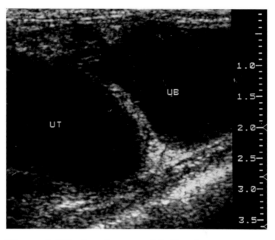

Figure 1.12b An ultrasound indicating gross enlargement of Lucy's uterus (UT), which is comparable in size to the full urinary bladder (UB).

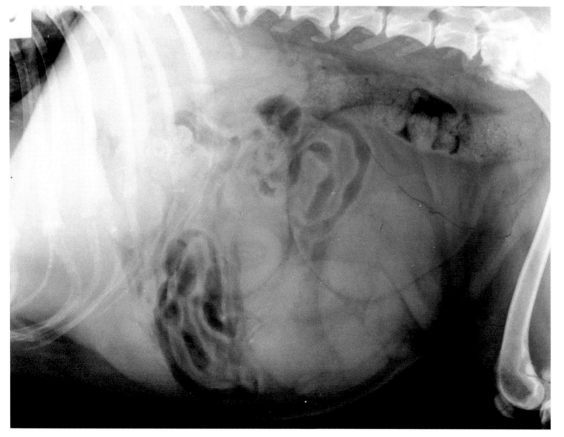

Figure 1.12a Right lateral radiograph of Lucy. Note the grossly enlarged uterine horns displacing the small intestines cranially. The bladder is full.

Table 1.12 **Lucy's venous blood test results**

PARAMETER	LUCY'S RESULTS	REFERENCE RANGE
pH	7.20	7.35–7.45
HCO_3^-	12.8	15.0–23.0 mmol/L
pCO_2	30	35.0–38.0 mmHg

a) How would you classify Lucy's acid–base disorder, and why?
b) What are the implications for ongoing stabilisation pre-surgery?
c) When should Lucy be taken to surgery?

1.13 Speed, 2-yo ME Australian Cattle Dog: hips

A recently qualified colleague working at a branch practice has just emailed you two radiographs for a second opinion (Figure 1.13a,b). Speed fell off a moving truck. Your colleague's message says, 'Apologies, these were the best pictures we could manage!'

a) Comment on the diagnostic quality of the images.
b) What can you see?
c) Is there anything unusual about Speed's problem?
d) What would be the first line of treatment for the most obvious injury?
e) Outline the treatment options if first-line methods fail.

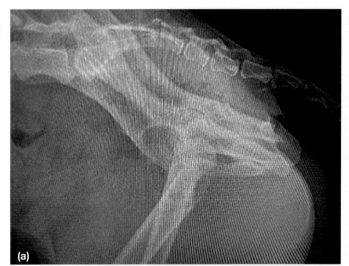

(a)

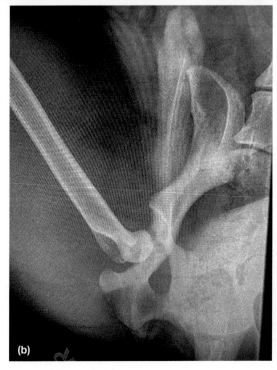

(b)

Figure 1.13a,b **Your colleague emails you these radiographs of the hips of Speed, who fell off a moving truck, and asks for an opinion.**

1.14 Paddy, 4-mo ME Cross-breed: another parvo? *in car*

Your practice has seen a number of cases of parvovirus in recent weeks, several of them sadly fatal. You examine newly rehomed Paddy in the practice car park, before admitting him through the side door straight to isolation. He is very depressed, 8–10% dehydrated, with subnormal temperature, and has been vomiting (6× this morning) and passing small, patchy amounts of diarrhoea (2× this morning). When you try to palpate his abdomen, he vocalises, guards his abdominal muscles, and retches. Shortly afterwards, he defaecates profuse bloody mucus. He looks thoroughly miserable in his kennel (Figure 1.14a).

Paddy's vaccination status is unclear. It seems he might have been given something by the breeder, but there is no certificate. Paddy was handed over to the owners at a motorway service station and the breeder has subsequently been uncontactable. You suspect they are a puppy farmer. Paddy is not yet insured and his owners are on a tight budget.

You perform a packed cell volume (PCV)/ total protein (TP) and blood glucose (Table 1.14) and begin IV fluids (Hartmann's solution), as well as SC amoxycillin-clavulanic acid, and IV maropitant.

Table 1.14 **Paddy's blood results (reference ranges in parentheses)**

PCV	TP	BLOOD GLUCOSE
0.65 (0.37–0.55)	8.8 g/dL (5.2–8.0)	4.0 mmol/L (4.3–6.7)

a) Comment on the above results and the general utility of these tests in the emergency context. What can they tell us?
b) What is the difference between 'total protein' and 'total solids', and when could this be clinically significant?
c) What are your parvovirus testing options and how might results be interpreted in terms of false positives/negatives? Would it be useful to test Paddy for parvovirus?
d) Paddy tests negative for parvovirus with a cage-side faecal antigen test (Figure 1.14b). What should you do?
e) What other viruses may cause signs similar to Paddy's?
f) What would be an important non-infectious differential in a young dog with Paddy's symptoms? How would you try to rule this out?

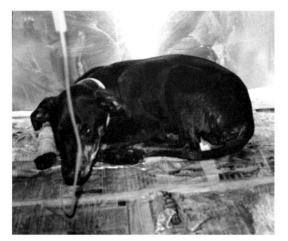

Figure 1.14a **Paddy produced severe bloody diarrhoea shortly after admission to an isolation kennel.**

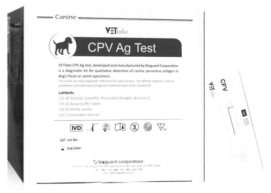

Figure 1.14b **Cage-side faecal antigen test for parvovirus in dogs.**

g) Assuming parvovirus, what other medications/treatments might you consider adding in?

h) When would you consider euthanasia, regardless of the final diagnosis?

1.15 Lady, 7-yo FN Greyhound: still lame

Lady has a severe, progressive left thoracic limb lameness, worse on hard ground, together with a depressed demeanour and reluctance to exercise. Initial clinical examination 1 week ago was unremarkable. Meloxicam was dispensed for a presumed sprain or strain, but on presentation today, Lady is still very lame. She will pull up on hard ground and refuse to move, sometimes holding up the affected limb.

Lady is insured and her owner requests 'a scan' as she has heard that Greyhounds are prone to bone tumours.

a) What are the common differential diagnoses for lameness in adult sighthounds?
b) You carry out a repeat clinical examination on Lady and find a hard focal area of hyperkeratosis on digital pad 3 (Figure 1.15). What is the aetiology here and how is this condition recognised on clinical exam?
c) What is the aim of rational treatment and how is this achieved?
d) What are the distal insertion points and actions of the superficial and deep digital flexor tendons?
e) Why might this condition recur after initial successful treatment by tendonectomy?
f) If recurrence takes place, revision surgery is possible, this time taking the form of a tenotomy of both superficial and deep digital flexors. This resolves the lameness. What might the effect occasionally be on stance?

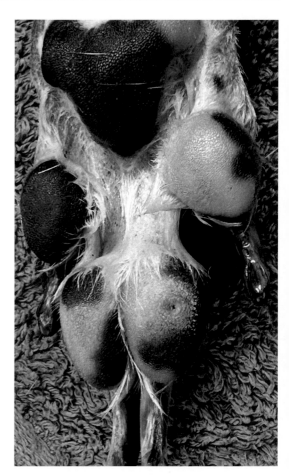

Figure 1.15 **Focal hyperkeratosis on digital pad 3.**

1.16 Mac, 1-yo ME Cross-breed: broken tooth, *heart murmur*

Mac, weighing 25 kg, presents at your clinic as he has been chewing stones and has fractured his right mandibular canine tooth (tooth 404; Figure 1.16). He is otherwise a healthy dog with no abnormalities noted by the owner. You are able to examine the mouth and determine that pulp is exposed. The owners are on a restricted budget and opt to have the tooth

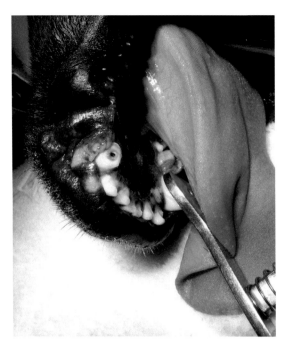

Figure 1.16 Mac's fractured 404 at the time of surgery, showing pulp exposure.

removed rather than progress to endodontic treatment.

On clinical examination, Mac is bouncy with a HR of 120 bpm and he is panting. You detect a grade II/VI systolic murmur on thoracic auscultation, although there are no other abnormalities present. After discussion with the owners, they decline further investigation of the heart murmur or referral to a cardiologist, reporting that Mac is very fit and active.

a) A note in Mac's clinical record mentions an American Society of Anesthesiologists (ASA) score of 2. What does this mean in terms of anaesthetic planning?
b) What premedication drugs could you administer IM for this patient?
c) Which breathing system would you select for Mac?

The premedication has a good effect and an IV cannula is placed in Mac's right cephalic vein. The breathing system and anaesthetic machine are checked, revealing no problems. General anaesthesia is induced with propofol given to effect and the trachea intubated.

d) After induction, you want to place Mac on IV fluids. Which fluid do you select and at what rate will you administer it?
e) As you are performing an extraction, you decide to perform a dental nerve block. Which nerve block is the most appropriate for this extraction? And how would this be performed?
f) You have bupivacaine 0.5% for the nerve block. The dose is up to 1 mg/kg. What is the maximum volume you can use for Mac?

1.17 Sam, 12-yo MN Airedale Terrier: very sore

Sam has had a 6-week history of hindlimb stiffness and back pain, which responded well to meloxicam prescribed by a colleague. This morning, Sam had an episode of unprovoked yelping after he got up out of his bed, and he remains very sore on any movement. You admit him for sedation and X-rays (Figure 1.17). Sam's owner has cost constraints.

a) Explain the radiological diagnosis and prognosis.
b) Are any further imaging studies indicated?
c) What might you expect to find on physical examination?
d) On being given the diagnosis, Sam's owner expresses concern that Sam should have been X-rayed sooner. How might you handle the owner's concerns?
e) Are neutered dogs predisposed to this condition?

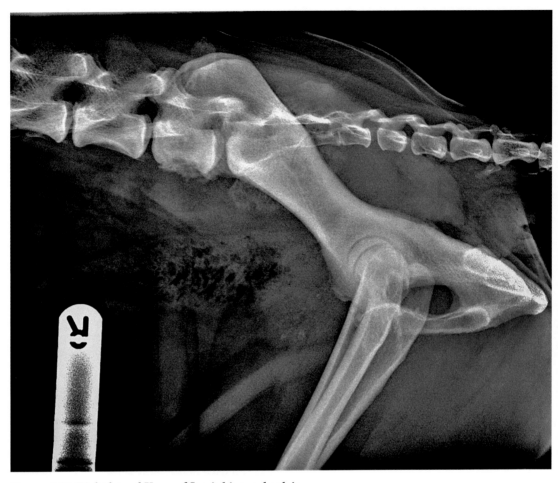

Figure 1.17 **Right lateral X-ray of Sam's hips and pelvis.**

1.18 Xena, 6-yo FN SBT: skin problem getting worse

Xena presents for skin irritation that has become markedly worse over the past week (Figure 1.18a). She is pruritic with poor hair-coat quality. She has numerous small pustules and papules over her dorsum and ventrum. She is otherwise well, bright and as energetic as usual. She lives indoors with regular outdoor access and is up to date with vaccinations. She is on a monthly oral tablet that is active against fleas, ticks, heartworm, and also mites such as demodex. She lives in a hot tropical area and enjoys swimming (Figure 1.18b).

a) What are the most likely causes of Xena's skin irritation?
b) Are there specific questions you wish to ask the owners?
c) What diagnostic tests would you recommend?
d) What treatment might you offer?
e) If there is not complete resolution after 2–3 weeks, what further treatment or diagnostic tests would you recommend?
f) What other condition may be complicating the resolution of Xena's skin irritation?

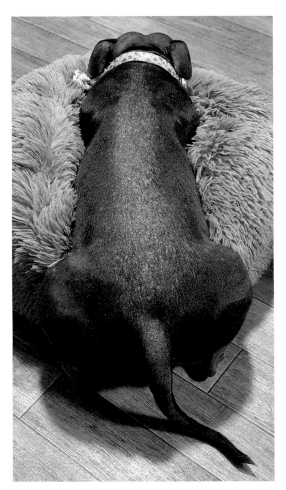

Figure 1.18a Loss of hair coat, particularly on Xena's dorsum.

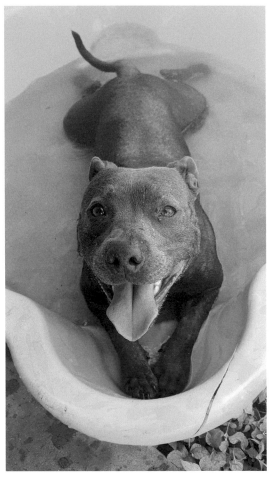

Figure 1.18b Xena is an otherwise happy and healthy dog who enjoys swimming.

1.19 Minty, 9-mo MN Bengal: biting owners

Minty (Figure 1.19) is presented for intermittent aggressive behaviour towards his owners. They report that he will be happily sitting on their lap one minute and then biting their hands or arms the next. There are no other pets in the household and Minty does not have access to the outdoors.

a) What are the most common differentials for owner-directed aggressive behaviour in cats?

A clinical examination does not reveal any evidence of medical/physical problems, but the clients mention that their work schedules have changed and that they are not at home as often as they used to be.

b) What would be your next steps with this case?

c) What behavioural first-aid advice would you give to the clients?

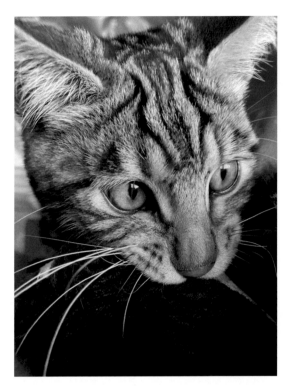

Figure 1.19 Minty has been biting his owners.

1.20 Greyson, 4-yo MN SBT x Boxer: O considering euth

You are busy catching up on notes when one of your nurses asks if you can take a phone call. A client wants to discuss the euthanasia of their dog due to behavioural concerns. You first open Greyson's file and have a quick read through. Greyson has visited the clinic for his annual vaccinations since he was 16 weeks old. He was seen for a torn dewclaw a year ago, and he was noted to be highly anxious. A muzzle was used when handling him.

a) How will you approach this conversation? What are the specific questions you wish to ask the owner?
b) What ethical challenges do you need to consider?
c) If the owner is to proceed with euthanasia, how can we best ensure the safety and wellbeing of all involved?

1.21 Staff meeting

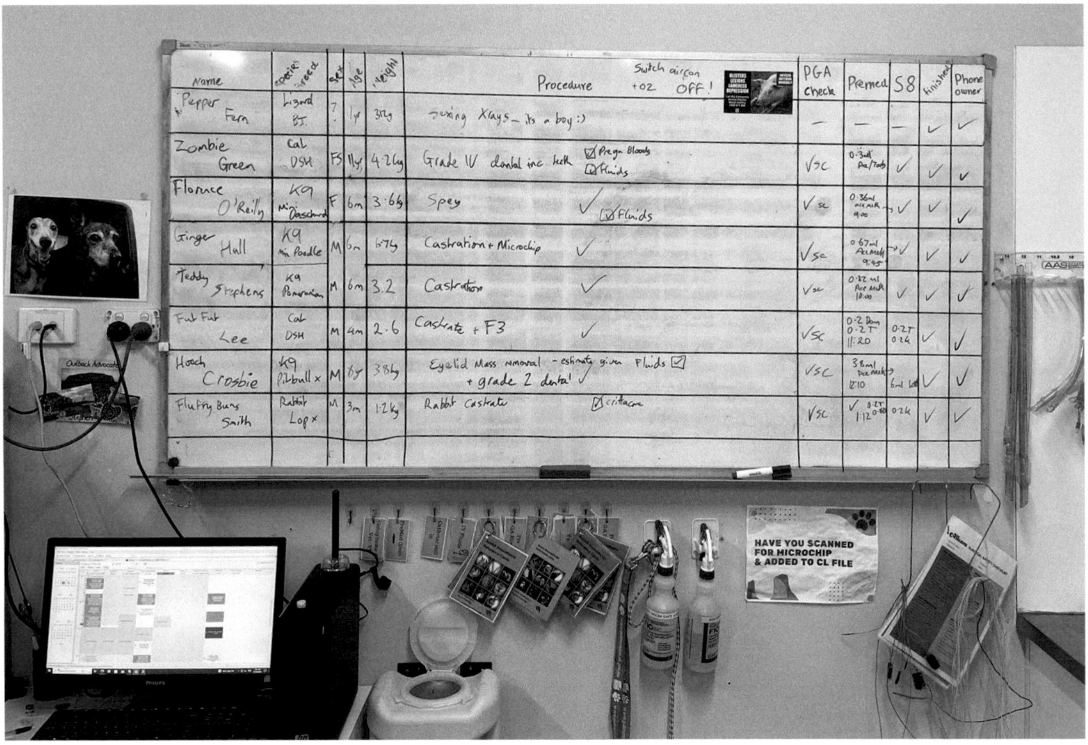

Figure 1.21a **Scheduling of appointments and procedures is a key modifiable workplace factor to control workload.**

Resilience is often portrayed as a characteristic of individuals, but even the most resilient veterinary team member can be negatively impacted by their workplace. At the staff meeting, one team member reports that several colleagues have confided that they feel 'burnt out'.

a) What is burnout?
b) Taking as long as you want (perhaps this is something to think about over the course of a day or two as you examine your own feelings and/or discuss with colleagues), ask yourself what are possible work-related factors associated with burnout in veterinary workplaces.

c) Workload is one workplace factor that could be modified to help minimise burnout, improve mental wellbeing, increase job satisfaction and reduce intention to leave (Figure 1.21a,b). Are there specific changes that could be implemented in your own workplace in the short term, and in the longer term, to help manage workload?

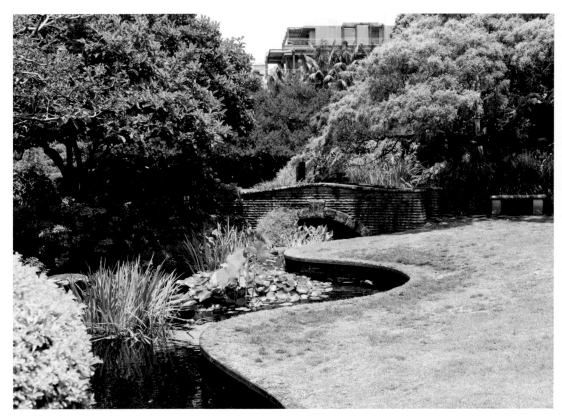

Figure 1.21b Work overload is one factor that contributes to burnout. It is important that all team members have a sustainable workload and are able to refuel and recharge.

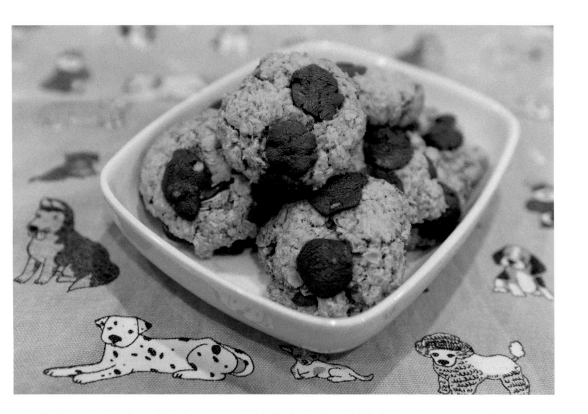

BANANA AND OAT CHOCOLATE CHIP COOKIES

These filling cookies are easy to make for a healthy snack for morning or afternoon tea, or as a between-consult pick-me-up.

Ingredients

1 large, over-ripe, peeled banana (if you have frozen a banana to preserve it, you can thaw it for this purpose)
75 g white sugar
60 g brown sugar
80 mL canola or grapeseed oil
1 teaspoon vanilla extract
125 g plain flour
170 g rolled oats
½ teaspoon bicarbonate of soda
½ teaspoon ground cinnamon
¼ teaspoon salt
85 g dark chocolate chips
4 tablespoons desiccated coconut
Optional: 1–2 tablespoons finely chopped nuts of your choice (e.g. walnuts, cashews)

Equipment needed

Baking trays and baking paper
Mixing bowl and wooden spoon
Spoon for scooping mix
Oven
Wire cooling rack

Instructions

1. Preheat the oven to 180 °C.
2. Line one or two large baking trays with baking paper.
3. In a medium to large bowl, mash the banana together with white and brown sugar, oil and vanilla extract, until the mixture is lump-free and smooth.

4. Mix in the flour, oats, bicarbonate of soda, cinnamon, salt, chocolate chips, and coconut, and stir. This will give your forearms quite a workout! If you are adding chopped nuts, do so at this stage.

5. Using a soup spoon or similar, scoop balls of dough (3.5–4.0 cm) onto the baking tray, and space cookies about 5 cm apart. Gently compress the balls until they are approximately 1 cm thick and 5 cm in diameter (you can use a piece of baking paper between the ball and your hand to avoid the mix sticking to you). Round up any stray chocolate chips and embed these back into the cookies.

6. Bake for 12–14 minutes, or until golden.

7. Cool for 5 minutes on trays, then gently place the cookies on a cooling rack. (Ensure that they cannot be accessed by companion animals, as the chocolate is potentially toxic – see Case 1.6!).

8. These are wonderful served fresh, when the chocolate is a bit gooey. However, they will last in an airtight container for 3–5 days.

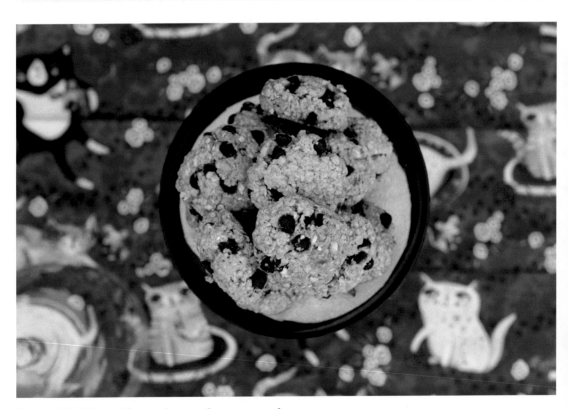

Figure 1.22 **Your mid-morning or afternoon snack.**

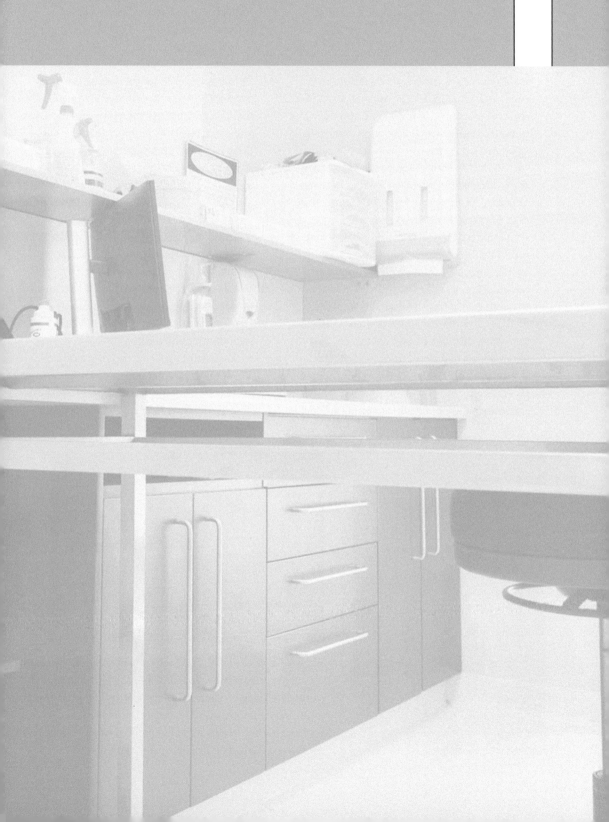

1.1 Tony, 1-yo ME Toy Poodle: sutures out

a) 206 (the upper, or maxillary, left second premolar) *https://avdc.org/PDF/Triadan_Tooth_Numbering_System.pdf*.

b) Papillomaviruses are ubiquitous in dogs, with most oral warts caused by canine papillomavirus 1 (CPV1) (Munday et al. 2022a). Papillomas are one of the most common tumours seen in young dogs; transmission is facilitated via damage to the oral epithelium, such as occurs with being mouthed by other dogs, or chewing sharp objects such as sticks or bones. As Tony was segregated from other dogs in hospital, and neutering is not associated with oral trauma, it is very unlikely that the papilloma was a result of surgery.

c) While surgical removal of papillomas is possible, spontaneous regression is likely to occur due to cell-mediated immunity (usually in 4–8 weeks, but oral warts may take up to 12 months and cutaneous warts may take up to 2 years to regress in the dog) (Munday et al. 2022a). Humoral immunity protects affected dogs from reinfection with the same papillomavirus. Surgical removal is indicated only if warts cause discomfort or interfere with eating (Figure A1.1a,b). There is no compelling reason to recommend surgery in this case.

d) While there are reports of squamous cell carcinomas (SCCs) developing in oral warts, malignant transformation appears to be rare and is currently thought to occur only in dogs that have an underlying genetic defect that prevents a normal immune reaction to a papillomavirus infection (Munday et al. 2022b). For this reason, it is important to monitor the wart. If it does not regress within 6 months and additional warts continue to develop over this time, biopsy and histopathology should be considered.

e) While there are rare reports of 'outbreaks' of warts in doggy day-care facilities, there are several factors to consider. These include the following:
- **Exposure risk.** Papillomaviruses are ubiquitous, and young dogs may carry the virus without developing visible lesions. It is not clear how long symptomatic

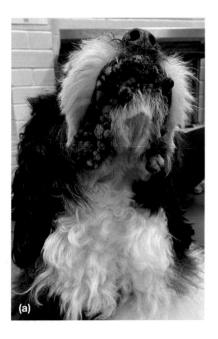

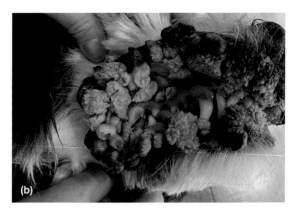

Figure A1.1a,b Florid papillomatosis in a 2-yo St Bernard × Cavalier × Miniature Poodle. This dog had concurrent stable IRIS stage 1 chronic kidney disease. Because these warts were causing oral discomfort, ulceration, and a foul smell, they were surgically removed in a two-staged procedure. This is an extreme presentation.

dogs shed the virus, so it is difficult to determine an appropriate and effective isolation period. Furthermore, isolating Tony will not necessarily reduce the risk of exposure of other dogs at day care (in fact, Tony could have contracted the virus *at* day care).

- **Availability of a screening test.** There are no easily available screening tests that can be used to isolate affected animals in the group.
- **Route of transmission.** Papillomaviruses may be transmitted through mouthing of other dogs (a frequent behaviour in young dogs), as well as via fomites (e.g. chew toys).
- **Severity of disease.** This is low, as infected dogs may be asymptomatic, and those with symptoms are likely to develop self-limiting papilloma(s).
- **Risk/benefit.** The consequences of isolation of young dogs from other dogs may be more severe (e.g. behavioural challenges due to poor socialisation) than the disease itself.

Therefore, this is a decision that needs to be made by the owner in consultation with the day-care facility.

REFERENCES

Munday, J. S., Knight, C. G. & Luff, J. A. (2022a) Papillomaviral skin diseases of humans, dogs, cats and horses: a comparative review. Part 1: Papillomavirus biology and hyperplastic lesions. *Veterinary Journal* **288**:105897. doi: 10.1016/j.tvjl.2022.105897.

Munday, J. S., Knight, C. G. & Luff, J. A (2022b) Papillomaviral skin diseases of humans, dogs, cats and horses: a comparative review. Part 2: Pre-neoplastic and neoplastic diseases. *Veterinary Journal* **288**:105898. doi: 10.1016/j.tvjl.2022.105898.

1.2 Caramel, 15-yo FN DSH: *fit in*, arthritis injection

a) Medication errors are among the most common types of errors reported in veterinary medicine (Wallis et al. 2019), and medications with similar-sounding names may be confused (Paul et al. 2008). The first step is to work out the dose the patient has been exposed to in mg/kg, and establish what the likely effects of such a dose would be. In this case, you gave 0.12 mL of a 100 mg/mL solution, or 12 mg (3 mg/kg). This is at the low end of the dose range you normally use for this drug (2.5–10 mg/kg) for sedation.

b) In some cases, you may be able to reverse the drug (e.g. naloxone can be used to reverse opioids; atipamezole reverses alpha-2 adrenergic drugs) or a component of the drug (the benzodiazepine component of the combination drug used in this case) – see Table A1.2. Alternatively, an antidote may be available. Depending on the drug and route of administration, decontamination may be indicated. In this case, Caramel should be admitted for supportive care and close monitoring until the effects of the drug wear off.

Table A1.2 **Examples of drug classes and their reversal agents**

DRUG CLASS	REVERSAL AGENT
Opioids	Naloxone
Alpha-2 agonists (medetomidine, dexmedetomidine, xylazine)	Alpha-2 antagonists (atipamezole, tolazoline, yohimbine)
Benzodiazepines	Flumazenil
Non-depolarising muscle relaxants	Cholinergic agents (edrophonium, neostigmine, physostigmine, pyridostigmine)

c) It is helpful to talk to a senior or more experienced colleague, practice manager, or even insurer. The earlier you do so, the better.

d) Error disclosure can be daunting, but in the initial stages the client has a right to know what happened, what are the likely effects, and what is being done to help Caramel as soon as possible. In time, it is also important for a client to understand why this error happened. It is important not to rush to be open with clients and share information that is inaccurate or speculative, as this can destroy trust (Gallagher & Kachalia 2024). Thus, it is useful to jot down notes before talking to the client, and only make statements about what is known. If the animal is likely to make a full recovery, this should be stated at the outset.

In this case, it was a human error made because the clinician was multitasking.

A response might incorporate the following, though it is important to pause to allow the client to respond:

- 'Unfortunately, I gave Caramel the wrong medication. A powerful sedative was given instead of the arthritis medication intended. This was a human error on my part.'
- 'I can understand that this must be incredibly distressing for you. This sedative, while long-acting, wears off and is unlikely to have any long-term effects.'
- 'To ensure the best possible outcome, with your permission, we would like to monitor Caramel here until the medication has worn off.'

It is important to make detailed contemporaneous records both for ongoing patient management and in case of a complaint.

e) It is commonly believed that an apology is an admission of liability, but studies have shown that apologies may help clients, and reduce the risk of litigation. You can say, 'I am so sorry that this has happened' and reassure the client that you have taken and will take steps to support both the client and the patient.

f) Errors can negatively impact those responsible for them, leading to feelings of guilt, distress, and shaken confidence. Those negative feelings can skew perspective and may inhibit our ability to learn from an error. In this case, discussion with other veterinarians within and outside the team revealed that the same error had been made by other clinicians previously. Discussing this error in a morbidity and mortality meeting, or debriefing with a trusted team member about what happened and how, can help us learn and brainstorm strategies to prevent similar errors in future, e.g. storage of different drugs by mode of action rather than alphabetically; a policy of not asking a question until medication has been drawn up and dispensed (Pang et al. 2018). It can be useful to jot down notes of what happened, and read about errors (Powell et al. 2010). Discussing cases like this with a mentor, who can share their experiences of making an error, can lend perspective. Physician Arthur L. Bloomfield said, 'There are some patients whom we cannot help, there are none whom we cannot harm' (Cox et al. 1962). What is important is that we investigate the source of error, take steps to prevent errors, and learn from errors that do occur.

REFERENCES

Cox, A. J., Hilgard, E. R. & Rytand, D. A. (1962) Arthur L. Bloomfield 1888–1962. *California Medicine* **97**:191–192.

Gallagher, T. H. & Kachalia, A. (2024) Responding to medical errors – implementing the modern ethical paradigm. *New England Journal of Medicine* **390**:193–197. doi: 10.1056/NEJMp2309554.

Pang, D. S. J., Rousseau-Blass, F. & Pang, J. M. (2018) Morbidity and mortality conferences: a mini review and illustrated application in veterinary medicine. *Frontiers in Veterinary Science* **5**(43). doi: 10.3389/fvets.2018.00043.

Paul, A. L., Shaw, S. P. & Bandt, C. (2008) Aplastic anemia in two kittens following a prescription error. *Journal of the American Animal Hospital Association* **44**:25–31. doi: 10.5326/0440025.

Powell, L., Rozanski, E. A. & Rush, J. E. (2010) *Small Animal Emergency and Critical Care: Case Studies in Client Communication, Morbidity and Mortality.* Oxford: Wiley-Blackwell.

Wallis, J., Fletcher, D., Bentley, A. & Ludders, J. (2019) Medical errors cause harm in veterinary hospitals. *Frontiers in Veterinary Science* **6**. doi: 10.3389/fvets.2019.00012.

1.3 Xanthe, 14-mo FE Mexican Hairless Dog: health check & vacc

a) Xanthe is missing teeth from both sides of her mouth. Premolars, molars, and possibly canine teeth appear to be missing. On this limited oral examination, there is no obvious evidence of gingivitis or periodontal disease.

b) The most common causes of 'missing' teeth in dogs are as follows:

- Unerupted teeth (Figure A1.3)
- Teeth lost or extracted due to, e.g. periodontal disease, trauma or tooth resorption
- Teeth that were never present in the mouth, i.e. congenitally missing

Xanthe's young age and lack of any history of trauma or obvious signs of periodontal disease would suggest her missing teeth are unerupted or congenitally missing.

c) Dental disease cannot be completely excluded without a comprehensive oral health assessment including examination of both sides of the mouth. This will include periodontal probing and dental radiographs (performed under general anaesthesia). Unerupted teeth and dentigerous cysts are visible on radiographs. If the owner cannot afford this investigation, or does not wish to go down this route, then periodic monitoring together with advice on signs of oral pain could be given (but see below).

d) Xanthe has congenitally missing teeth. Interestingly, Mexican Hairless Dogs have a phenotype labelled as canine ectodermal dysplasia (CED), characterised by a sparse or absent hair coat and missing or abnormally shaped permanent teeth (Drögemüller et al. 2008, Kupczik et al. 2017). This phenotype is the result of an

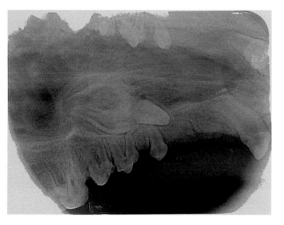

Figure A1.3 An unerupted right permanent maxillary canine (104) in a puppy with a 'missing' tooth. This dog had several 'missing' teeth, with no clinical signs.

While it is impossible for a single veterinarian to know about every inherited condition in companion animals, it can be useful to research breed predispositions when confronted with an individual patient showing particular signs. In Xanthe's case, a brief online search – together with the examination and history – reassured the veterinarian of the likely explanation for her unusual dentition. Of course, knowing the breed predisposition could give the veterinarian confidence in adopting a pragmatic response to part c) above, avoiding general anaesthesia and X-rays, but the principle of X-raying for 'missing' teeth is a sound one.

inherited mutation in the *FOXI3* gene (Kupczik et al. 2017). Aside from Mexican Hairless Dogs, CED affects Peruvian Hairless and Chinese Crested Dogs. These breeds have missing or misshapen permanent teeth.

e) Xanthe has fewer teeth, so it is important to ensure that they last a long time. Active home care includes daily tooth-brushing, which has thus far proven unsuccessful with Xanthe. Nonetheless, it may be a question of technique – some dogs will not tolerate a toothbrush, but may be conditioned to accept the use of a thimble-style brush or dental wipes. It is common for owners to start tooth-brushing in too rushed a manner. The first stages may simply involve rewarding the dog for allowing the face to be gently touched, then the lip raised, then the gum pressed, and so forth, with each step undergoing many (rewarded) repetitions before progressing to the introduction of the toothbrush itself. With nervous dogs, this whole process might take several weeks, but it is worth it. Passive home care may consist of feeding dental chews or the use of products such as water additives that have received the seal of approval from the Veterinary Oral

Health Council (VOHC) for demonstrating efficacy in decreasing plaque and calculus accumulation (*www.vohc.org/*). There is a risk that chewing on bones could lead to tooth damage, including fractures (Bellows et al. 2019); the owner should be informed of this risk. Xanthe's teeth should be checked at least annually, or if her owner has any concerns, e.g. if Xanthe fractures a tooth; if there are signs of gingivitis, periodontal disease or halitosis; or if Xanthe experiences any difficulty eating.

REFERENCES

Bellows, J., Berg, M. L., Dennis, S. et al. (2019) AAHA dental care guidelines for dogs and cats. *Journal of the American Animal Hospital Association* **55**(2):49–69. doi:10.5326/jaaha-ms-6933.

Drögemüller, C., Karlsson, E. K., Hytönen, M. K. et al. (2008) Mutation in hairless dogs implicates FOXI3 in ectodermal development. *Science (American Association for the Advancement of Science)* **321**(5895):1462–1462. doi:10.1126/science.1162525.

Kupczik, K., Cagan, A., Brauer, S., & Fischer, M. S. (2017) The dental phenotype of hairless dogs with FOXI3 haploinsufficiency. *Scientific Reports* **7**(1):5459. doi: 10.1038/s41598-017-05764-5.

1.4 Chanel, 12-mo FE Pomeranian: mated by accident

a) The canine gestation period is commonly considered to be 63 days. Quoted ranges are 57–72 days post-mating or 64–66 days post-luteinising hormone (LH) surge, if this is known (Lamm & Makloski 2012). Note that, in a small-breed dog like Chanel, 12 months seems a little late for a first heat. It is possible that this is Chanel's second heat and the first was clinically silent with minimal bleeding and vulval swelling, which the owners missed.

b) While there are many tests described for pregnancy detection in a bitch, key tests used in practice are abdominal palpation,

ultrasonography, radiography (Figure A1.4a,b) and relaxin assay (Table A1.4). As a rule of thumb, pregnancy detection is most reliable 4 weeks post-mating. Therefore, it may be useful to recheck Chanel in 10 days.

c) Caesarean sections are typically indicated for the treatment of dystocia, but may also be used to prevent dystocia. There is currently no consensus on which bitches would benefit from elective C-sections (Schrank et al. 2022). The maternal mortality rate associated with dystocia was 1.7%, while puppy mortality rates of 20% have been reported (O'Neill et al. 2019). While the

Table A1.4 Methods used to confirm pregnancy in the bitch (adapted from Lamm & Makloski 2012)

METHOD	IDEAL TIME TO PERFORM	COMMENTS
Abdominal palpation	3–4 weeks (21–30 days) post-mating	It may be possible to palpate small ovoid swellings along the uterine horns during this time, but the sensitivity of this technique depends on the operator and the dog. Palpation cannot be used to determine the number or viability of fetuses
Blood relaxin levels	From 3 weeks (21 days) post-breeding; peaks around days 40–50	Relaxin cannot be used to determine the number or viability of fetuses. False-negative results can occur with small litter sizes
Abdominal ultrasonography	3–4 weeks (21–30 days) post-LH surge	Ultrasonography can detect fetal heartbeats (should be >220 bpm; rates >180 and <220 indicate moderate fetal distress and those <180 indicate severe fetal distress); fetal movement can be detected from day 31. Ultrasonography is unreliable in assessing the number of fetuses
Abdominal radiography	More sensitive approximately 6.5 weeks (>47 days) post-breeding or 42–45 days post-LH surge, if known	Radiographs can be used to estimate the number of fetuses (count number of skulls). Visible radiographic structures can be used to estimate gestational age based on mineralisation, though not all structures are visible until late in gestation: 1. Skull: days 43–46 2. Scapula, humerus, femur: days 46–51 3. Radius, ulna, tibia: days 50–53 4. Pelvis and all ribs: days 53–59 5. Coccygeal vertebrae, fibula, calcaneus, distal extremities: days 55–64 6. Teeth: days 58–63 Radiographs are unreliable in estimating fetal viability. Note that it may not be possible to take diagnostic quality radiographs without sedation. Appropriate radiation safety precautions should be taken if patients are manually restrained for radiographs. Manual restraint may be forbidden by local regulation

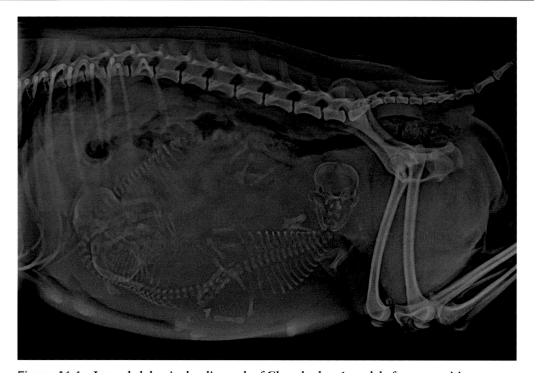

Figure A1.4a Lateral abdominal radiograph of Chanel taken 1 week before parturition.

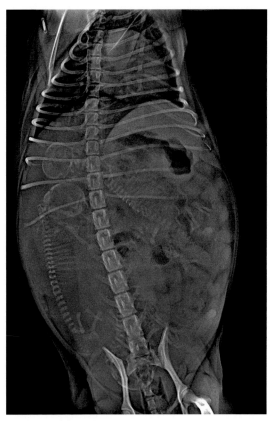

Figure A1.4b Ventrodorsal abdominal radiograph of Chanel 1 week before parturition.

rates of stillbirths were lower with elective C-sections than with emergency C-sections, having a C-section was associated with a fourfold increase in the risk of needing a C-section in future whelpings (Schrank et al. 2022). As the risk of dystocia is increased in cases of feto-maternal disproportion, which in turn may be more likely in single-fetus pregnancies or small litters (Figure A1.4c), it may be helpful to reserve judgement until you are able to take a radiograph. Owners need to be counselled about the risks of general anaesthesia and surgery, risks to the patient and puppies, and potential impact on subsequent breeding.

d) Eclampsia, caused by hypocalcaemia, most commonly occurs post-partum when pups have started nursing, increasing demands on the maternal calcium supply. It is particularly common in smaller breeds (Figure A1.4d). It can also occur during pregnancy. Clinical signs include restlessness, panting, stiffness, and muscle tremors and fasciculations. Clinical signs can be confused with Stage 2 labour if eclampsia occurs pre-partum. The

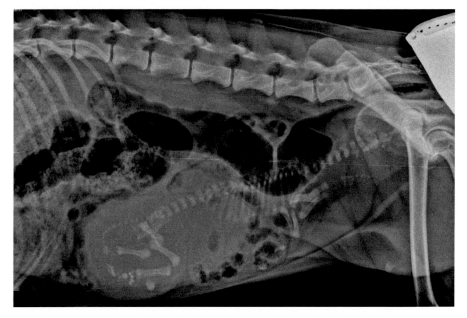

Figure A1.4c A case of dystocia in a feline patient associated with a single fetus.

condition can be fatal if not treated. Low calcium concentrations (<6.5 mg/dL of serum calcium or <2.4 mg/dL of ionised calcium) are diagnostic (Lamm & Makloski 2012). Treatment requires IV administration of 10% calcium gluconate.

REFERENCES

Lamm, C. G. & Makloski, C. L. (2012) Current advances in gestation and parturition in cats and dogs. *Veterinary Clinics of North America Small Animal Practice* **42**:445–456. doi: 10.1016/j. cvsm.2012.01.010.

O'Neill, D. G., O'Sullivan, A. M., Manson, E. A. et al. (2019) Canine dystocia in 50 UK first-opinion emergency care veterinary practices: clinical management and outcomes. *Veterinary Record* **184**:409. doi: 10.1136/vr.104944.

Schrank, M., Contiero, B. & Mollo, A. (2022) Incidence and concomitant factors of Caesarean sections in the bitch: a questionnaire study. *Frontiers in Veterinary Science* **9**:934273. doi: 10.3389/fvets.2022.934273.

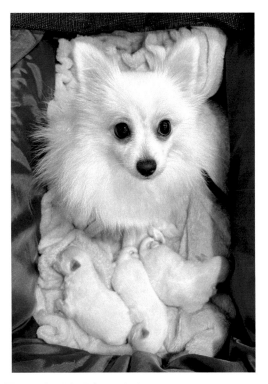

Figure A1.4d Eclampsia is commonest post-partum in small-breed dogs.

1.5 Miso, 12-yo FN DSH (inpatient): not eating

a) The potential causes of inappetence are listed in Table A1.5a. There are probably many more causes here than you thought of in a few minutes, but this is just to remind you of how susceptible cats are to being put off their food.

b) The first thing you can do is repeat the physical examination. This is inexpensive and minimally invasive, and allows you to assess Miso's condition (including the presence of pain), her hydration, and any change in her physical status that might help focus further investigations, if needed. A full dietary history should be taken and Miso's preferred food can be offered. Her hospital cage should be set up to allow her a space to hide, and she should be housed well away from other animals. Blood work can be performed, but, to minimise costs, could be run in a staged fashion. It would be useful to assess hydration (PCV/TP) and electrolytes, which can also be useful in guiding fluid therapy. A complete blood count (CBC) and blood smear will help identify and characterise anaemia, or an increased white cell count, which may be indicative of inflammation or infection. Blood smears can be screened for infectious organisms. A biochemistry panel, along with a urine specific gravity (USG) and dipstick, may indicate hepatobiliary or renal disease, diabetes mellitus, and screen for pancreatitis. If pancreatitis is suspected, feline pancreatic lipase may provide support. Imaging may be useful and should be staged according to the physical examination findings. Three-view thoracic radiographs are useful in screening for cardiovascular, lower respiratory and thoracic disease (such as congestive heart

Table A1.5a **Factors associated with inappetence in cats, and potential causes (adapted from Taylor et al. 2022)**

FACTOR THAT MAY CAUSE INAPPETENCE	EXAMPLE(S)
Pain	Secondary to primary gastrointestinal disease (such as a foreign body or neoplastic disease) or pain outside the GIT (orthopaedic pain, dermatological pain), pain associated with IV catheter
Pyrexia	Infectious disease, inflammatory or immune-mediated disease
Nausea	May be related directly to underlying disease or medication
Ileus	May be associated with pancreatitis, gastrointestinal foreign bodies, and electrolyte derangements (such as hypokalaemia)
Constipation	Megacolon, pelvic fractures, osteoarthritis, dehydration
Distress	Transport to vet and removal from familiar environment and people, proximity to dogs or other cats in hospital, being handled and examined by unfamiliar people, unfamiliar routines, dietary change, lack of agency, restricted movement (e.g. that caused by the presence of bandages or dressings, IV fluid giving sets, Elizabethan collars), unfamiliar auditory and olfactory stimulation
Dietary	Food preference not available, food aversion, reduced food palatability
Gastrointestinal disease	Oral/dental disease, oesophagitis, inflammatory bowel disease, gastrointestinal foreign body
Pancreatic disease	Pancreatitis (acute or chronic), pancreatic abscess or neoplasia
Liver disease	Cholangitis
Urinary tract disease	Acute or chronic kidney disease, ureteral obstruction, feline lower urinary tract disease
Endocrinopathy	Diabetic ketoacidosis, hyperaldosteronism
Immune-mediated disease	Immune-mediated haemolytic anaemia (IMHA)
Haematological	Anaemia – acute or chronic
Neoplastic disease	Primary GIT, or extra-GIT (e.g. lymphoma)
Respiratory disease	Upper respiratory tract inflammation or infection, pneumonia
Cardiovascular disease	Congestive heart failure
Neurological disease	Intracranial disease, diseases impacting prehension and/or swallowing of food
Medication	Bitter taste of medication, adverse effect of medication, interaction of medications, aversion to handling associated with medication administration

failure, neoplastic disease), while abdominal radiographs may provide a useful screen for organomegaly, gastrointestinal foreign bodies, and to evaluate the severity of constipation, when present. Abdominal ultrasonography is a more useful modality to screen for hepatobiliary disease, intestinal disease, and disease involving the kidneys and ureters.

c) Appetite stimulants are contraindicated in patients with nausea or acute vomiting, those unable to ingest food properly, where analgesia is inadequate or ineffective, in the presence of ileus and when patients are otherwise critically ill (Taylor et al. 2022).

d) Appetite stimulants used in feline patients are outlined in Table A1.5b.

REFERENCES

Pardo, M., Spencer, E., Odunayo, A. et al. (2024) AAHA fluid therapy guidelines for dogs and cats. *Journal of the American Animal Hospital Association.* **60**(4):131-163. doi: 10.5326/JAAHA-MS-7444. PMID: 38885492.

Taylor, S., Chan, D. L., Villaverde, C. et al. (2022) ISFM consensus guidelines on management of the inappetent hospitalised cat. *Journal of Feline Medicine and Surgery* **24**:614–640. doi: 10.1177/1098612X221106353.

Table A1.5b Agents used to stimulate appetite in feline patients (adapted from Taylor et al. 2022)

DRUG	DOSE, FREQUENCY, AND ROUTE OF ADMINISTRATION	POSSIBLE ADVERSE EFFECTS	CONTRAINDICATIONS/ INTERACTIONS
Mirtazapine	2 mg per cat every 24 hours (q24h) per os (PO) or transdermal (NB reduce frequency to q48h in patients with renal/hepatic disease)	• Vocalisation • Agitation • Erythema at site of application (if transdermal administration)	Do not use concurrently with cyproheptadine
Capromorelin	2 mg/kg q24h PO	• Vomiting • Hypersalivation • Lethargy • Hyperglycaemia • Bradycardia • Hypotension	• Do not use in cats with diabetes mellitus, acromegaly • Avoid in systemically compromised patients
Cyproheptadine	1–4 mg per cat q12–14h	• Sedation	• Do not use concurrently with mirtazapine • Avoid in cats with hepatic lipidosis

1.6 Bosca, 2-yo MN Wolfhound: *phone call*, ate choc muffins

a) Where toxic exposure is suspected, it helps to know the animal's weight, type of chocolate (Table A1.6), and the maximum amount in g/kg ingested, as well as an approximate time frame during which the ingestion took place. As these muffins were home-made, it would help to know the recipe, as they may contain other potential toxins. There are several free, online chocolate toxicity calculators that can be useful in suggesting whether a dog has consumed a potentially toxic dose. These include those published in the MSD Manual and Vets Now:

- *www.msdvetmanual.com/multimedia/ clinical-calculator/chocolate-toxicity-calculator*
- *www.vets-now.com/dog-chocolate-toxicity-calculator/*

b) The artificial sweetener, xylitol, may lead to hypoglycaemia or hepatic injury (DuHadway et al. 2015); raisins or sultanas may lead to acute kidney injury and neurological signs (Schweighauser et al. 2020); macadamia nuts may lead to gastrointestinal and neurological signs (Cortinovis & Caloni 2016). In addition, fatty foods can trigger gastroenteritis or pancreatitis (Weingart et al. 2021).

c) Documented signs include agitation, tremors, seizures, muscle stiffness, ataxia, loss of consciousness, vomiting, panting, PU/PD, diarrhoea, tachycardia, and hyperthermia.

d) Bring Bosca in as soon as possible to induce vomiting. Dogs should be observed once emesis is induced, as some patients will re-ingest the vomitus. Once the offending

Table A1.6 Theobromine and caffeine content in different types of chocolate (adapted from Weingart et al. 2021 and Martínez-Pinilla et al. 2015)

TYPE OF CHOCOLATE	THEOBROMINE	CAFFEINE
White chocolate	Negligible	Negligible
Milk chocolate	0.5–2.0 mg/g	0.1–0.9 mg/g
Dark chocolate (>55% cocoa)	5.0–8.5 mg/g	0.5–2.6 mg/g
Bitter chocolate (>70% cocoa)	5.5–12.7 mg/g	0.7–3.0 mg/g
Cocoa powder	5.0 mg/g	2.6 mg/g

chocolate is expelled, an anti-emetic such as maropitant can be given to treat residual nausea. Following emesis, dogs can be given activated charcoal (1–4 g/kg PO). As methylxanthines undergo extrahepatic recirculation, it may be helpful to administer charcoal every 12 hours over a 72-hour period.

e) The onset of toxicity can be delayed in dogs, and while the mortality rate is low (<3%; Weingart et al. 2021), chocolate toxicity is a known cause of death in dogs. It is easier (and less costly) to treat ingestion than potentially life-threatening effects of toxicity.

f) Treatment is supportive and symptomatic, and may include fluid therapy to replace losses and maintain blood pressure (BP), a cardioselective beta-1 adrenergic antagonist for tachycardia (e.g. esmolol 25 µg/kg/minute IV), benzodiazepines (e.g. midazolam 0.2–0.5 mg/kg) for dogs exhibiting agitation, tremors or seizures, anti-emetics (e.g. maropitant 1 mg/kg SC or IV q24h) and close monitoring (Weingart et al. 2021).

REFERENCES

Cortinovis, C. & Caloni, F. (2016) Household food items toxic to dogs and cats. *Frontiers in Veterinary Science* 3:26. doi: 10.3389/fvets.2016.00026.

DuHadway, M. R., Sharp, C. R., Meyers, K. E. & Koenigshof, A. M. (2015) Retrospective evaluation of xylitol ingestion in dogs: 192 cases (2007–2012). *Journal of Veterinary Emergency and Critical Care* 25(5):646–654. doi: 10.1111/vec.12350.

Martínez-Pinilla, E., Oñatiba-Astibia, A. & Franco, R. (2015) The relevance of theobromine for the beneficial effects of cocoa consumption. *Frontiers in Pharmacology* 6:30. doi: 10.3389/fphar.2015.00030.

Schweighauser, A., Henke, D., Oevermann, A. et al. (2020) Toxicosis with grapes or raisins causing acute kidney injury and neurological signs in dogs. *Journal of Veterinary Internal Medicine* 34(5):1957–1966. doi: 10.1111/jvim.15884.

Weingart, C., Hartmann, A. & Kohn, B. (2021) Chocolate ingestion in dogs: 156 events (2015–2019). *Journal of Small Animal Practice* 62(11):979–983. doi: 10.1111/jsap.13329.

1.7 Kenya, 6-yo FN Jack Russell Terrier: smells bad!

a) There are many reasons why a dog may 'smell bad'. Kenya is exhibiting three of them: dental disease, full anal glands, and otitis externa. Encouraging the owner to describe the smell may help localise it (anal gland secretion can have a 'fishy' odour, ears can smell 'yeasty', and bad teeth can smell 'like a sewer'), but human sensitivities to smell do vary! Other common reasons for bad smells can include nasal disease and sinusitis, foreign bodies in the mouth or nose, skin disease (including skin fold dermatitis), wet and matted coat, flystrike, pseudocoprostasis, urinary incontinence/infection, discharge from an open pyometra (or stump pyometra in a neutered dog), uraemic breath and flatulence.

b) Kenya has some telltale signs of serious dental disease: cementum exposure on the left upper canine (requiring a difficult, probably surgical, extraction), furcation exposure on left lower carnassial (requiring a difficult, probably surgical, extraction). Going on the basis that dental disease is often worse than it looks on cursory inspection, there is a strong possibility that deposits of tartar/calculus are masking similar problems in other teeth. So this looks like a major procedure that might need to be staged into more than one operation for Kenya.

c) Clinical examination has itself revealed a possible explanation for Kenya's ill-defined weight loss. There are both advantages and disadvantages to comprehensive blood screens in a dog like Kenya (see also Case 2.10 which concerns pre-anaesthetic blood screening). Looking at the abnormal values, the challenge is attaching significance to them in the light of Kenya's presenting signs and clinical examination.

The absolute values for lymphocytes and eosinophils are within the normal ranges and the pathologist noted no abnormalities on the smear, so these slight changes can be 'parked' for the moment.

Globulin, ALT and ALP are slightly elevated, but liver enzyme elevations, when clinically significant, occur in orders of magnitude.

The calcium values are low. This is what triggered Kenya's owner's anxiety, except she appears to have misunderstood what she read on the internet, or read from an unreliable source, because high calcium, not low, has an association with cancer. Calcium is susceptible to delays in sample processing and other artefacts and Kenya's sample did have to wait overnight to be assayed. Kenya's value of 0.80 mmol/L for ionised calcium sits on the cusp of a hypocalcaemia diagnosis; however, she had no signs attributable to this problem and 'the need for treatment of hypocalcaemia is dependent on the presence of clinical signs, rather than a specific cut-off of serum concentration of iCa itself' (Poli 2018). The main approach here would be to correct the owner on calcium and cancer and explain the probably artefactual low result.

The cholesterol and triglyceride changes are marginal and hard to interpret with no clinical suspicion of relevant disease.

The raised C-reactive protein is only slightly above the reference range and, being a marker for inflammation, may reflect Kenya's periodontitis or could be inconsequential.

Regarding the other 'abnormalities',
the best approach would be to talk the owner through the principles of laboratory reference ranges, how they are based on a normal distribution curve, and how, if you measure enough parameters in any dog, it is likely that some will lie outside the 'normal' range. This is one of the perils of using blood screens as a 'net' to go fishing for abnormalities: they can result in blind alleys being pursued at further expense to the owner, and are sometimes detrimental to the client–vet relationship (McKenzie 2016). You cannot, of course, say that Kenya definitely does not have cancer, merely that these bloods show no cause for concern regarding cancer given Kenya's current history and physical exam.

In terms of the weight loss and the owner's worry, it is possible that even though Kenya is in good body condition, she may have been overweight. Dental disease may be associated with weight loss in some dogs. Because the owner is concerned, it is worth ensuring that Kenya revisits for weighing in subsequent weeks and months. It is also worth revisiting the history regarding the weight loss. Is it possible that Kenya is exercising a bit more, e.g. in better weather, for longer or additional walks?

d) Kenya should be booked in for her dentistry, which is a clear clinical problem and likely to be causing her pain. At the same time, her ears can be thoroughly examined, cleaned and treated if necessary, and another check made of those anal glands.

REFERENCES

McKenzie, B. A. (2016) Overdiagnosis. *Journal of the American Veterinary Medical Association* **249**:884–889. doi: 10.2460/javma.249.8.884.

Poli, G. (2024) Ionised hypocalcaemia, part 3: acute treatment and management. *Veterinary Times* 13 February. Available at: www.vettimes.co.uk/ionised-hypocalcaemia-pt-3-acute-treatment-and-management/.

1.8 Charles, 5-yo MN Cocker Spaniel: licking left paw+++

a) Grass-seed foreign-body disease can be associated with a range of presentations, from relatively uncomplicated cases, such as that of Charles, to highly complex clinical presentations involving the lungs and pleural space, retroperitoneal space, vertebral column, spinal cord, brain and lower urinary tract (Combs et al. 2017). Clinical signs relate to the location of the seed, as per Table A1.8.

    Factors influencing presentation are as follows:

i) **Site of entry** (e.g. through the skin, nose, external ear canal, conjunctiva or penile urethra).

ii) **Pathogens** that may be translocated with the migrating grass seed (e.g. saprophytic organisms such as *Nocardia* spp., skin flora such as *Staphylococcus pseudintermedius* or oropharyngeal flora such as *Pasteurella multocida* or *Streptococcus* spp.

iii) **Path of migration**, as pointed barbs and angled serrations of awns cause unidirectional passage of the seed with body movement. Thus grass seeds may migrate between fascial planes, between muscles or along airways and into the pleural space, leading to inflammation, infection and perforation of structures.

iv) **Drainage** of the site of septic focus, e.g. via a sinus in the skin.

b) A needle could be inserted into the skin proximal to the sinus, and the sinus flushed with sterile saline from the inside out, to ensure that foreign material is not inadvertently forced deeper into the wound. It may be beneficial to heavily sedate or anaesthetise Charles to permit clipping of the fur to facilitate visualisation and thorough exploration of the sinus. The sinus could be bluntly enlarged and gently lavaged to flush foreign material out. In some cases, it may be

Table A1.8 **Common clinical signs associated with grass seeds or awns, depending on location (adapted from Philp et al. 2022)**

LOCATION OF GRASS SEED/AWN	COMMON CLINICAL SIGNS
Cutaneous, subcutaneous or intramuscular	Localised swelling, with or without a draining sinus
Aural canal	Head shaking, head tilt, otitis externa with purulent discharge
Oral cavity	Dysphagia, tongue swelling, gagging
Nasal cavity	Persistent sneezing, epistaxis
Ocular (often conjunctival fornix)	Blepharospasm, ocular swelling, corneal ulceration
Airways/thoracic cavity	Coughing, tachypnoea, pneumothorax or pyothorax
Urogenital tract	Discharge
Sublumbar	Lethargy, regional pain

useful to make a small incision to extend the sinus dorsally and follow the tract.

c) Foreign bodies can be challenging to locate, even in the presence of a sinus. Owners should always be warned that a foreign body may not be located on the first attempt. Radiography may be beneficial in locating radiopaque foreign bodies or accumulation of gas, but has low sensitivity for detecting plant material. The injection of radiopaque dye into a sinus tract may be helpful in locating foreign bodies in more chronic cases. Ultrasonography may be helpful in detecting subcutaneous grass seeds. If a foreign body is not found, it may be useful to take a swab for culture, and consider other differentials such as an insect bite or sting, or neoplasia. As long as the dog remains systemically well, it may be helpful to re-examine in 24–48 hours. In some (often more chronic) cases, referral for computerised tomography (CT) or ultrasonography may be required to localise a grass seed (Figure A1.8a,b).

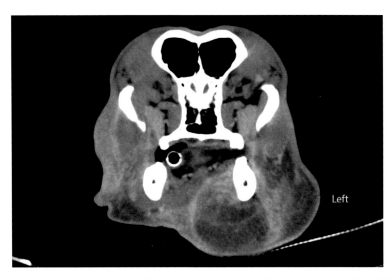

Figure A1.8a A CT scan of a 1.5-year-old Boxer puppy presented for severe facial swelling with a focus around the left mandible. The puppy had recently undergone surgical exploration of the area, during which a single grass seed was retrieved.

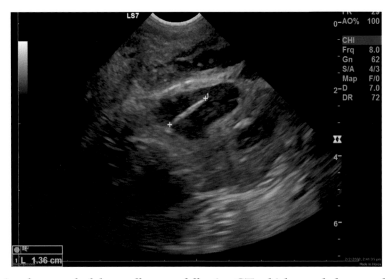

Figure A1.8b An ultrasound of the swollen area following CT, which revealed a second grass-seed foreign body that was subsequently removed.

d) The aim of treatment is to remove the foreign material and (if required) resect diseased tissue. As this presentation is acute and superficial, flushing of the wound with sterile saline can be performed to minimise contamination. It is important to check Charles for other potential sinuses and ensure the coat is clear of grass seeds.

Charles is sore and probably requires analgesia. As he is systemically well with a normal appetite, a non-steroidal anti-inflammatory drug (NSAID) may be suitable. In addition, he may require an Elizabethan collar to minimise self-trauma during recovery. Once the foreign body has been removed and the wound flushed, the sinus should heal and the cellulitis should resolve rapidly. If the wound does not substantially improve in 24 hours, or if it worsens, Charles should be reassessed.

REFERENCES

Combs, M., Hicks, A., Young, P. et al. (2017) Grass seed foreign body-related disease in dogs and cats: a wide spectrum of clinical presentations. *Australian Veterinary Practitioner* **47**(1):13–24.

Philp, H. S., Epstein, S. E. & Hopper, K. (2022) Clinical and clinicopathological characteristics, treatment, and outcome for dogs and cats with confirmed foxtail foreign body lesions: 791 cases (2009–2018). *Journal of Veterinary Emergency and Critical Care (San Antonio)* **32**(5):653–662. doi: 10.1111/vec.13209.

1.9 Felix, 8-yo MN Sphynx: swelling on flank

a) Cellulitis is a diffuse bacterial infection of the skin and subcutaneous tissues. Unlike an abscess, which is localised, cellulitis can move through tissue planes and, if serious, can enter the bloodstream, causing sepsis. Cellulitis will make an animal systemically unwell, and is often associated with pyrexia.

b) When lancing and draining an abscess, choose an area that is dependent, i.e. where gravity will allow the fluid/pus to drain of its own accord. A common mistake is to make the drainage incision too small so that it closes up again before drainage is complete; the abscess then reforms. A drainage incision of around 1.0 cm should be enough.

c) Flushing with warm sterile saline is sufficient. Alternatives are dilute chlorhexidine and proprietary flush solutions, but saline is fine. Just make sure the flushing is copious (50–100 mL) and gentle.

d) Antibiotics are not indicated. Australian Veterinary Prescribing Guidelines (University of Melbourne) state that systemic antimicrobials are required only for a surgically managed abscess when one or all of the following criteria are met:
   i) The animal is systemically unwell, e.g. true pyrexia
   ii) There is evidence of diffuse tissue involvement
   iii) There is potential joint involvement
   iv) The patient is immunosuppressed

If any of these apply, it is recommended to give amoxicillin, 11–15 mg/kg q8–12 hours, for 5–10 days.

In a healthy cat such as Felix, with no history of renal disease, a dose of NSAIDs should be given for pain relief. The most important thing is to keep the abscess draining and clean. If the owner, Lizzie, can keep Felix indoors and gently wipe the crust from his abscess wounds once or twice daily, this is likely to be sufficient. She could use boiled and cooled water and cotton swabs. Ideally, you would provide Lizzie with a handout clearly explaining what to do and when, and perhaps prompt her to think about people she can call upon if she finds wound care difficult on her own. Ensure the owner realises that the purpose of the bathing is to keep the wound open for a few days to allow it to 'heal from the inside' since this is a counter-intuitive concept for many owners, who expect all wounds to be stitched up.

e) Few people feel comfortable contradicting what their boss has said and done, but this is a different situation from the last bite. To avoid awkwardness, if Felix does not need antibiotics, you might say something like the following:
   - 'I'm guessing that last time, the situation was a bit different. For example, the abscess might have been closer to a joint, or there could have been signs that Felix

was developing a more serious infection, so antibiotics were given. But the good news is that, this time, I am confident that he doesn't need antibiotics.'

- 'Antibiotics are great when they are needed, but I don't think that's the case this time around. We avoid antibiotics whenever we can, because they come with some downsides, for example, they will also kill good bacteria in Felix's gut. Too many antibiotics can also encourage superbugs inside Felix that could cause bigger problems for him down the track.'

If you do need to use antibiotics, e.g. due to associated cellulitis or other patient factors, such as immune compromise, you might try the following:

- 'I'm going to need you to keep Felix inside for the next 5 days and give him these amoxycillin tablets to sort out the cellulitis. That long-acting injection can be a useful antibiotic, but it lasts for longer than Felix needs for this particular abscess, and we really don't want to treat him for longer than he needs because … [dysbiosis, superbugs, adverse effects]'
- 'I've been reading some recent research/ heard at a conference that amoxycillin is the best antibiotic for this situation – it's a bit more work to give than the injection, but it's a better match for the bacteria involved so it's what we should give Felix. The other antibiotic he had last time is one we should really keep in reserve for if and when he really needs it.'
- 'I'm going to show you two really good ways to give a cat a tablet and then I'll give you a handout of the steps and send a link to a video to your phone, so you can review it at home. If you find it really difficult, give us a call, and we'll figure something out.'

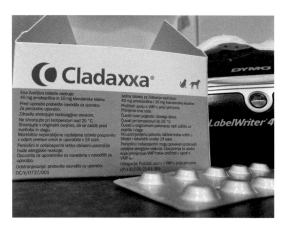

Figure A1.9 While many veterinarians may prescribe amoxycillin–clavulanate (as shown here) for cat-bite abscess, amoxycillin alone is a more guideline-concordant choice for uncomplicated cellulitis in cats.

If tableting is genuinely not feasible, consider long-acting amoxycillin injections q48h.

Finally, involve your veterinary nurses in your antibiotic stewardship efforts! Qualitative research with Australian veterinarians has found that doing so enables the team to find innovative ways to provide antibiotic guideline-concordant care (Scarborough et al. 2023) (Figure A1.9).

REFERENCES

Scarborough, R. O., Sri, A. E., Browning, G. F. et al. (2023) 'Brave enough': a qualitative study of veterinary decisions to withhold or delay antimicrobial treatment in pets. *Antibiotics* **12**(3):540. doi: 10.3390/antibiotics12030540.

University of Melbourne (2019) *Australian Veterinary Prescribing Guidelines, Dogs and Cats* (version 2). Melbourne, VIC: The University of Melbourne. Available at: https://vetantibiotics.science.unimelb.edu.au/.

1.10 Lucy, 15-mo FN DSH: vomiting

a) Vomiting and inappetence may be signs of primary GIT disease or systemic disease (McGrotty 2010). The acute onset of both vomiting and inappetence in a young cat are most suggestive of primary GIT disease, with gastrointestinal foreign body, acute gastritis secondary to diet, or ingestion of a toxin high on the index of suspicion. Very occasionally, an oral foreign body may cause similar signs (Figure A1.10a).

b) *Does Lucy play with toys? Have you seen her chew on or eat non-food items?* This can suggest exposure to potential foreign bodies. (In this case, the owners said Lucy frequently chews hair ties.)

   What is Lucy's normal diet? Has this changed? Dietary change, contamination, or food intolerance can lead to acute vomiting.

   Has Lucy had exposure to potential toxins such as plants, pesticides, cleaning products or medications? Exposure to these can cause irritation and acute inflammation of the GIT, leading to vomiting. These patients may have oral ulcers and ptyalism. In

addition, toxins may lead to acute kidney or hepatic injury, which can also cause vomiting. In such cases, animals usually present with other signs (e.g. in the case of acute kidney injury, polydipsia, polyuria, or even anuria may be reported; in the case of hepatic injury, animals may be jaundiced or present with signs of a coagulopathy such as petechiae or bruising).

c) These should be guided by the specific patient history and physical examination. Often, the 'minimum database' for the vomiting patient undergoing investigations includes a CBC, biochemistry panel, and urinalysis. In a young healthy animal, this rarely yields a diagnosis, but may rule out systemic disease and inform fluid therapy. Because the owners revealed that Lucy chews hair ties (i.e. potential foreign bodies), plain radiography was performed.

d) As the cause is not known, supportive care is recommended. Fluid therapy can be used to restore and maintain hydration, while analgesia may be indicated. Clinicians may vary somewhat in their use of anti-emetics in a case like Lucy's. Some may argue that these drugs should not be used until a cause for the vomiting is established; others are happy to treat in suitably assessed cases and would consider continued vomiting following administration of anti-emetics a prompt for investigation (usually imaging). In one study, the use of anti-emetics in dogs and cats subsequently diagnosed with a gastrointestinal foreign body was associated with increased time to definitive treatment and increased length of hospitalisation, but was not associated with an increased risk of foreign body-associated complications. The authors conclude that 'antiemetics are not inherently contraindicated in patients for whom [gastrointestinal foreign-body obstruction] is a differential, but clients

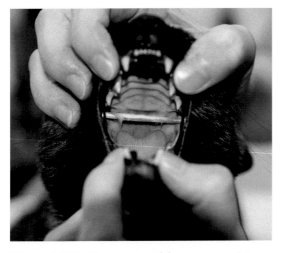

Figure A1.10a Cat presented for acute vomiting and inappetence after eating a feather. Oral examination revealed the shaft of a feather lodged between the upper teeth.

should be counselled to monitor for progression of clinical signs and follow up accordingly' (Puzio et al. 2023). This does not guide the *timing* of diagnostic evaluations, however, which is left to clinical judgement in individual cases. If in doubt, recommend (and record) the investigations and ensure that the owner understands your reasons even if they decline and opt to 'wait and see'. Antibiotics are not recommended for the treatment of acute vomiting.

e) In cats, linear foreign bodies may become anchored around the base of the tongue, so oral examination is particularly important. Similarly, foreign bodies are often located in the stomach, pylorus, and ileocolic junction (Bebchuk 2002). Abdominal palpation may reveal a mass effect. In a fractious cat like this patient, sedation or even anaesthesia may be required to perform an oral examination and abdominal palpation. Fractious patients can often appear healthier than they really are, but can deteriorate quickly.

f) Given the position of the foreign body (distal to the stomach – see Figure 1.10 in the question), surgical removal via exploratory laparotomy is the treatment of choice. This allows removal by enterotomy if the intestine is viable, which it is likely to be given the recent acute onset of signs, or resection and anastomosis if the gut is compromised. A foreign body was removed from Lucy (Figure A1.10b). The gut was

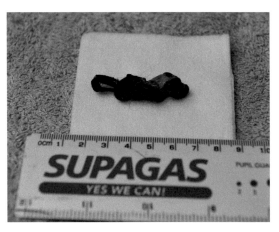

Figure A1.10b **The hair tie that was removed from Lucy via enterotomy following an exploratory laparotomy.**

thoroughly explored for additional foreign bodies. Gastric foreign bodies may be able to be removed by endoscopy.

Lucy was also treated with IV fluids, analgesia (methadone every 4 hours), maropitant, and meloxicam. Food was introduced 6 hours post-surgery to promote early enteral nutrition. The owners were advised to be vigilant in case Lucy ingested further foreign bodies.

- Antibiotics are not recommended for the treatment of acute vomiting.
- Fractious patients can often appear healthier than they really are, but can deteriorate quickly.
- Anti-emetics are not contraindicated when the cause of vomiting is uncertain, but should be used with care when foreign-body obstruction is a differential.

REFERENCES

Bebchuk, T. N. (2002) Feline gastrointestinal foreign bodies. *Veterinary Clinics of North America: Small Animal Practice* **32**(4):861–880. doi: 10.1016/s0195-5616(02)00030-x.

McGrotty, Y. (2010) Medical management of acute and chronic vomiting in dogs and cats. *In Practice* **32**(10):478–483. doi: 10.1136/inp.c6670.

Puzio, C. E., Rudloff, E. & Pigott, A. M. (2023) Delay of definitive care in cats and dogs with gastrointestinal foreign body obstruction following antiemetic administration: 537 cases (2012–2020). *Journal of Veterinary Emergency and Critical Care (San Antonio)* **33**(4):442–446. doi: 10.1111/vec.13315.

1.11 Ariel, 18-mo MN DSH: rehomed – sneezing & snorting

a) Ariel's nostril and philtrum deviate to the left side and there seems to be a defect in the upper right lip. The right lower canine (404) is visible rostrally and the crown is sitting in front of the right nares. Three symmetrical and widely spaced lower incisors are present, suggesting that some teeth are missing in between. Apart from this, Ariel looks healthy and alert, with no ocular, nasal, or oral discharges.

b) There is communication between the nasal and oral cavities rostrally caused by deviation and loss of bone (premaxilla) and soft tissue between right upper incisors 1 and 2 (101, 102). In addition, tooth alignment is disrupted. The lateral part of the right nostril and a section of upper lip are missing. Three lower incisors (probably 301, 302, and 402) are absent. Functionally, the problem is the rostral communication between nasal and oral cavities, creating an oronasal fistula. There is little sign of inflammation or infection currently.

c) One option is a fuller history to check Ariel's overall health status, quality of life (QOL), and signs of oral discomfort. If QOL is good, then an option is to do nothing and monitor the situation. Advice from a veterinary dentist or surgery specialist could be sought regarding costs and the owner could perhaps start saving for reconstructive surgery. You do not want to end up making the situation worse ('first, do no harm'); however, it is possible problems may develop that will push surgery further up the agenda. It is also possible that referral costs or practicalities (e.g. travel) may be prohibitive at any stage. If going to surgery, informed consent is necessary, including the possibility of additional costs associated with complications with this type of surgery.

d) In Ariel's case, the main principles would be to try to restore separation and continuity of the oral and nasal cavities and ensure good function with no discomfort. The simplest procedure to attain this would likely have the best chance of success. Common problems when operating in this area include lack of tissue for mobilisation and consequent tension on suture lines leading to dehiscence. The oral cavity is an awkward place in which to operate: small, sharp instruments, good lighting, magnification if needed, a comfortable seating position, and plenty of time are required. Preparation and rehearsal will help, e.g. drawing out intended procedures on paper or using plasticine on a skull if available. Research will be necessary, even if Ariel's specific problem is unlikely to be covered in standard texts, but surgery is often about adapting techniques while following general principles (e.g. Niemiec 2012, Kirpensteijn & ter Haar 2013, Radlinsky & Fossum 2018). Specialists may be able to help by conference call or email. Procedures might need to be staged, requiring more than one anaesthetic, e.g. an initial procedure might be to remove some teeth in order to mobilise gingiva or mucosa later, once the extraction sites have fully healed, since removing teeth and creating flaps at the same time might increase the risk of wound breakdown. Tension on the suture line is the enemy in this type of procedure. Part of the planning should involve intra-oral X-rays, as these will help give you a better picture of what is going on. Appropriate suture material, cat-sized instruments (especially a sharp periosteal elevator), and a plan B, if possible, will increase the chances of success. Fully informed consent and good owner communication are vital in cases like Ariel's to manage expectations.

Halsted's principles

William Stewart Halsted (1852–1922) was an American surgeon who developed some core principles for surgery:
- Handle tissues gently
- Create excellent haemostasis
- Preserve the blood supply
- Use aseptic technique
- Close tissues without tension
- Avoid creating dead space

Aseptic technique is not possible in the oral cavity, but the other principles all apply.

REFERENCES

Kirpensteijn, J. & ter Haar, G. (2013) *Reconstructive Surgery and Wound Management of the Dog and Cat*. London: Manson Publishing.

Niemiec, B. A. (2012) Pathologies of the Oral Mucosa. In: Niemiec, B. A. (ed.) *A Colour Handbook of Small Animal Dental, Oral and Maxillofacial Disease*. Boca Raton, FL: CRC Press. pp. 183–198.

Radlinsky, M. & Fossum, T. W. (2018) 'Chapter 18, The Digestive System', in Fossum, T.W. (ed) *Small Animal Surgery*, 5th edition. St Louis, MO: Mosby.

1.12 Lucy, 10-yo FE Lab (inpatient): pre-pyo, *review bloods*

a) Acidaemia is defined as a blood pH of <7.35 and alkalaemia as a blood pH of >7.45, so Lucy is acidotic.

There are a few rules to bear in mind when interpreting acid–base results and compensations:
- A change in the respiratory or metabolic dimension induces an opposite response in the other in an effort to normalise the pH and regain homoeostasis
- Respiratory compensations occur quickly through ventilation
- Metabolic compensations occur much more slowly, via the kidney's function, starting within a few hours and maximising metabolic compensation after 4–5 days (overcompensation does not occur)
- The presence of compensation can therefore provide some information about the duration of the underlying condition

In Lucy's case, the low bicarbonate indicates metabolic acidosis and the low pCO_2 indicates respiratory alkalosis as the body tries to correct the metabolic acidosis by 'blowing off' CO_2. The bicarbonate buffering equation is helpful to remember here:

$$CO_2 + H_2O \rightleftarrows H_2CO_3 \rightleftarrows HCO_3^- + H^+$$

In Lucy's case, 'blowing off' CO_2 helps pull the equation to the left, removing the excess hydrogen ions (and attempting to correct acidosis).

b) Lucy is currently receiving normal saline, an acidifying solution. By helping to correct dehydration, saline will contribute to normalisation of her acid–base status, but Hartmann's, an alkalising solution, is the more rational choice in this case and is often the best empirical choice of fluid.

c) Lucy should be taken to surgery as soon as she is clinically stable for anaesthesia. This could be before her blood parameters have completely normalised. 'Never let the sun set on a pyometra' (i.e. do not unnecessarily delay operating) is an old adage that, like all adages, contains a lot of truth but is not universally true (see Case 5.21).

REFERENCE

Monnig, A. A. (2013) Practical acid-base in veterinary patients. *Veterinary Clinics of North America: Small Animal Practice* **43**(6):1273–1286. doi: 10.1016/j.cvsm.2013.07.009.

1.13 Speed, 2-yo ME Australian Cattle Dog: hips

a) The radiographs are low resolution, apparently having been 'screenshotted' rather than emailed directly as files. In addition, the positioning is suboptimal, possibly because Speed was not sufficiently sedated at the time of obtaining the X-rays. Often, general anaesthesia is needed for accurate positioning in trauma cases due to pain associated with manipulation and restraint. A clinical note should be made of these technical issues, and the owner informed, in case something is missed. However, some diagnostic information can be obtained from these pictures.

b) There is a lateral and dorsal–ventral (DV) or ventral–dorsal (VD) view. The lateral view appears to show an empty acetabulum consistent with hip luxation. The DV or VD view tells us Speed is a male dog as the bony os penis and soft tissue of the penis are visible. It is a partial view of the right hemipelvis and is very tilted. It confirms luxation of the right hip. No other fractures are immediately evident, but this is an incomplete survey of the pelvis, and trauma sufficient to luxate a hip could also cause fractures elsewhere or fracture-separations of the sacroiliac joints. A straight view of the entire hip and pelvic region is needed. The bladder is not visible, and bladder rupture is always a possibility with hindquarter trauma. In trauma cases like this, thoracic radiographs should also be taken to screen for pneumothorax and diaphragmatic hernia.

c) The hip luxation appears to be caudoventral. Most hip luxations are craniodorsal.

d) Closed reduction of the luxated hip should be attempted first, but always advise owners that this may fail and ultimately require surgery (Table A1.13). Closed reduction requires general anaesthesia and, importantly, cage rest for 1 week followed by strict confinement (e.g. crate, small room, no jumping) and short toileting walks for 3–4 weeks to allow the replaced hip to stabilise. An Ehmer sling is a possibility for craniodorsal luxations, but can be poorly tolerated and may cause more harm than good. In one study, 50% of dogs suffered soft tissue injury secondary to use of an Ehmer sling due to technical difficulties with sling application and retention; one dog required amputation of the limb (Schlag et al. 2019). Re-luxation after successful closed reduction suggests that surgery will be required; however, caudoventral luxations re-luxate less frequently than craniodorsal after closed reduction, so Speed has a better prognosis. Your colleague can use the opportunity provided by general anaesthesia for reduction to take better-quality hip radiographs, and also thoracic radiographs if not already done.

e) Surgical options for canine hip luxation include iliofemoral suture, transarticular pin, and joint reconstruction/replacement. Femoral head and neck excision (excision arthroplasty) may be cost-effective for clients unable to afford advanced procedures, and can provide good outcomes, especially in smaller and medium-sized dogs who are not overweight.

REFERENCE

Schlag, A.N., Hayes, G.M., Taylor, A.Q. et al. (2019) Analysis of outcomes following treatment of craniodorsal hip luxation with closed reduction and Ehmer sling application in dogs. *Journal of the American Veterinary Medical Association* **254**(12):1436–1440. doi: 10.2460/javma.254.12.1436.

Table A1.13 **Closed or manual reduction of hip luxations**	
DIRECTION OF LUXATION	**REDUCTION TECHNIQUE**
Craniodorsal	• Induce general anaesthesia (sedation is not sufficient) • Place the dog with affected leg uppermost • Ensure the table is at a comfortable operating height • Use countertraction to keep the dog still against the table (one operator) • Externally rotate and distract the femur against the countertraction (second operator) – in doing this, imagine the head of the femur being pulled ventrally so that it crosses the lip and overlies the depression of the acetabulum • Internally rotate and adduct the femur – imagine the head of the femur regaining the acetabulum (this is often felt as the hip 'clunks' back into place) • Extend and abduct the limb and take the joint through the full range of motion to confirm reduction and dispel clots from the acetabulum • ***Important***: Provide cage/crate rest (1 week) then small-room or crate rest with toileting lead exercise only for 3–4 weeks • Note that surgical stabilisation following reluxation may be required • Ehmer slings are reported to cause bandage injury in 50% of cases and re-luxation occurred in 43% of cases (Schlag et al. 2019)
Caudoventral	• Induce general anaesthesia (sedation is not sufficient) • Place the dog with affected leg uppermost • Ensure the table is at a comfortable operating height • Use countertraction to keep the dog still against the table (one operator) • Externally rotate the hip while abducting the hip and adducting the stifle ('hip out, stifle in') • Push dorsally against the countertraction • Relocate the head of the femur in the acetabulum • Note: you may convert the luxation into a craniodorsal one, in which case follow the above method • Extend and abduct the limb and take the joint through the full range of motion to confirm reduction and dispel clots from the acetabulum • ***Important***: Provide cage/crate rest (1 week) then small-room or crate rest with toileting lead exercise only for 3–4 weeks • *Consider* hobbles if tolerated • Caudoventral luxations are less likely to reluxate than craniodorsal luxations

1.14 Paddy, 4-mo ME Cross-breed: another parvo? *in car*

a) These tests are cheap and quick to carry out in-house and can be combined with a blood smear, and, if appropriate, a strip test for blood urea nitrogen (BUN). They are appropriate for cases where there are economic constraints and can give valuable information/confirmation (Table A1.14). In Paddy's case, the tests confirm dehydration and reveal that he is marginally hypoglycaemic.

b) Protein is the main contributor to the refractive index of plasma, but the refractometer measures all substances dissolved in plasma, including some non-protein substances such as glucose, urea, cholesterol, and triglycerides. Modern refractometers are calibrated to subtract 2.0 g/dL to account for these non-protein substances, so are measuring the (estimated) total protein, not the total solids. This slightly 'nerdy' point may be relevant if, for example, an animal had an unusually high concentration of non-protein solids, e.g. a highly lipaemic sample from an animal

Table A1.14 **Interpreting the combined PCV and TP in several different clinical contexts: the important thing is to understand the possibilities of changing values of PCV and TP**

PCV	TP	POSSIBLE INTERPRETATION
↑	↑	• Dehydration
↓	↓	• Haemodilution from IV fluid overload • [Post-haemorrhage: hours later]
↑	Normal	• Dehydration with hypoproteinaemia • Splenic contraction • [Polycythaemia]
↓	Normal	• Red blood cell destruction or reduced production • Anaemia of chronic disease
Normal	↓	• Early haemorrhage (with splenic contraction) • Loss of protein (gastrointestinal, renal) or low production (liver)
↓	↑	• Lymphoproliferative disease • Anaemia of chronic disease

with pancreatitis. This would result in an erroneously high total protein reading. This demonstrates the importance of 'reading' laboratory values in conjunction with the whole clinical picture and not in isolation.

c) Cage-side immunoassays for parvovirus incorporate a parvovirus-specific antibody that binds to the viral antigen in a faecal sample, resulting in colour change. They are economical and useful tests, best employed when results may change the diagnosis and treatment. The test depends on antigen being shed in the faeces.

- **False negatives** can result from failure of the test kit (e.g. manufacturing or storage problem) or lack of antigen-shedding in faeces, either because shedding lags behind clinical signs or because antigen has already been bound by mucosal antibody in the gut. If you return a negative test yet clinical signs lead you to suspect parvovirus, you should treat the animal as if positive pending re-testing with the same or another test.
- **False positives** can result from recent (1–2 weeks) vaccination using modified live vaccines or from test malfunction.

Polymerase chain reaction (PCR) tests detect virus, even when bound with antibody, and are therefore more sensitive tests (the current 'gold standard'), but are not cage-side and need to be sent to a commercial laboratory, delaying diagnosis. These tests are also more costly.

d) An assumption of false negative should be made while Paddy is being monitored as he is displaying signs very typical of parvovirus. PCR testing could be performed, but carries additional cost. A pragmatic response is to continue therapy if Paddy is stabilising.

e) Other viruses that can resemble parvovirus (but usually with less severe signs) include canine coronavirus and rotavirus.

f) An important differential for these signs in a young dog is a gastrointestinal obstruction due to a foreign body. Dogs in isolation are in danger of being less closely monitored and examined because of the necessity to don protective clothing and because isolation spaces may be cramped and awkward to work in. There is much to be said for the repeated basic clinical exam in emergency and critical cases. By repeatedly examining Paddy, especially after analgesia hopefully makes abdominal palpation more tolerable for him and more productive for you, a mass effect or foreign body may be detected. Paying careful attention to his basic clinical parameters and response to therapy will also help assess his general status. Ultimately, though, if you are suspicious, imaging may be needed to rule out a foreign body. In performing these tests, considerable precautions will be needed if moving Paddy temporarily into the main hospital. Associated costs will have to be discussed with the owners. In cases like this, regular updates are needed to keep the owners on board. Bear in mind it is possible to be 'tricked' into thinking a young dog with a foreign body has parvovirus (especially if you have seen a recent run of infectious cases, as here), but also vice versa: a young dog with a suspected radiolucent foreign body actually has parvovirus. If a dog with parvovirus undergoes exploratory laparotomy for a suspected foreign body, this would compromise their health and recovery, and also produce a major incident for operating theatre hygiene. With the best will in the world, these situations may occur due to the complexity of diagnosis and the fact that not all foreign bodies are seen on X-ray, prompting exploratory surgery.

g) Finances are limited, but meaningful initial stabilisation and treatment has taken place and repeated assessments can be made now that Paddy is hospitalised. Analgesia should be provided if Paddy is in pain; buprenorphine has the advantage of a long duration of action and is economical. Gut antispasmodics (e.g. hyoscine butylbromide, Buscopan™) and ongoing anti-emetics could also be considered. If Paddy is not deteriorating, keeping him on fluids for 24 hours would be rational, with careful attention to his overall status. Early nutritional support and empirical deworming are recommended (Mazzaferro 2020). If a foreign body is detected, then discussions would need to be started about possible surgery.

h) Euthanasia should be considered in the clinically deteriorating patient with poor prognosis where there is no scope for additional therapy, or where additional investigation or treatment has been ruled out on cost grounds, or if pain cannot be controlled. Repeating diagnostic tests can help in making this decision, but this will increase costs even more, so the judgement may be made on clinical grounds. Asking colleagues for an opinion relieves the burden on one individual and helps with owner communication. Note that outpatient treatment of dogs with parvovirus has been described (Perley et al. 2020a,b). This has been historically practised in charity animal clinics (outpatient 'drip clinics') and may be helpful to reduce hospitalisation costs in suitable cases.

REFERENCES

Mazzaferro, E. M. (2020) Update on canine parvoviral enteritis. *Veterinary Clinics of North America: Small Animal Practice* **50**(6):1307–1325. doi: 10.1016/j.cvsm.2020.07.008.

Perley, K., Burns, C. C., Maguire, C. et al. (2020a) Retrospective evaluation of outpatient canine parvovirus treatment in a shelter-based low-cost urban clinic. *Journal of Veterinary Emergency and Critical Care* **30**(2):202–208. doi: 10.1111/vec.12941.

Perley, K., Burns, C. C., Maguire, C. et al. (2020b) Erratum. *Journal of Veterinary Emergency and Critical Care* **30**(2):501–503. doi: 10.1111/vec.12962.

1.15 Lady, 7-yo FN Greyhound: still lame

a) Corns are the commonest cause of lameness in adult sighthounds. The main differential diagnoses are foreign-body penetration and osteosarcoma. Long-bone osteosarcoma is **common** in older Greyhounds and needs to be ruled out. Radiographs will help to eliminate bone tumours and radiopaque foreign bodies, but cannot completely exclude them. A thorough examination of the foot is mandatory, as corns should always be suspected in these dogs.

b) Hyperkeratisation (corn) is a protective response to trauma to the integument. In the digital pad, it results from excessive loading pressure. Causes of corns are multifactorial, including abnormal weight-bearing from previous injury, foreign-body penetration, foot conformation, and a genetic predisposition. Corns are diagnosed by observation of the lesion, palpable mediolateral thickening of the pad, and a pain response from orthogonal digital pressure. Corns in other pads of the same or a different limb are common.

c) The aim is to achieve pressure reduction over the corn. This is possible by removing a section of the superficial digital flexor (SDF) tendon. With the affected digit held in hyperextension, an incision is made over the SDF tendon at the distal third of the metacarpus/tarsus, the tendon is isolated with curved fine mosquito forceps, and about 1 cm is excised (Figure A1.15a). This allows the corn to exfoliate and rapidly resolves lameness. Other treatments, including surgical excision of the corn and hulling, do not address the underlying issue and frequently fail.

d) The SDFT inserts on the proximal second phalanx, flexing the proximal interphalangeal joint, and the deep digital flexor (DDF) tendon inserts on the third phalanx, flexing the distal interphalangeal joint. The surgery works through biomechanical reduction of loading of the digital pad.

e) The tendon may rejoin, recreating the original problem.

f) Rarely, the SDF/DDF tenotomy can cause hyperextension of the proximal interphalangeal joint (Figure A1.15b).

REFERENCES

Guilliard, M. (2023) Tendon cutting procedures for the treatment of corns in dogs. *Journal of Veterinary Sciences* **7**:001.

Guilliard, M. J. & Doughty, R. W. (2021) Digital flexor tenotomy for the treatment of digital pad corns in sighthounds. *Australian Veterinary Practitioner* **51**:151–159.

Guilliard, M. J. & Doughty, R. W. (2022) Superficial digital flexor tendonectomy for the treatment of corns in sighthounds. *Veterinary Dermatology* **33**(6):581–586. doi: 10.1111/vde.13117.

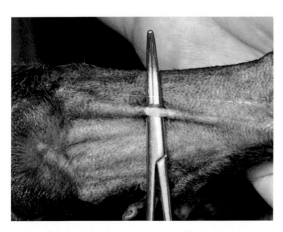

Figure A1.15a Isolation of the SDF tendon prior to tendonectomy.

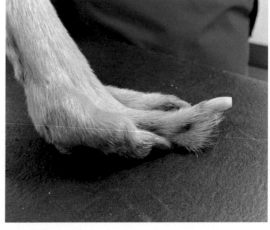

Figure A1.15b Hyperextension of the proximal interphalangeal joint after SDF and DDF tenotomy revision surgery.

1.16 Mac, 1-yo ME Cross-breed: broken tooth, *heart murmur*

a) The ASA provides a subjective assessment of a patient's overall health, from I (healthy) to V (moribund). While clinicians may vary in ASA scoring of the same patient, taking a few moments to apply this simple and practical system is valuable in helping us to slow down and identify elevated risk. Patients with higher ASA scores have higher risks of anaesthetic morbidity and mortality (Table A1.16).

While Mac does have a low-grade heart murmur, he is a young, asymptomatic animal, hence the subjective score of 2. The main point is that the act of scoring makes us stop and think about risk categories in a useful way.

The following steps can be taken to minimise risks to all patients:

- Provide an ASA score for all patients and, when possible, address identified risk factors prior to procedures (e.g. correcting dehydration prior to anaesthesia)
- Calculate drug doses based on lean body mass in obese patients
- Customise anaesthetic plans for each patient
- Use alpha-2 agonists, phenothiazines, and local anaesthetics perioperatively to reduce required doses of anaesthesia, and to minimise pre-surgical stress
- Increase post-operative monitoring, e.g. keep recovering animals in a highly visible location where staff can easily see them

b) As Mac is young, has no reported exercise intolerance, and is bouncy, an alpha-2 agonist would be an appropriate choice, despite the presence of the heart murmur. Acepromazine could be used; however, it probably would not give the required level of sedation in Mac. Alpha-2 agonists are usually combined with an opioid for pre-emptive analgesia and additional sedation. As this procedure is painful, methadone would be the most appropriate choice.

c) For a 25-kg dog, the most appropriate breathing system would be a circle as it requires a lower fresh gas flow, and thus less inhalational anaesthetic agent, than non-rebreathing systems. A Bain, Lack or Humphrey ADE system could be used; however, these would be less efficient in terms of anaesthetic gas usage

ASA SCORE	DESCRIPTION	MORTALITY % (95% CONFIDENCE INTERVAL)
I	Normal healthy animal; no underlying disease	0.08 (0.04–0.16)
II	Minor disease present; animals with slight to mild systemic disturbance; animal able to compensate	0.24 (0.19–0.30)
III	Evident disease present; animal with moderate systemic disease or disturbances; mild clinical signs, e.g. anaemia, moderate dehydration, fever, low-grade heart murmur, or cardiac disease	1.00 (0.84–1.20)
IV	Significantly compromised by disease; animals with pre-existing systemic disease or disturbances of a severe nature, e.g. severe dehydration, shock, uraemia, toxaemia, high fever, uncompensated heart disease, uncompensated diabetes, pulmonary disease, or emaciation	6.47 (5.46–7.65)
V	Moribund; surgery is often performed in desperation on animals with life-threatening systemic diseases; advanced heart, kidney, liver or endocrine disease cases, profound shock, severe trauma, pulmonary embolus, or terminal malignancy	15.73 (11.69–20.78)

Table A1.16 **Anaesthetic death associated with different ASA classifications from an international multicentre study (n = 405) involving 55,022 dogs (Redondo et al. 2023)**

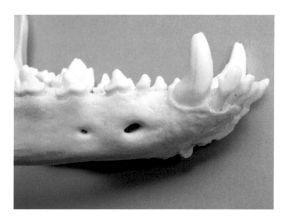

Figure A1.16a The middle mental foramen block is usually not sufficient for mandibular canine extraction, which can involve considerable bone removal.

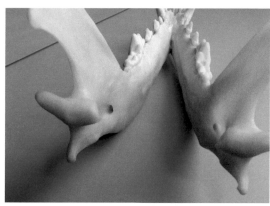

Figure A1.16b The mandibular foramen on the caudomedial mandible. The extraoral approach described in the text is technically easy. Blocking at this point anaesthetises the whole quadrant.

(a consideration in terms of improving environmental sustainability of veterinary practice). It would not be appropriate to use a T-piece or Mini Lack for this size of dog, unless it was an emergency situation, because the fresh gas flow rate would be unacceptably high.

d) As Mac has no clinical disease, Hartmann's solution would be a good choice of fluid because it is isotonic. Normal saline (0.9% NaCl) could also be used; however, it is acidifying. For a dental procedure in a dog with a single extraction, fluid therapy would usually be started at 5 mL/kg/h (5 mL/kg/h × 25 kg = 125 mL/h for Mac) and adjusted as required.

e) For a canine tooth extraction, sometimes the mental nerve block is adequate, particularly in dolichocephalic breeds such as Greyhounds. In most dogs, however, a mandibular nerve block is the best choice. This block should be performed on only one side due to the risk of self-trauma in recovery. The mandibular foramen is located on the inner surface of the caudal mandible and can be palpated intra-orally

(Figure A1.16b). A needle is then inserted at the ventral surface of the mandible and directed dorsally up the medial surface of the mandible until it can be palpated submucosally beside the foramen. A good guide for needle insertion point is to imagine a plumb line dropping down to the mandible from the lateral canthus of the eye. Insert the needle at the medial surface of the mandible at this point. The plunger should be withdrawn to ensure that there is no IV injection, and then the drug injected.

f) Bupivacaine 0.5% contains 5 mg/mL of drug (because 0.5% = 0.5 g/100 mL = 0.005 g per mL = 5 mg/mL). The dose is up to 1 mg/kg; therefore, 1 mg/kg × 25 kg = 25 mg can be used in Mac. 25 mg ÷ 5 mg/mL = 5 mL maximum; however, in practice, it is rare to use >1 mL for a single dental block.

REFERENCE

Redondo, J. I., Otero, P. E., Martínez-Taboada, F. et al. (2023) Anaesthetic mortality in dogs: a worldwide analysis and risk assessment. *Veterinary Record* e3604. doi: 10.1002/vetr.3604.

1.17 Sam, 12-yo MN Airedale Terrier: very sore

a) There is prostatic enlargement with areas of calcification evident within the parenchyma. The descending colon is full of faeces and displaced ventrally. The ventral border of L7 is irregular or 'moth-eaten' and there is enlargement of sublumbar lymph nodes. The radiological diagnosis is prostatic neoplasia with local metastasis. Prostatic carcinomas are androgen-independent, and, in the majority of cases (70–80%), metastasise rapidly to sites including regional lymph nodes, pelvic muscles, lumbar vertebrae, urinary bladder, kidney, adrenal glands, colon and rectum, liver, and spleen, as well as more distal sites including the lung, heart, and distant lymph nodes (Palmieri et al. 2022). The use of NSAIDs, chemotherapy, radiation therapy, and surgery (prostatectomy) have been reported to increase survival time, but these (with the exception of NSAIDs) involve considerable expense and may be associated with significant complications (Clerc-Renaud et al. 2021). The prognosis is very poor.

b) Chest X-rays may show thoracic metastasis.

c) Physical examination per rectum will reveal an enlarged and often painful prostate, typically irregular in shape, hard, and fixed in position, with irregular nodules sometimes detectable. It may be possible to feel enlarged sublumbar lymph nodes. Lumbar and/or abdominal pain may be noted. On questioning, the owner may have noticed stranguria, dysuria, pigmenturia (probably from haematuria), constipation, dyschezia, or weight loss leading up to Sam's presentation (Palmieri et al. 2022).

d) You will need to show good empathy when delivering this diagnosis. It is useful to retrace Sam's history and presenting signs, explaining how two conditions, one common and one rare, present in similar ways and that old, stiff dogs are frequently treated symptomatically with NSAIDs to good effect. This provides the owner with a narrative to aid understanding. You can add that, as NSAIDs have been reported to modestly improve survival time in dogs with prostatic carcinoma, their use may have benefitted Sam (Sorenmo et al. 2004). It appears that Sam's prostate was not checked before – always a useful exam to remember in older male dogs, especially those with back pain or hindlimb lameness, but patient compliance is necessary when the test is carried out in the conscious patient. Prostatic examination might have revealed the problem sooner, although the outcome would not change. Because the prostate-specific antigen (PSA) test is used to screen for prostate diseases in humans in some jurisdictions, owners of dogs may expect veterinarians to use similar tests. It can be helpful, therefore, to explain that there are no commercially available canine-specific prostate markers, so disease is often detected late in its course (Palmieri et al. 2022). This all needs to be explained in a careful way, focusing on what is best for Sam going forward (imminent euthanasia, most cases being euthanased soon after diagnosis), and will test veterinary communication skills to the full.

e) Prostatic neoplasia is the commonest prostate disease in neutered males and finding prostatic mineralisation is highly indicative of neoplasia (but take care not to confuse tiny bone fragments in the colon or stool with prostatic calcification – ask about diet and consider serial radiographs if required). Castration is considered to be a risk factor for prostatic carcinoma, but note that prostatic neoplasia is uncommon overall (and extremely rare in cats). Airedales are one of a number of dog breeds that seem predisposed.

REFERENCES

Clerc-Renaud, B., Geiger, T. L., Larue, S. M. & Nolan, M. W. (2021) Treatment of genitourinary carcinoma in dogs using nonsteroidal anti-inflammatory drugs, mitoxantrone, and radiation therapy: a retrospective study. *Journal of Veterinary Internal Medicine* **35**(2):1052–1061. doi: 10.1111/jvim.16078.

Palmieri, C., Fonesca-Alves, C. E. & Laufer-Amorim, R. (2022) A review on canine and feline prostate pathology. *Frontiers in Veterinary Science* **9**. doi: 10.3389/fvets.2022.881232.

Sorenmo, K. U., Goldschmidt, M. H., Shofer, F. S. et al. (2004) Evaluation of cyclooxygenase-1 and cyclooxygenase-2 expression and the effect of cyclooxygenase inhibitors in canine prostatic carcinoma. *Veterinary & Comparative Oncology* **2**(1):13–23. doi: 10.1111/j.1476-5810.2004.00035.x.

1.18 Xena, 6-yo FN SBT: skin problem getting worse

a) If good-quality parasite prevention is being given appropriately to prevent ectoparasites such as fleas and mites, then the most likely cause of skin irritation in this case is allergic skin disease, and may include atopy, food allergy, or contact allergy. However, these conditions can be complicated by secondary infections. Note that it is good practice to employ parasiticides strategically based on individual risk assessment rather than blanket use, because of the residual environmental effects of these products (Perkins et al. 2024).

b) Suitable questions include the following:
   - Has this happened before?
   - What is Xena's history in relation to skin conditions?
   - Are there any known triggers?
   - Have other tests or treatments been used in the past? How has Xena responded?
   - What is her current diet?
   - Does she have access to any known irritant plants (e.g. Moses-in-the-cradle; Figure A1.18)?
   - Has anything changed with her diet or location or routine recently?

c) These should be guided by the specific patient history and physical examination. A thorough history and good client communication to manage expectations is critical with any dermatology case – allergic skin disease often requires lifelong

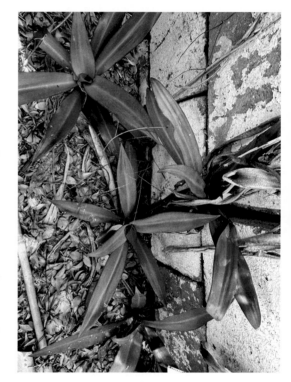

Figure A1.18 Moses-in-the-cradle (*Tradescantia spathacea*), also known as Moses-in-a-basket, oyster plant or boatlily, is a herb of the Commelinaceae family. It is a common ornamental, semi-succulent plant, with fleshy rhizomes and rosettes of waxy, pointed leaves that are dark green above and purple below. It is increasingly popular as it is seen as an easy-to-grow, low-maintenance plant.

management. Impression or acetate tape preparations of the affected areas can be performed and material from pustules can be expressed onto a slide for examination. In Xena's case, a small number of neutrophils with intracellular cocci were noted. A sticky tape squeeze test was performed to check for demodex mites; this was negative (Barillas et al. 2019). If Xena had severe pruritus, the distribution was around the face, ears, or elbows, and she was not on strategic, risk-assessed parasite prevention, scabies mite could be considered and superficial skin scrapes performed; however, this is less common with the use of isoxazoline antiparasitic medications.

d) Superficial pyodermas can be treated by topical therapy alone, which helps to prevent the development of antimicrobial resistance from long courses of oral antibiotics. In Xena's case, a twice-weekly medicated shampoo and medicated conditioner containing chlorhexidine were recommended for the first 2 weeks along with a topical lipid barrier agent for ongoing maintenance of the skin barrier after the shampoo and conditioner treatment had been completed.

It can be helpful to make time for future discussion with the owner or consider providing some information handouts about possible causes and management of allergic skin disease and diagnostic and treatment options. Often, there is too much information to present at the time of initial presentation and owners can become overwhelmed.

e) If there is not complete resolution of the pyoderma after 2–3 weeks, it is recommended to repeat cytology of pustule contents and perform a microbial culture and sensitivity (C&S) test to determine if systemic antimicrobials are required. A longer duration of topical antimicrobial therapy may still be appropriate without the need to use systemic antimicrobials. Underlying allergic skin disease may be complicating treatment and may need to be addressed concurrently. In the short term, this typically involves medicating to reduce pruritus and skin inflammation, but in the longer term this will require avoiding known flare factors including skin infections, taking steps to restore skin barrier function and integrity, and possibly desensitisation to allergens via allergen-specific immunotherapy (ASIT) (Outerbridge & Jordan 2021).

f) Xena has a superficial bacterial pyoderma, secondary to atopy, as well as colour dilution alopecia (CDA). CDA is a congenital alopecia caused by a genetic mutation (Welle et al. 2009). Affected animals may have a normal coat at birth but then develop loss of hair and broken hair as they age. Generally, the dorsum is most affected. Secondary bacterial pyoderma can be a complication of CDA due to the disruption in normal hair coat and skin barrier.

> At the initial consultation, it can be helpful to make time for future discussion with the owner or consider providing some handouts about possible causes and management of allergic skin disease and diagnostic and treatment options. Often, there is too much information to present at the time of initial presentation and owners can become overwhelmed.

REFERENCES

Barillas, O. F., Bajwa, J., Guillot, J. & Arcique, A. (2019) Comparison of acetate tape impression, deep skin scraping, and microscopic examination of hair for therapeutic monitoring of dogs with juvenile generalized demodicosis: a pilot study. *Canadian Veterinary Journal* **60**(6):596–600.

Outerbridge, C. A. & Jordan, T. J. M. (2021) Current knowledge on canine atopic dermatitis: pathogenesis and treatment. *Advances in*

Small Animal Care **2**:101–115. doi: 10.1016/j.yasa.2021.07.004.

Perkins, R., Barron, L., Gäeten, G. et al. (2024) Down the drain pathways for fipronil and imidacloprid applied as spot-on parasiticides to dogs: estimating aquatic pollution. *Science of the Total Environment* **917**:170175. doi: 10.1016/j.scitotenv.2024.170175.

Welle, M., Philipp, U., Rüfenacht, S. et al. (2009) *MLPH* genotype – melanin phenotype correlation in dilute dogs. *Journal of Heredity* **100**(1):S75–S79. doi: 10.1093/jhered/esp010.

For antibiotic prescribing guidelines, see https://vetantibiotics.science.unimelb.edu.au/companion-animal-guidelines/medical-guidelines/skin/.

1.19 Minty, 9-mo MN Bengal: biting owners

a) Common differentials for biting like this include the following:

Physical problems
- Musculoskeletal pain
- Dental pain
- Gastrointestinal issues
- Skin disease
- Bladder pain (feline lower urinary tract disease [FLUTD])
- Hyperthyroidism (in older cats)

Social/environmental differentials
- Misdirected predatory behaviour
- Social fear/anxiety
- Frustration (lack of control over environment and lack of appropriate outlets for species-specific behaviour)
- Attention-seeking/learned behaviour

In addition, Bengal cats are a hybrid of an Asian Leopard Cat (*Prionailurus bengalensis*) and a domestic breed (a European or American Shorthair or Egyptian Mau). Asian leopard cats are considered 'one of the least tameable of all of the wild felids' due to a lack of display of social behaviour towards keepers and other felids in captive environments (Martos Martinez-Caja et al. 2021). Some reports suggest that this breed of cat may exhibit more problem behaviours, including aggression toward animals, than domestic cats.

b) After investigating potential medical/physical causes for the behaviour, the next step is to evaluate the cat's social and physical environment, including provision of key resources. There are questionnaires available that can help with this (e.g. Ohio State University 2024). You can then ask about the specific context, precursors, and outcomes to the behaviour to see if motivation can be ascertained.

c) It is important that Minty is not punished for biting behaviour. Instead, the clients should respond to this behaviour by giving Minty space. Advise the clients to allow Minty to decide when he does or does not want physical interaction and to pause stroking him every few seconds and then allow him to reinitiate contact. You can also ensure that the clients are aware of feline handling preferences and body language and that they can spot any potential precursors to the biting behaviour and withdraw contact sooner, e.g. flick of the tail; change in ear position; tensing of the body; wide, darting eyes.

It is important to ensure that species-specific needs are being met and that sufficient outlets for predatory behaviour are provided. This is likely to involve a combination of self-directed activities, e.g. hunting for food around the home, and short and frequent interactive play sessions with the clients. Biting of hands during play should never be encouraged. Bengal cats often have a high predatory drive and it can be challenging for clients to meet their needs in an indoor environment. It may be possible to consider controlled access to the outdoors, e.g. enclosed garden or outdoor run.

Psychotropic medication may be indicated when physical problems have been ruled out and the cat's emotional response is considered to be abnormal and/or the behaviour is maintained even after all social and environmental factors contributing to the behaviour have been addressed.

REFERENCES

Ackerman, L. J. & Landsberg, G. M. (2023) Chapter 24, 'Feline Aggression'. In Ackerman, L. J. & Landsberg, G. M. (eds) *Behavior Problems of the Dog and Cat*, 4th edition. Philadelphia, PA: Saunders.

Martos Martinez-Caja, A., Rosseau, J., Vervaecke, H. & Moons, C. P. H. (2021) Behavior and health issues in Bengal cats as perceived by their owners: a descriptive study. *Journal of Veterinary Behavior* **41**:12–21. *doi: 10.1016/j.jveb.2020.10.007.*

Ohio State University (2024) Indoor cat home checklist. Available at: https://indoorpet.osu.edu/sites/indoorpet.osu.edu/files/imce/2017_Household%20Resource%20Checklist.docx.

1.20 Greyson, 4-yo MN SBT x Boxer: O considering euth

a) It is important to approach the conversation with an open mind and to give the owner time to tell their story. The decision to euthanise is never easy. While some owners may view animals as disposable, the vast majority agonise over this choice. It's important not to jump to conclusions before understanding the full story and context. Start the conversation by empathising with the owner. Acknowledge that they are in an awful position and that you are there to help. Invite them to speak by asking open-ended questions such as, 'Tell me what's happening at the moment.' You can then ask some targeted questions:

- Has a specific event pushed them to make the decision?
- Has Greyson attacked or come close to attacking a person or animal?
- Is there a new baby in the family, children in the household, or children visiting regularly?
- Is Greyson destructive to the point that he is harming himself and/or the property?

It is important to find out what the trigger for this conversation is and to then discuss the development of the behaviour that has led to this, such as signs of anxiety or resource guarding. Acknowledge any attempts the owner has made to manage the behaviour and give them space to talk about how the behaviour has impacted Greyson's QOL, as well as their own. It is important to get the whole story, to really understand what kind of life Greyson is living and how his behaviour is affecting the owner and other household members. Greyson may be a candidate for a behavioural consultation, referral, and or/medication, but you need to understand the situation (and the owner's limitations) to make appropriate recommendations.

b) Behavioural euthanasia is considered when the QOL of the pet or other stakeholders – including humans and other animals – is compromised. While physical health may not be the issue, many animals suffer from poor mental health, anxiety, or emotional distress. These factors can deeply impact their overall well-being. Acknowledging the importance of both physical and emotional health makes it easier for veterinarians to advocate for the patient and the client simultaneously. The decision to euthanase for behavioural reasons is often based on an 'overall risk assessment', which factors in patient size, their behavioural history, including any bites or incidents of aggression, the perceived predictability and manageability of that behaviour, the risk status of household members (including children, vulnerable household members and other animals), and the feasibility of preventing contact between the animal and at-risk persons or animals (Pachel 2023). The owners may be feeling a tremendous amount of guilt over the situation and you may have your own opinions on how they have dealt with the situation up until now. It is important not to assume that euthanasia is an 'easy' or 'convenient' decision for the owners; the vast majority will not see it that way. Dealing with a pet with behavioural concerns can take over people's lives, and often families are unable to go through all the steps of medication, referral, and training due to financial, physical, practical, or emotional constraints. Successfully rehoming a pet with behavioural concerns, particularly aggression, may not be feasible. In some countries, there may be legislation regarding indications for euthanasia that need to be considered. A consultation will allow you to assess Greyson, take a behavioural history, understand the caregiver burden of his owners, and develop a more detailed understanding of the risks presented by this behaviour in the current context, as well as any potential future context (rehoming).

c) If euthanasia is agreed to be the best course of action for Greyson, it should be performed in a manner that minimises fear, anxiety, and distress in Greyson, and, where possible, maximises his comfort and wellbeing. Providing a peaceful death and supporting the family through their grief will protect his welfare while also protecting the wellbeing of his owners and veterinary team members involved. Talk to the owners about their wishes and previous experience with euthanasia.

A young, anxious animal in an unfamiliar environment may be more highly aroused – this is why starting the sedation process in the home where Greyson is relaxed is ideal, if safe to do so. Alternatively, home euthanasia may help reduce Greyson's stress. Make sure you are comfortable with sedation options and have clear communication with the owners before attempting this; there is greater potential for you or the owners to be injured without the support of your team. You may seek advice from behavioural specialists or home euthanasia vets or refer the case. Safety is paramount, followed by the stress-free handling of Greyson.

If Greyson is highly anxious/aggressive leaving the home, oral sedation is warranted. For example, you may be able to dispense a combination of oral medications that the owners can administer 2 hours prior to the visit. An example might be gabapentin at 40–80 mg/kg (note a much higher dose is used prior to euthanasia than for other indications), combined with trazodone (4–8 mg/kg) or acepromazine (2 mg/kg). Note that the effects of oral sedation are variable and depend heavily on an animal's mentation, physical health, age, and anxiety levels. Discussion should be had with owners regarding the variability and potential adverse reactions (and possible death) in frail and compromised animals. Trazodone can reduce blood pressure and may have adverse effects on the pet (i.e. increase anxiety/aggression or result in serotonin syndrome if used with other behavioural medications such as fluoxetine).

The aim is to ensure the safety of the owners and staff by relying on medication rather than manual restraint. Allow a longer appointment time – oral sedation will take longer to work. A quiet, dark space that encourages Greyson to relax is beneficial. You may need to provide additional oral medication in the clinic if you cannot approach Greyson. This can

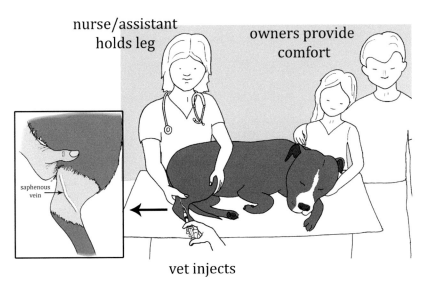

nurse/assistant holds leg

owners provide comfort

saphenous vein

vet injects

Figure A1.20 The lateral saphenous vein, though more mobile and 'wobbly' than the cephalic, may be useful, as this allows the veterinarian and assistant to work at the caudal end of the dog, while the family remain near the head, with minimal intrusion. It is important to ensure that aggressive animals are adequately immobilised under reliably deep sedation or anaesthesia. Bear in mind that apparently well-sedated animals may still respond to stimulation, so cautiously testing the depth of sedation is wise.

be hidden in food, treats, or squirted into his mouth if it is safe to do so. Examples include tiletamine/zolazepam (10 mg/kg), butorphanol (0.3 mg/kg), and acepromazine (2 mg/kg). If tiletamine/zolazepam is not available, consider ketamine (5–10 mg/kg) instead. When it is safe to approach, SC or IM sedation can be given. For example, butorphanol (0.1–0.3 mg/kg) and acepromazine (0.1–1 mg/kg), combined SC, followed (once patient is sedated) by one of the following:

- Tiletamine/zolazepam (10 mg/kg SC)
- Alfaxalone CD (2–5 mg/kg IM)
- Ketamine (10 mg/kg SC)

Common side effects of sedation include heavy breathing and twitching of limbs and face (discuss this with owners prior to administration to avoid alarm). A muzzle can be used if appropriate and removed once Greyson is confirmed to be heavily sedated (Figure A1.20). It is better to be

overcautious and prevent harm. Once you are sure that Greyson is safely immobilised, you can administer pentobarbital intravenously. It is important that clear, compassionate communication is had with the owners to signpost what each step involves and how plans may change. This helps to set expectations and avoid distress and confusion. Despite the situation, even if you know there are no better options, behavioural euthanasia may still not sit right with you. If this is the case, you can refer the clients to a colleague who feels more comfortable. Performing a euthanasia that goes against your values can lead to moral distress.

REFERENCE

Pachel, C. 2023. *Considerations for Behavioural Euthanasia in Dogs*. Clinician's Brief. Available at: www.cliniciansbrief.com/article/behavioral-euthanasia-injury-risk-assessment.

1.21 Staff meeting

a) Burnout is defined by the World Health Organization (WHO) as a syndrome (not a medical diagnosis) resulting from chronic workplace stress that has not been successfully managed (WHO 2023). According to the WHO, burnout is characterised by three dimensions:
   i) Feelings of energy depletion or exhaustion
   ii) Increased mental distance from one's job, or feelings of negativism or cynicism related to one's job
   iii) A sense of ineffectiveness and lack of accomplishment (WHO 2023)

While, in veterinary and other settings, burnout has historically been viewed as a problem of individuals, simply focusing on improving individual wellbeing or trying to 'fix' the burnt-out person does not resolve it. Indeed, seeing burnout in this way 'is an antiquated misconception that affects its prevention and is therefore harmful' (Steffey et al. 2023). Christina Maslach, who developed the Maslach Burnout Inventory, has written that burnout occurs when there is a 'mismatch' between the conditions and requirements of a workplace, and the resources and needs of those working within it.

b) Maslach identified six types of mismatch that can occur between working conditions and job requirements and the people within a certain workplace. These mismatches are sources of burnout (Table A1.21a).

c) According to Maslach, the ideal job–person match is characterised by six features:
   i) Sustainable workload
   ii) Ample choice and control
   iii) Gratifying recognition and rewards
   iv) Supportive work community
   v) Norms of fairness, respect, and social justice
   vi) Well-aligned values and meaningful work (Maslach & Leiter 2022)

Some modifiable workplace factors that may reduce work overload are listed in Table A1.21b. The features in this table highlight factors that you might make inquiries about when looking for a job.

Table A1.21a **Sources of burnout and examples (adapted from Hilton et al. 2022 and Maslach & Leiter 2022)**

SOURCE OF BURNOUT	EXAMPLES
Work overload	• Long hours, overtime, overbooking, not enough staff
Lack of control	• Team members have no control over the order in which they complete tasks, or they feel they are being micromanaged
Insufficient reward (intrinsic or extrinsic)	• Work does not feel meaningful or of value to the person undertaking it (lack of intrinsic reward) • Poor remuneration, poor recognition of work well done (lack of extrinsic reward)
Value conflicts	• Team members feel they are being asked to assist with or perform tasks that compromise animal welfare or the wellbeing of clients
Feeling at odds with colleagues/ breakdown of community	• Interpersonal conflict or feeling excluded by team members or management • Workers feel ineffective in a team environment
Feeling of unfairness/ absence of fairness	• A team member may feel that they have been overlooked for promotion or recognition in favour of a colleague less deserving

Table A1.21b Modifiable workplace factors that may reduce work overload in veterinary settings, and examples of modifications

MODIFIABLE WORKPLACE FACTOR	EXAMPLE MODIFICATIONS
Total weekly hours worked by each team member	• Reduce total number of hours by employing additional team members • Reduce opening hours
Number of consults scheduled each day	• Reduce total number of consults scheduled each day • Increase appointment length
Daily hours in surgery	• Reduce the number of surgical procedures booked each day • Minimise total surgery time by minimising the number of major procedures that can be booked each day relative to team members available
Working beyond rostered hours	• Provide time in lieu of overtime worked • Provide adequate remuneration for working overtime • Schedule time to catch up (on hospital cases, correspondence and telephone calls, record-keeping) each day • Employ adequate staff so that people can complete their work and leave on time
Take regular breaks	• Schedule regular breaks • Provide an inviting space for staff to take breaks
Sacrificed lunch breaks	• Do not disturb team members during breaks (Figure A1.21) • Do not schedule appointments during breaks • Employ adequate staff to ensure that staff on duty can take a break
Allocated time to catch up and do administration	• Schedule time throughout the day for team members to catch up on hospital cases, correspondence, telephone calls, record-keeping, and other tasks, including writing and reviewing practice policy, attending staff meetings, and so on
Walk-ins	• Minimise walk-in appointments: if not urgent, schedule for a more convenient time • Leave space in the schedule for emergencies (especially where these are most likely to occur, e.g. first or last appointments of the day), or reschedule routine appointments to accommodate emergencies • Refer urgent cases to an emergency facility
Interruptions	• Minimise frequency of interruptions, e.g. by scheduling time to follow up non-urgent queries or 'batching' requests (e.g. for scripts and dispensing medication) • Improve internal communications and record-keeping to minimise the need for interruptions
Ability to take holidays	• Employ adequate staff to ensure that annual leave can be covered • Establish a relationship with locum staff or a locum agency
Ability to take sick leave	• Employ adequate staff to ensure that sick leave can be covered • Establish a relationship with locum staff or a locum agency
Sense of control over the working day	• Allow team members to determine the order in which they complete tasks where possible

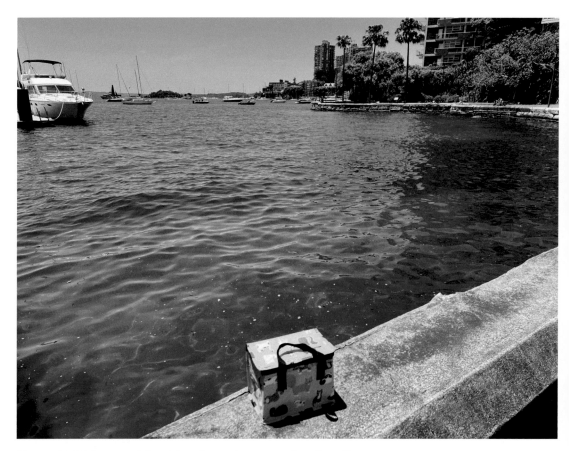

Figure A1.21 Protected lunch breaks are important for all staff.

REFERENCES

Hilton, K. R., Burke, K. J. & Signal, T. (2022) Mental health in the veterinary profession: an individual or organisational focus? *Australian Veterinary Journal* **101**(1–2):41–48. doi: 10.1111/avj.13215.

Maslach, C. & Leiter, M. P. (2022) *The Burnout Challenge: Managing People's Relationships with Their Jobs.* Cambridge, MA: Harvard University Press.

Steffey, M. A., Griffon, D. J., Risselada, M. et al. (2023) A narrative review of the physiology and health effects of burnout associated with veterinarian-pertinent occupational stressors. *Frontiers in Veterinary Science* **10**. doi: 10.3389/fvets.2023.1184525.

WHO (2023) Burnout. *International Classification of Diseases (ICD-11)*, 11th edition. Geneva: WHO. Available at: www.who.int/news/item/28-05-2019-burn-out-an-occupational-phenomenon-international-classification-of-diseases.

TODAY'S CASE LIST

2.1 Betty Blue, 5-yo FN Affenpinscher: walk-in, no appt

2.2 Benji, 2-yo MN Pointer: stealing & guarding things

2.3 Poppy, 12-yo FN DSH: not eating, face different?

2.4 Rocco, 5-yo MN Cocker Spaniel: red eye

2.5 Carlos, 8-mo MN guinea pig: had a fit

2.6 Joey, 18-mo ME Cross-breed: ear flush

2.7 Tabitha, 5-mo FE DSH: flank cat spay

2.8 Gemima, 10-mo FN Springer Spaniel: spay wound burst

2.9 Rikki, 4-mo ME Golden Retriever: ?stung on face

2.10 Dotty, 4-yo MN DSH: dental prophy

2.11 Chuck, 17-yo MN DSH: 'gone downhill'

2.12 Busy, 4-yo MN DSH: rash on chin

2.13 Benji, 5-yo MN Cockerpoo: check, seen OOH

2.14 Henry, 6-yo MN CKCS: dental, *murmur*

2.15 Smithers, 13-yo MN DSH: recheck throat

2.16 Maggie, 6-yo FN Doberman Pinscher: freq urination

2.17 Spaghetti, 9-mo ME rat: bleeding nose & eyes

2.18 Pat, 7-yo MN Shetland Sheepdog: licking bottom ++

2.19 Spot, 5-yo FN Lagotto: ate fishing line

2.20 Confidential meeting with T

Recipe: Chickpea curry

DOI: 10.1201/9781003278306-2

2.1 Betty Blue, 5-yo FN Affenpinscher: walk-in, no appt

Betty Blue's owner reports that Betty Blue has become profoundly lethargic and weak over the previous 24 hours. Betty Blue vomited twice overnight; the vomitus contained digested food and some green material. She has since shown no interest in food. She has a history of being an indiscriminate eater, and did escape for a short period unsupervised into the bushes in a public park about 48 hours ago.

Pertinent physical findings:

- Demeanour: quiet, rousable but flat
- BCS: 3/5
- HR = 200 = PR, with a weak, thready pulse
- MMs: white, CRT delayed >2 seconds
- Tender on abdominal palpation, but cannot palpate mass or foreign-body effect
- Temp: 36.4 °C

You perform a CBC and biochemistry panel (Table 2.1a). A blood smear reveals varied staining (polychromasia) and varying size of red blood cells (anisocytosis).

Table 2.1a **Results of in-house haematology and biochemistry tests for Betty Blue. Results highlighted in red lie outside reference ranges**

PARAMETER	RESULT	REFERENCE RANGE
RBC	4.51	$5.65–8.87 \times 10^{12}$/L
Haematocrit	0.323	0.373–0.616 L/L
Hb	128	131–205 g/L
MCV	71.6	61.6–73.5 fL
MCH	28.4	21.2–25.9 pg
MCHC	397	320–379 g/L
RDW	13.6	13.6–21.7%
% reticulocyte	3.1	–
Reticulocytes	140.6	10.0–110 K/µL
WBC	26.51	$5.05–16.76 \times 10^9$/L
% Neutrophils	87.2	–
% Lymphocytes	3.5	–
% Monocytes	9.3	–
% Eosinophils	0.0	–
% Basophils	0.0	–
Neutrophils	23.11	$2.95–11.64 \times 10^9$/L
Lymphocytes	0.92	$1.05–5.10 \times 10^9$/L
Monocytes	2.47	$0.16–1.12 \times 10^9$/L
Eosinophils	0.01	$0.06–1.23 \times 10^9$/L
Basophils	0.0	$0.0–0.10 \times 10^9$/L
Platelets	347	$148–484 \times 10^9$/L
Platelet distribution width (PDW)	11.6	9.1–19.4 fL
Mean platelet volume (MPV)	10.6	8.7–13.2 fL
Plateletcrit	0.37	0.14–0.46%
Glucose	10.34	4.11–7.95 mmol/L
Creatinine	53	44–159 µmol/L

PARAMETER	RESULT	REFERENCE RANGE
Urea	8.5	2.5–9.6 mmol/L
BUN:creatinine ratio	40	–
Phosphorus	1.51	0.81–2.20 mmol/L
Calcium	2.17	1.98–3.00 mmol/L
Sodium	144	144–160 mmol/L
Potassium	3.9	3.5–5.8 mmol/L
Na:K ratio	37	–
Chloride	100	109–122 mmol/L
TP	58	52–82 g/L
Albumin	30	23–40 g/L
Globulin	28	25–45 g/L
Albumin:globulin ratio	1.1	–
ALT	57	10–125 U/L
ALP	218	23–212 U/L
Gamma-glutamyl transferase (GGT)	4	0–11 U/L
Bilirubin – total	<2	0–15 µmol/L
Cholesterol	4.94	2.84–8.26 mmol/L
Osmolality	294	mmol/kg

You explain to the client that Betty Blue is very unwell, and is likely suffering from haemorrhage (due to a coagulopathy, bleeding mass, or gastrointestinal blood loss). Given the history and clinical signs, you strongly suspect that Betty Blue is suffering from a coagulopathy secondary to ingestion of an anticoagulant rodenticide. The owner consents to sending a blood sample to an external laboratory to perform coagulation studies (Table 2.1b).

Table 2.1b **Results of coagulation studies for Betty Blue**

PARAMETER	RESULT	REFERENCE RANGE
Prothrombin time (PT)	111.0 s	5.4–10.7 s
Activated partial thromboplastin time (APTT)	41.7 s	10.7–18.4 s
Thrombin time	16.4 s	14.7–23.9 s
Fibrinogen	5.4 g/L	1.8–2.7 g/L

The prolonged PT and APTT are consistent with rodenticide toxicity (more than one clotting factor involved), while the increased fibrinogen is likely to be related to an acute phase protein reaction to severe clinical illness.

The owner consents to point-of-care abdominal and thoracic ultrasonography to investigate potential haemorrhage. The abdominal scan is unremarkable, but the thoracic one suggests a right-sided pleural effusion, which is confirmed on radiographs. The heart appears to be normal size and shape.

You recommend referral for intensive care, further workup, including sampling of the pleural fluid, and blood transfusion if required, but the client declines due to cost constraints.

a) What features of the CBC support your assessment of regenerative anaemia?
b) What is your interpretation of the other abnormalities?
c) What are the most common sites of haemorrhage in dogs with anticoagulant rodenticide intoxication?

d) How would you treat this patient given the owner's cost constraints?
e) The suspected bait was concealed within bushes in a public park, thus the type and amount of rodenticide ingested are unknown. Therefore, for how long would you treat this patient with vitamin K_1?

2.2 Benji, 2-yo MN Pointer: stealing & guarding things

PART 1

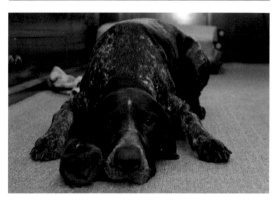

Figure 2.2 Benji has been stealing and guarding random objects.

Benji has been booked in for an extended consultation to discuss his behaviour. At his annual health check and booster, his owners reported that Benji has been stealing a variety of objects, then guarding them aggressively (Figure 2.2). He also becomes aggressive if told to get off the sofa. Benji's previous medical history includes investigation for a suspected gastrointestinal foreign body. Benji's owners were very concerned at the time of the foreign-body investigations, as they were given a potentially guarded prognosis, and now exercise great vigilance in case he should pick up and swallow something. Benji was neutered at the age of 8 months.

a) Can you think of four or five general background questions you would ask of Benji's owners to start off the consultation?
b) Can you think of five or six specific questions you would ask regarding the aggressive episodes?

Please look at the answers for Part 1 before going on to Part 2.

PART 2

a) Can you relate Benji's past medical history to the current behavioural problem?
b) Can you identify any misconceptions in the owners' response to Benji's behaviour from their answers to the questions raised in Part 1?
c) It emerges that Benji has received some gun-dog training. What are the implications for Benji and his behaviour?
d) How might the owners work on encouraging Benji to give up items in his mouth and modify Benji's aggressive behaviour on the sofa?
e) What do you think of the owners' explanation that the sofa is giving Benji 'ideas above his station'?
f) Benji seems more responsive to his male owner's commands. How would you approach this subject with the owners?
g) Is the fact that Benji was neutered when young, and possibly before social maturity, relevant?

2.3 Poppy, 12-yo FN DSH: not eating, face different?

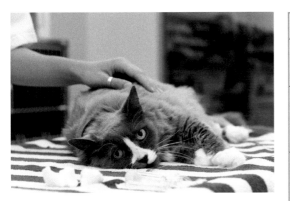

Figure 2.3 Poppy's elderly owner was in hospital and is now worried about her cat.

Table 2.3 **Clinical signs of dehydration**	
DEGREE OF DEHYDRATION	**CLINICAL SIGNS**
5–8%	
8–10%	
10–12%	
>12%	

Poppy, an indoor-only cat, comes in with her elderly owner (Figure 2.3). Miss Syme has been in hospital for 10 days and Poppy was being looked after by a neighbour. Since Miss Syme returned home 2 days ago, Poppy has barely touched her food. The neighbour remarked to Miss Syme that Poppy was 'not much of an eater'. Previously, Poppy had cleared her bowl each day. Miss Syme also thinks Poppy's face looks different but cannot say how. 'Just different', she says to you.

a) What simple clinical signs are often used to test for an animal's hydration status?

b) Complete Table 2.3 to give a quick, rule-of-thumb estimate as to degrees of dehydration based on common clinical signs.

c) You estimate Poppy to be 8–10% dehydrated. She purrs constantly during your examination, but you find her HR is slightly low for a cat in a clinical setting, at around 145 bpm. Her MMs are pale pink with a CRT of 3 seconds and Poppy's matching femoral pulses are thready. Might Poppy be in shock? Explain your thinking.

d) Miss Syme does not want to leave Poppy with you; however, you manage to persuade her that Poppy needs some help. What are your immediate priorities for this morning?

e) Your practice is running short of IV fluids but there is plenty of glucose saline in stock (sodium chloride 0.18% and glucose 4%). Could this be used for Poppy? Explain your answer.

f) Suggest a few 'old cat' differentials you might consider for Poppy in the absence of a good recent clinical history.

g) Miss Syme seems concerned that Poppy 'looks different'. Why might Poppy's face appear different?

h) Poppy weighs 3.2 kg. Assume she is 10% dehydrated. You decide to fully rehydrate her over 24 hours. Show your workings for the amount of IV fluids Poppy should be given per hour for the 24-hour period.

2.4 Rocco, 5-yo MN Cocker Spaniel: red eye

Rocco presents with a red left eye (Figure 2.4). The owner reports that he 'woke up this way' this morning and seems a bit subdued. Rocco was at the off-leash dog park last night; nothing out of the ordinary occurred. The eye is partly closed. The third eyelid is protruding and it is difficult to see the cornea properly. Rocco is reluctant to have his head handled.

a) What are the possible causes of an acute 'red eye' in an otherwise healthy dog?
b) Which, if any, of these could potentially threaten the dog's vision?
c) For any of these possible causes, are there any breed predispositions to take into account?
d) What diagnostic tests would you recommend?
e) Which tests are particularly important and in which order should they be performed?

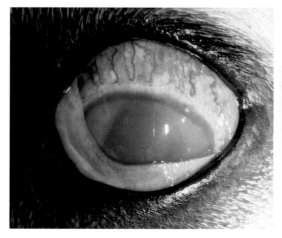

Figure 2.4 Rocco's eye is red and apparently painful and the third eyelid is protruding.

f) What would you recommend if you are not able to identify a likely cause?

2.5 Carlos, 8-mo MN guinea pig: had a fit

Carlos presents as an emergency after having what sounds like a seizure at home. On physical exam, you note that Carlos is missing patches of fur and has severe crusting on his flanks and dorsum (Figure 2.5). Every time you touch him, he tries to scratch and nibble at himself. As you examine Carlos, he falls over on his side and shows paroxysms of itching. The owner tells you that this is the behaviour that prompted her to come to the clinic.

a) What are your differential diagnoses for Carlos?
b) What diagnostic tests would you recommend?
c) What are your treatment options?
d) What would you recommend for at-home care?

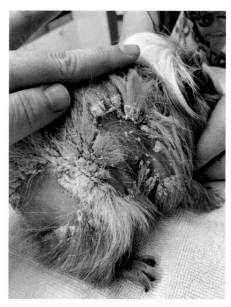

Figure 2.5 Carlos has patches of fur loss and scabby wounds.

2.6 Joey, 18-mo ME Cross-breed: ear flush

Joey, who has not been seen in your practice before, has been sedated for an ear flush when you notice a problem with his mouth (Figure 2.6a,b).

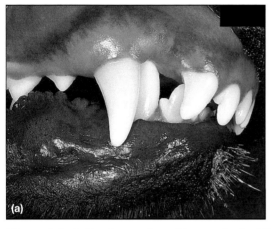 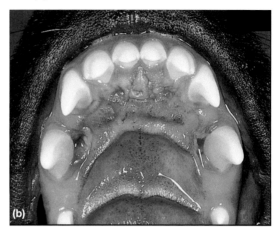

Figure 2.6a,b **Joey's mouth problem noticed while under sedation.**

a) Describe the features of normal, anatomical dental occlusion in dogs.
b) What abnormalities are visible in Joey's case?
c) How has this appearance come about?
d) How common is this type of malocclusion?
e) What are the treatment options in (i) puppies and young dogs presenting with this malocclusion and (ii) an older dog, like Joey?

2.7 Tabitha, 5-mo FE DSH: flank cat spay

Tabitha presents for a left flank spay (Figure 2.7).

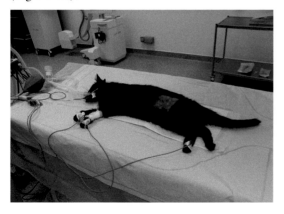

Figure 2.7 **Tabitha being prepared for her spay operation.**

a) Describe the surgical anatomy of the flank laparotomy, from skin to peritoneal cavity. How is entry to the abdomen achieved through the muscle layers?
b) List three advantages and three disadvantages of flank spays in cats.
c) The flank technique relies on accurate positioning of the initial skin incision. Describe how to locate this point using easy anatomical landmarks.
d) The incision made by experienced surgeons is typically small. How do you locate the uterine horn through such a tiny hole and, crucially, how do you ensure you have isolated the correct structure before you start placing ligatures and cutting tissues?

e) A colleague says they prefer the flank approach because it causes less post-operative pain. What is a counterargument to this position?

f) During the breeding season, why can it be difficult to schedule a cat for spaying while avoiding oestrus?

g) You begin a flank spay and discover the cat is in oestrus. What are some surgical tips to avoid disintegration of friable tissue and consequent haemorrhage?

h) Does it have to be the left flank?

2.8 Gemima, 10-mo FN Springer Spaniel: spay wound burst

Gemima was spayed 2 days ago and has re-presented because the wound is open (Figure 2.8). The owner followed practice telephone advice to cover the wound with a clean moistened pillowcase before attending the clinic immediately.

a) What is the holding layer for sutures closing a coeliotomy (midline laparotomy) incision? Should muscle be included?

b) What suture material, patterns, and knot throws are required for midline closure?

c) Describe factors that may lead to a coeliotomy dehiscence.

d) How would you now manage Gemima going forward?

e) Should the owner pay for costs associated with the wound dehiscence?

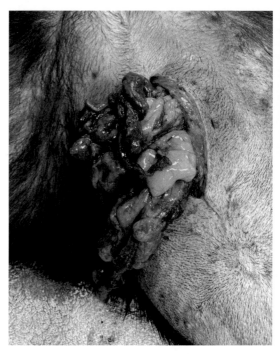

Figure 2.8 Gemima's spay wound opened after 2 days.

2.9 Rikki, 4-mo ME Golden Retriever: ?stung on face

Rikki is presented with a swollen face (Figure 2.9a). The owner reports that Rikki was sniffing in the garden when he yelped and ran inside, frantically rubbing his face on the carpet. The owner suspects a bee sting as the insects have been very active and are seen buzzing around the area Rikki had been exploring.

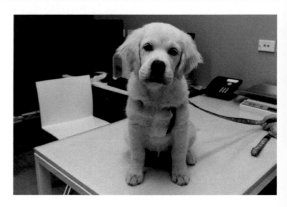

Figure 2.9a Rikki, with facial swelling following an episode in the garden.

On physical examination, Rikki's lips are swollen and oedematous, and feel warm and tender to touch. You see a small brown foreign body embedded in the buccal mucosa on the right side of Rikki's mouth, and remove this with tweezers (Figure 2.9b,c). Rikki's HR is elevated (176 bpm), but there are no other abnormalities on physical examination.

a) Describe the pathophysiology of bee sting in the dog.

b) How would you treat Rikki? Explain how this treatment addresses the pathophysiology.

c) What are the most serious sequelae of bee stings, and how would you address these?

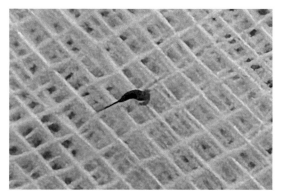

Figure 2.9b A bee sting, removed from Rikki, on a piece of gauze. The venom sac is to the right of the sting.

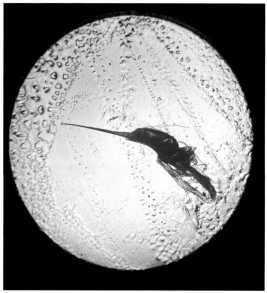

Figure 2.9c The bee sting as viewed under a microscope (4× objective), again with venom sac visible on the right.

2.10 Dotty, 4-yo MN DSH: dental prophy

Dotty, weighing 4.6 kg, presents for a dental scale and polish due to grade 2/4 periodontal disease (Figure 2.10).

He has significant tartar deposits on his molars, but otherwise his clinical examination is normal with an HR of 150 bpm and an RR of 24 breaths per minute. A routine history reveals nothing of concern. His owner has declined pre-operative blood work due to cost concerns.

a) Would you have recommended pre-operative blood work in this case?

b) Which breathing system would be appropriate for Dotty?

c) Calculate the fresh gas flow required for Dotty's anaesthetic.

d) Induction of general anaesthesia is smooth; however, Dotty coughs while being intubated, necessitating a bolus of induction agent. After this, Dotty becomes apnoeic. What course of action do you take?

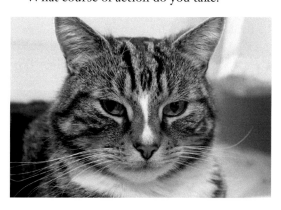

Figure 2.10 Dotty is a young healthy cat scheduled for dental prophylaxis.

2.11 Chuck, 17-yo MN DSH: 'gone downhill'

Chuck is a long-term patient usually seen by one of the senior vets. He has been managed for chronic kidney disease (CKD) for the past 3 years. Chuck has been vomiting for the past 2 days and is now refusing food, which means that the owners cannot administer his medications (ondansetron and mirtazapine). He is very dehydrated and the owners, who have been trying to give him 50 mL of SC fluids every 2 days, are now struggling. Chuck, who usually objects to being handled in a veterinary setting, looks miserable and offers none of his usual fuss as he is removed from the carrier and placed in front of you on the exam table (Figure 2.11).

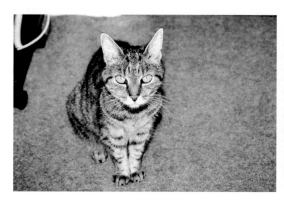

Figure 2.11 Chuck has deteriorated over the course of a few days.

a) What specific questions do you wish to ask the owner to help gauge the whole situation?

b) What diagnostics, if any, do you want to offer?

c) You are concerned about Chuck's QOL. How can you express this to the owners without causing offence?

d) Is euthanasia an acceptable treatment option in this case? How can you bring this up with the owners?

e) If the owners elect for euthanasia, how would you perform the procedure with a cat like Chuck?

2.12 Busy, 4-yo MN DSH: rash on chin

Busy's owner is concerned about a 'rash' on his chin. One month ago, Busy was rehomed into a multi-pet household following the separation of his previous owners, with whom he lived as the sole pet in a small apartment.

Examination of Busy's head reveals a large region of black comedones and crusts rostrally and around the lip margins, and a smaller region of alopecia caudally (Figure 2.12). Busy is not pruritic, and the site is not painful to examine. Busy is an otherwise healthy cat. His vaccinations are up to date, and the new owners have treated Busy and the other animals in the household (one cat and two dogs) with flea treatment.

a) What is this condition and how might it have arisen?

b) How would you treat this condition?

c) What if the lesions progress?

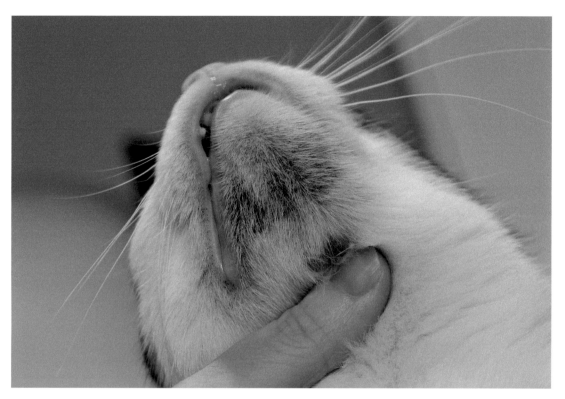

Figure 2.12 **A large region of black comedones and crusts rostrally and around the lip margins, and a smaller region of alopecia caudally (adjacent to the thumb of the handler).**

2.13 Benji, 5-yo MN Cockerpoo: check, seen OOH

Benji was seen out of hours (OOH) at an emergency clinic yesterday evening, 1 hour after he was attacked by another dog. There are bite wounds on the hindquarters (Figure 2.13a). The emergency vets clipped the area as much as Benji would tolerate, flushed the wounds with saline, and used staples to achieve primary closure where suitable. After injections of methadone and meloxicam, Benji was discharged with owner instructions to seek further veterinary treatment today.

a) Describe the injury.
b) What are your immediate considerations for Benji?

You recheck Benji after 24 hours (Figure 2.13b).

c) The owner remarks that the wound looks different today. How would you explain the change in appearance to the owner?

The owner consents to surgical wound management.

d) Describe and justify the steps you would take to prepare the wound for surgery once Benji has been stabilised under general anaesthetic.
e) What surgical considerations are important when approaching wounds such as these?
f) Describe and justify the steps you would take in the surgical management of Benji's wound.

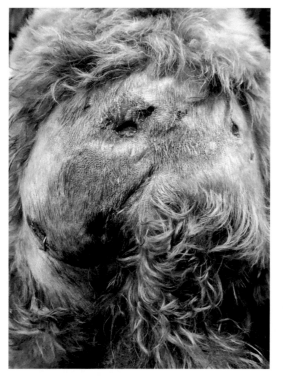

Figure 2.13a Benji presents having been seen OOH for bite wounds.

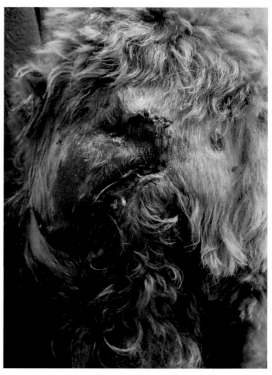

Figure 2.13b Benji's bite wound, day 2.

2.14 Henry, 6-yo MN CKCS: dental, *murmur*

Henry (Figure 2.14) presents with grade 2 periodontal disease, with a query about the potential need to extract some upper and lower incisors. This was picked up at his recent annual vaccination. Six months ago, he was diagnosed with stage B2 myxomatous mitral valve disease (MMVD) and prescribed pimobendan and benazepril by your colleague. His heart murmur on examination today is grade III/VI left apical systolic – unchanged from your colleague's initial assessment. He is reportedly exercising normally, with a resting RR of 16 breaths per minute. You propose to perform oral examination, dental radiographs, and necessary treatment under general anaesthesia.

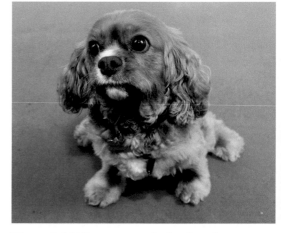

Figure 2.14 Henry comes in for dental treatment. He has a heart murmur.

a) The staging system for MMVD describes four basic stages of heart disease and heart failure. How is each stage characterised and what are the general recommendations for each stage? (You don't have to recall this in parrot-fashion, but it is useful to have a good working knowledge of how to stage patients you see on a daily basis.)

b) Are there any investigations that you would recommend prior to undertaking anaesthesia in Henry?

c) What recommendations would you give regarding Henry's heart medication around the time of anaesthesia?

d) What are your aims in terms of looking after Henry's cardiovascular system during anaesthesia?

e) What classes of analgesic would you consider for managing intra- and post-operative pain in Henry?

f) How might your management approach change if Henry behaved aggressively in the veterinary hospital?

2.15 Smithers, 13-yo MN DSH: recheck throat

You examine Smithers, who first presented a week ago with intermittent choking, poor appetite, and a history of 0.2 kg weight loss since a previous visit for vaccines 9 months ago. A colleague noticed an abnormality in his oral cavity under light sedation and took a photograph (Figure 2.15). A fine-needle aspirate examined in-house showed neutrophils and epithelial cells. The mandibular lymph nodes were not enlarged (nor were any other lymph nodes) and there were no lesions found beneath the tongue. Your colleague gave injections of a long-acting cephalosporin and a depot (long-acting) steroid, as well as a cautious prognosis.

Smithers now appears back to normal. His owner says he has been eating well, with no choking episodes. You attempt to examine his

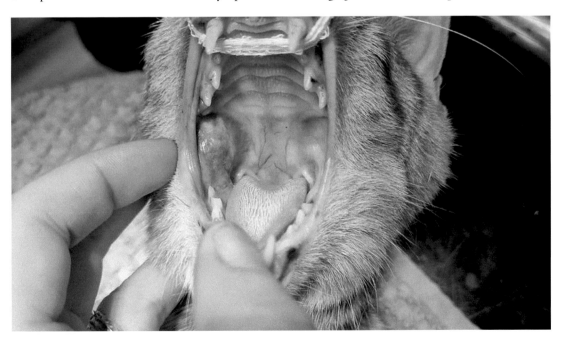

Figure 2.15 **Smithers's oral cavity at initial presentation 1 week ago.**

oral cavity conscious, but Smithers will not allow it. The lymph nodes are not palpable. You request permission for repeat sedation and examination, but the owner declines. They cannot afford the cost of repeat sedation, even at the practice's discounted rate for a second procedure. You do get a decent look at Smithers's teeth and, apart from moderate tartar accumulation, especially on the upper cheek teeth, they seem okay for a cat of his age.

a) Describe the oral cavity lesion on initial presentation (Figure 2.15).

b) What are possible diagnoses for a lesion such as this?

c) The owner requests ongoing treatment along the same lines as before and declines any more investigations. What will you offer in terms of treatment and how will you manage owner expectations going forward? How often would you like to see Smithers back in the clinic?

d) Should the owner be asked to sign a form stating that they are 'going against veterinary advice'?

2.16 Maggie, 6-yo FN Doberman Pinscher: freq urination

Maggie (Figure 2.16) is presented with a 3-day history of small, frequent, strained urination and intermittent vulval licking, which began 2 days after the urinary signs. There is mild inflammation of the vulval skin; physical examination is otherwise normal. The owner has brought a sample of cloudy urine (approximately 1 tablespoon), which she caught in a clean jar at home 20 minutes prior to the appointment. She also reports that Maggie has had a similar problem once before, approximately 3 years ago, which she said resolved with a course of antibiotic tablets.

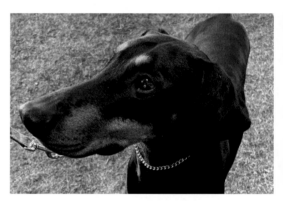

Figure 2.16 **Maggie has been straining to urinate for 3 days.**

a) What steps would you take before prescribing antibiotics in this case?

b) If treating empirically, which antimicrobial would you select?

c) What other treatment would you initiate?

d) What duration of antimicrobial therapy would you prescribe?

e) What are the benefits of following a guideline-recommended antimicrobial duration?

f) How would you determine whether the infection has resolved?

g) What if Maggie presents with the same clinical signs 2 weeks later?

2.17 Spaghetti, 9-mo ME rat: bleeding nose & eyes

Spaghetti presents for 'bleeding' from his nose and eyes (Figure 2.17). On physical examination, you notice that Spaghetti has dried red-tinged discharge on the medial forelimbs and he frequently sneezes. He has increased respiratory effort and auscultation reveals a mild increase in lung sounds bilaterally. Spaghetti's coat also appears unkempt, compared with that of his brother, Fettuccini.

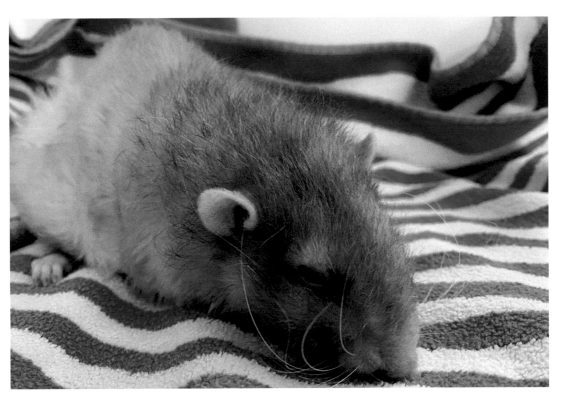

Figure 2.17 **Spaghetti on presentation for 'bleeding'.**

a) What is the bleeding noticed by the owner?
b) What is the most likely cause?
c) What diagnostic tests could you perform?

d) How would you treat Spaghetti?
e) Spaghetti's owner would like some tips on husbandry. What would you advise?

2.18 Pat, 7-yo MN Shetland Sheepdog: licking bottom ++

Pat is presented with a 48-hour history of 'chewing around his bottom all the time'. On physical examination, you observe and palpate a large, fluctuant mass associated with the left side of the anus, at approximately 8 o'clock (Figure 2.18). Pat's rectal temperature is 38.3 °C. You perform a rectal examination. There is a mass effect associated with the left anal sac, which is very painful to palpate. You are not able to express it without causing Pat discomfort. The right anal sac is moderately full but easily expressed. Otherwise, the rectal mucosa palpates normally. There is soft stool in the rectum. The rest of your physical examination is unremarkable.

a) What findings might you identify on a rectal examination?
b) What are your differential diagnoses?
c) What are the risk factors for non-neoplastic anal sac disease?
d) What treatment options would you offer?
e) What if the problem does not resolve?

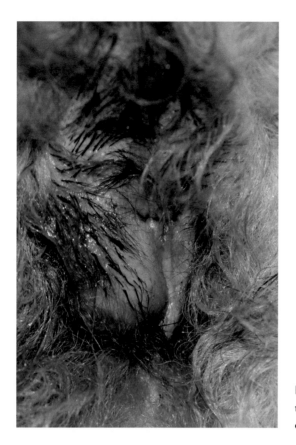

Figure 2.18 **A large, fluctuant, painful mass on the left-hand side of Pat's anus. Note the matting of perianal fur where Pat has been licking.**

2.19 Spot, 5-yo FN Lagotto: ate fishing line

Spot's owner, Meredith, had been walking Spot down near the local marina after work. While ranging off-lead, Spot ate something from the ground. Moments later, Meredith noticed what looked like fishing line emerging from Spot's mouth. As Meredith tried to take a better look in Spot's mouth, Spot swallowed the line.

Spot is a healthy dog with no pre-existing conditions, but does have a penchant for ingesting foreign bodies, which have in the past been retrieved successfully when emesis is induced. She is bright, highly excitable, and tends to bite when restrained.

Meredith asks if you can induce vomiting. You are worried about a fishing hook and

decide to take radiographs. Despite sedating Spot intramuscularly with a combination of medetomidine (20 µg/kg) and butorphanol (0.2 mg/kg), you only manage to take a single lateral radiograph of the thorax and cranial abdomen (Figure 2.19). She will need further sedation or general anaesthesia to facilitate positioning for additional views.

a) Under ideal circumstances, what radiographic views would you take in a case like this?
b) Outline different approaches for managing a foreign body, or bodies, like this, including potential advantages and disadvantages/complications.

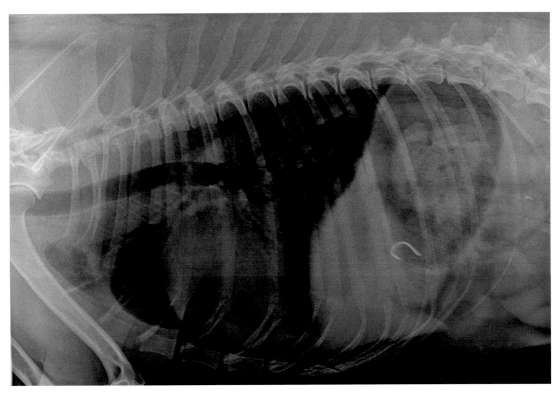

Figure 2.19 A right/left lateral radiograph with significant movement artefact. A radiopaque barbed metal hook is present in the ventral stomach, which also contains what appears to be a substantial amount of food.

You update Spot's owner at 6 p.m. and recommend referral to a nearby emergency facility. The veterinarian on duty requests that the medetomidine sedation is reversed to facilitate safe transport of Spot. You reverse the sedation with atipamezole, give the owner directions to the facility, and forward your records. The emergency veterinarian says they will update you on Wednesday morning (see Case 3.1).

2.20 Confidential meeting with T

You are an employer, manager, or supervisor in a veterinary practice. A colleague, T, requests a meeting with you to discuss a confidential matter. During this meeting, they seem very nervous but eventually tell you that they are transgender and wish to start transitioning at work. You ask them if there is anything you can do to help and they ask you to have a look at the Gender Identity Bill of Rights (GIBOR) in the veterinary workplace.

You talk to another senior vet who has had an employee transition gender at work. They tell you that their practice sent out a mass email to all their clients at the time and that they had an overwhelmingly positive response, including an uptick in new clients. Impressed by this, you draft a similar email, when a colleague tells you that T seems unhappy and anxious since they found out about the email idea.

PART 1

a) What general areas and issues do you think GIBOR might cover?
b) What should you do next to help support T?

PART 2

About 3 months later, T's coming out has been overall well accepted by staff and clients alike and T is feeling much happier. T mentions there have been a couple of offhand comments from other staff along the lines of 'He/she/they, whatever...' and 'Maybe I'll just change my name as well!' but, in T's words, 'it's not a big deal'.

a) What are these types of 'offhand comments' called and what should be done about them?

PART 3

It is now 6 months since T came out at work and things are going really well. You are passed an email from a client who has a high, regular monthly spend. In the email, the client complains that a staff member called them out and asked them to stop when the client said that they did not want to see T. The client had said that 'all this trans stuff is just woke nonsense' and that 'trans women are just pretending in order to gain an advantage over "real" women'. In the email, the client now threatens to take their business elsewhere unless they receive an apology from the staff member for calling them out.

a) How should you respond to this email?

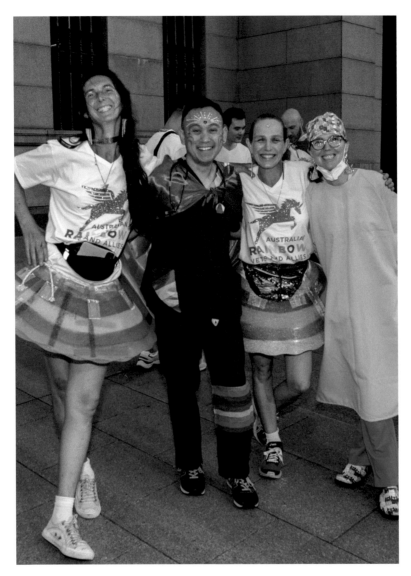

Figure 2.20 Veterinary medicine still has work to do to ensure a fully diverse and inclusive profession for all, but groups such as British Veterinary LGBT+, Pride VMC in the United States, and Australian Rainbow Vets and Allies (ARVA) welcome all members of the LGBTQIA+ community and their allies.

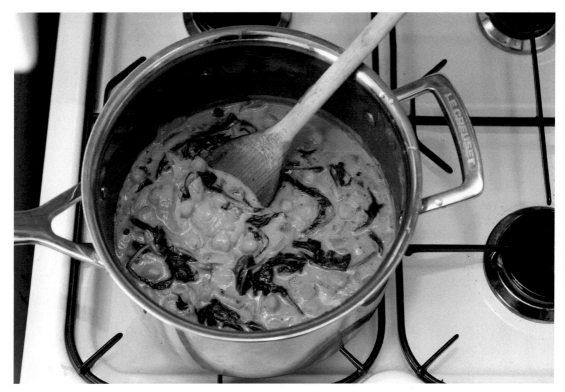

Figure 2.21a **Chickpea curry garnished with baby spinach.**

CHICKPEA CURRY

This very quick curry is a low-effort, nutritious meal. It is flexible, so can be extended with optional extras. When served with rice or similar, it makes about four meals. It can be consumed fresh, or as leftovers, and can be frozen, thawed, and reheated.

Ingredients
Oil for frying onion/garlic
1 onion, finely diced
2 cloves garlic, finely chopped
1 teaspoon ground cumin
½ teaspoon ground turmeric
½ teaspoon chilli flakes (or more, to taste)
2 heaped tablespoons mild curry paste (or hot, if preferred)
2 heaped tablespoons mango chutney
1 × 400 mL can full-fat coconut milk
2 × 400 g cans chickpeas (drained and rinsed)
2 heaped tablespoons coconut or plain vegan yoghurt
Rice, baked potatoes, or naan bread

Optional extras
- Handful of baby spinach leaves, handful of raw cashew nuts, handful of frozen peas, handful of cherry tomatoes
- Salt and pepper to taste
- Jalapeños
- Handful of coriander leaves, chopped, to garnish

Method

1. Preparation: chop the onion and garlic and set these aside together; drain and rinse the chickpeas. You can also put the cumin, turmeric, chilli flakes, curry paste, and mango chutney in a separate bowl.
2. Heat the oil and add onion and garlic and cook over medium high heat for 2 minutes.
3. Stir in cumin, turmeric, chilli flakes, curry paste, and mango chutney until the onion and garlic is thoroughly coated in this aromatic mix.
4. Add the chickpeas and coconut milk, and simmer for 8–10 minutes, stirring frequently until the sauce is creamy.
5. If you plan to add baby spinach, cashew nuts, frozen peas, or cherry tomatoes, do this about 3–5 minutes before you remove the saucepan from heat.
6. Remove from heat and stir in coconut yoghurt.
7. Season with salt and pepper and garnish with coriander and jalapeños if you wish. Serve with rice, baked potatoes, or naan bread.

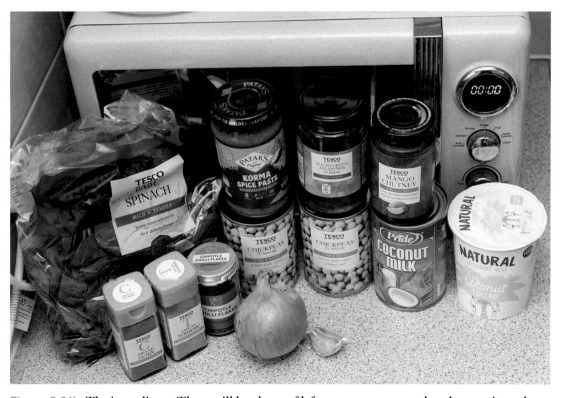

Figure 2.21b **The ingredients. There will be plenty of leftover curry sauce and yoghurt, so it can be economical to make this dish a few times in quick succession to use these up.**

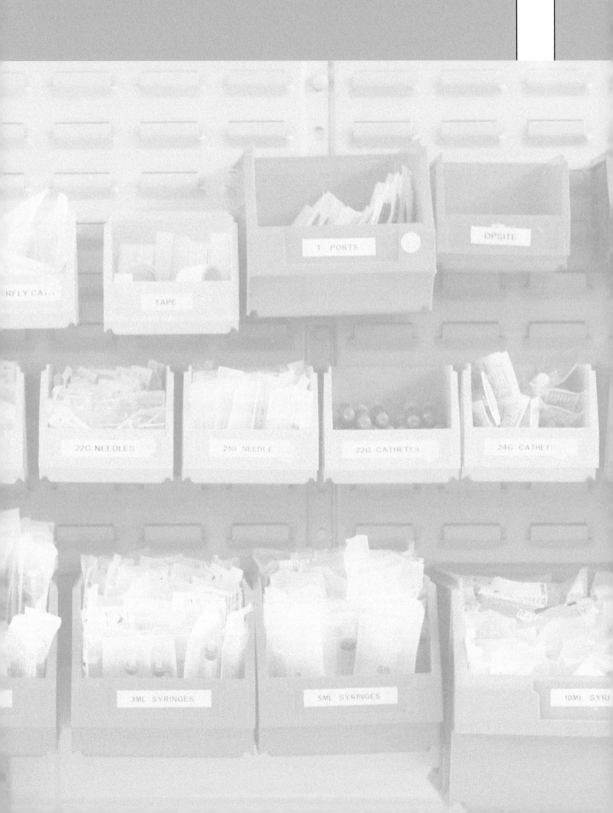

2.1 Betty Blue, 5-yo FN Affenpinscher: walk-in, no appt

a) Betty Blue's reduced haematocrit, Hb, and erythrocyte count, together with the presence of increased levels of reticulocytes, and polychromasia and anisocytosis on the blood smear, are all suggestive of regenerative anaemia. Other potential findings in regenerative anaemia include overall increased red blood cell size, evidenced by increased mean corpuscular volume (not shown in this case), and the presence of nucleated red blood cells, which are not specific for regenerative anaemia as increased circulating levels can be associated with erythroid neoplasia, toxicity, or splenic disease (Maddison 2015).

b) Other haematological alterations (leukocytosis, primarily due to neutrophilia accompanied by lymphocytopenia, monocytosis, and eosinopenia) are suggestive of a stress (corticosteroid-induced) leukogram. The elevated glucose level would also suggest stress. The other biochemical abnormalities detected, i.e. hypochloridaemia and mildly elevated alkaline phosphatase, could be explained by vomiting (chloride result) and hypoxia or stress (ALP result).

c) Bleeding can occur at any site in the body, but the most common sites of haemorrhage, in descending order of frequency, are shown in Figure A2.1.

   In an evaluation by Stroope et al. (2022), 55% of dogs had haemorrhage at more than one site. Importantly, neither location of haemorrhage nor number of haemorrhaging sites was associated with survival or requirement for transfusion (Stroope et al. 2022).

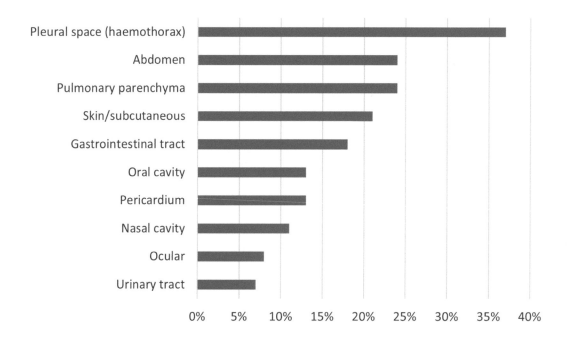

Figure A2.1 The most frequent sites of haemorrhage associated with anticoagulant rodenticides.
(Adapted from Stroope et al. 2022.)

d) Betty Blue is in a serious condition. The goals of treatment in this case are to prevent hypovolaemic shock (indicated by her hypothermia, tachycardia, and poor peripheral perfusion), and prevent further haemorrhage. To restore volume, you can administer fluids to correct hypovolaemia, followed by administration of fluids at 1.5–2.0 times maintenance until she is non-coagulopathic (Hommerding 2022). To address anaemia and prevent further haemorrhage, ideally, Betty Blue would undergo transfusion with whole blood or fresh frozen plasma after cross-matching, to replace red blood cells and active clotting factors. In one study, dogs who received a transfusion had a significantly increased rate of survival to discharge (Stroope et al. 2022). Serial monitoring of PCV/TP and coagulation parameters every 6–12 hours will give some indication of response to treatment (Hommerding 2022). Anticoagulant rodenticides antagonise vitamin K_1, leading to depletion of vitamin K_1-dependent clotting factors (II, VII, IX, and X) and prevent conversion of prothrombin to thrombin (Hommerding 2022, Stroope et al. 2022). Treatment with vitamin K_1 should be administered. This is available in injectable (2.5–5.0 mg SC, injected at several sites) and oral formulations. If given orally (usually at 1.0–2.5 mg/kg q12h or 5.0 mg/kg q24h), it is best absorbed with a fatty meal. As Betty Blue is not eating, it makes sense to initially treat her with an SC injection of vitamin K_1, being careful to minimise the risk of injection-associated haematoma formation. Treatment with vitamin K_1 should lead to production of coagulation factors within 6–12 hours, and Betty Blue's PT/APTT would be expected to improve within 12–24 hours (Hommerding 2022). The client should be advised that Betty Blue will be in hospital for a minimum of 24 hours, and possibly longer. She may also require oxygen supplementation, anti-emetics, and gastroprotectants. Betty Blue should be confined until she is non-coagulopathic, to minimise the risk of haemorrhage. It is important to inform the client of the risk that Betty Blue could die if left unmonitored overnight. This discussion should be documented in the clinical records.

e) This case is challenging because the dose, type of anticoagulant used, and time since ingestion are all important pieces of information when managing toxicity in animals, and they are unknown here. First-generation anticoagulant rodenticides are rarely used for public rodent control (Table A2.1). If the anticoagulant type is unknown, it is prudent to assume that the longest-acting toxin has been ingested. At a minimum, the patient should be treated for 21 days, repeating the PT test 2 days post-treatment and again 3 weeks later. If the client cannot afford further testing, the patient should be treated with vitamin K_1 tablets for a minimum of 30 days, and monitored carefully for further haemorrhage. In-house PT testing is relatively cheap and may be less costly than dispensing additional vitamin K_1 tablets.

Table A2.1 **Types of anticoagulant rodenticides, and recommended treatment and follow-up (adapted from Mensching & Volmer 2008 and Hommerding 2022)**

TYPE OF ANTICOAGULANT RODENTICIDE (AND ACTIVE INGREDIENT)	RECOMMENDED TREATMENT WITH VITAMIN K₁	FOLLOW-UP
Short-acting hydroxycoumarin (first-generation) agents (warfarin, dicoumarol)	• Initial treatment: 2.5 mg/kg SC (administered at several sites) • Ongoing treatment: 1.0–2.5 mg/kg PO q8–12h for 7–14 days	Re-evaluate PT 2 or 3 days following treatment. If abnormal, administer vitamin K₁ orally for an additional 1–2 weeks until post-treatment PT is normalised
Longer-acting hydroxycoumarin (second generation) agents (brodifacoum, bromadiolone, difenacoum)	• Initial treatment: 5 mg/kg SC (administered at several sites) • Ongoing treatment: 2.5 mg/kg PO q12h for 21 days	Re-evaluate PT at 21 days and 3 weeks after cessation of treatment
Indandione agents (pindone, diphacinone, difethialone, bromadiolone, chlorophacinone)	• Initial treatment: 2.5–5 mg/kg SC (administered at several sites) • Ongoing treatment: 2.5 mg/kg PO q12h for 30 days	Re-evaluate PT 2 days after cessation of treatment If prolonged, continue treatment for an additional week and repeat again 2 days after treatment

TIP: Response to vitamin K₁ within 24 hours is supportive of a diagnosis of anticoagulant rodenticide toxicity.

REFERENCES

Hommerding, H. (2022) 'Anticoagulant rodenticide (warfarin and congeners) poisoning in animals'. Reviewed March 2022. MSD. Available at: www.msdvetmanual.com/toxicology/rodenticide-poisoning/anticoagulant-rodenticide-warfarin-and-congeners-poisoning-in-animals.

Maddison, J. (2015) Anaemia. In: Maddison, J., Volk, H. A. & Church, D. B. (eds). *Clinical Reasoning in Small Animal Practice*. Hoboken, NJ: Wiley.

Mensching, D. & Volmer, P. A. (2008) Chapter 124: Rodenticides. In: Morgan, R. V. (ed) *Handbook of Small Animal Practice*, 5th edition. Philadelphia, PA: Saunders Elsevier.

Stroope, S., Walton, R., Mochel, J. P. et al. (2022) Retrospective evaluation of clinical bleeding in dogs with anticoagulant rodenticide toxicity. A multi-centre evaluation of 62 cases (2010–2020). *Frontiers in Veterinary Science* **23**(9). doi: 10.3389/fvets.2022.879179.

2.2 Benji, 2-yo MN Pointer: stealing & guarding things

PART 1

a) Suitable questions include the following:
  1. How has Benji been trained and by whom?
  2. What is the family set-up? Are there other pets in the household?
  3. What is Benji's daily routine/exercise?
  4. What are Benji's diet/feeding times?
  5. What does Benji steal?

As a result of your questions, you discover that Benji is the only pet in the household and there are no children. Relatives' children do, however, visit regularly. He is taken out twice daily, mainly by one or other owner (sometimes both), though it is the male owner who has been responsible for taking him to dog training with a 'balanced' trainer, who uses a combination of positive punishment and positive reward. The female owner is responsible for veterinary visits. Benji is fed twice daily with proprietary kibble. The owners have been led to believe that lying on the sofa will give Benji 'ideas above his station'.

b) Suitable questions include the following:
   1. Has Benji bitten someone? If so, what was the severity of the bite?
   2. Does Benji have a preferred retreat area?
   3. Does he have his own bed?
   4. What does Benji do with a stolen item?
   5. How do the owners try to retrieve the item?
   6. How do the owners try to remove the dog from the furniture?

As a result of your questions, you find out that Benji tends to steal socks, underwear, and tea towels if left within reach. He then retreats to his bed or under the dining table and growls if approached. As he becomes particularly ferocious if in possession of pig ears, he is no longer given them. You find out that the owners have tried (unsuccessfully) to use food 'treats' to swap for a stolen item. This has inevitably made them somewhat frustrated and angry with Benji at times, as they worry he could swallow dangerous items such as socks. Benji has nipped both owners,

> Regardless of reasons why Benji feels the need to become aggressive, human safety is paramount. In all likelihood, Benji will see no need to become aggressive in other more public contexts. However, this must be confirmed by tactful history-taking. How a dog behaves in the veterinary surgery, at the groomers, towards tradespeople, postal workers, or other visitors to the house may indicate a more wide-reaching problem with potential legal implications.

without breaking the skin, on being grabbed by the collar in attempts to retrieve items from his mouth and to remove him from the sofa. Benji is generally more responsive to the male owner's commands than to those of the female partner.

PART 2

a) It is highly likely that the previous suspicion of a foreign body and investigation required has resulted in owners who are hypervigilant regarding anything Benji may pick up and carry in his mouth. The attention the dog receives at such times gives added value to the stolen item and inadvertently reinforces the very behaviour they want to extinguish.

b) Although correctly used food rewards are becoming accepted as doing much more than just bribing a dog, human anger at canine 'naughtiness' is not generally thought of as a training method. Unfortunately, the false idea that aggressive dogs are being dominant in trying to exert their will over their human pack is still all too common, despite being debunked (e.g. American Veterinary Society of Animal Behaviour 2008). The result is escalation of aggression as threat is met with threat: the threatening behaviour of the dog is met with behaviour by the owner that the dog perceives as threatening.

c) Gun dogs are frequently trained by threat for getting a choice of behaviour wrong (positive punishment) and no threat (negative reward) for getting it right, often enacted via a slip lead (Figure A2.2). A 'balanced' trainer uses positive punishment for wrongdoing and positive reward for correct behaviour. Confirming how Benji's balanced trainer has altered Benji's choices, and whether this has been replicated at home, is fundamental. If punished for stealing, an inadvertently reinforced behaviour, Benji will have experienced

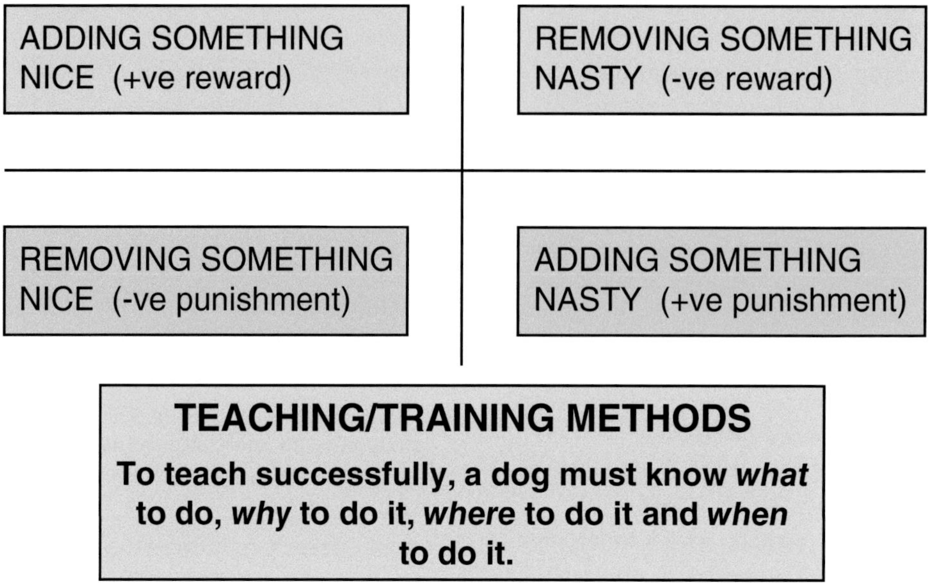

ADDING SOMETHING NICE (+ve reward)	REMOVING SOMETHING NASTY (-ve reward)
REMOVING SOMETHING NICE (-ve punishment)	ADDING SOMETHING NASTY (+ve punishment)

TEACHING/TRAINING METHODS

To teach successfully, a dog must know *what* to do, *why* to do it, *where* to do it and *when* to do it.

© Kendal Shepherd 2004

Figure A2.2 Positive and negative reinforcements of behaviour.

extreme emotional conflict, as his actions also herald threat and punishment.

d) Anything a human has in their possession is automatically desirable and therefore more valuable in a dog's eyes – even if the item in the owner's pocket is identical to that in the dog's mouth. Routinely practising the exchange of items, such as chew toys or rawhide chews, even socks, with items increasing in value, before Benji becomes aroused and defensive will help to persuade him that human hands give rather than take away. Plenty of rehearsal in advance of approaching the problem situation is essential. To reduce his need to defend aggressively, Benji needs to anticipate positive reward (generally in the form of tasty food) for dropping whatever is in his mouth and negative punishment (in the form of withdrawal of attention and the food) if he chooses not to. The latter is the opposite of the way a balanced trainer influences a dog's choice of behaviour.

If necessary, when Benji demonstrates aggressive behaviour, the owners should walk out of the room, closing the door behind them to clearly demonstrate their disapproval.

e) The sofa is simply an item that Benji thinks is his and needs to defend. There is no relationship whatsoever between a dog's spatial position and his perception of relative social standing. Banning areas at a height for such spurious reasons creates unnecessary conflict. A dog may lie anywhere he chooses, as long as the owners can successfully ask him to move away from it to other areas when needed. It is also worth checking the decor style and furnishings in the house and the quality and position of Benji's bed. The sofa is also often the only comfortable place to lie, giving the obvious reason for his choice. Supplying at least two comfortable dog beds and rewarding Benji whenever he chooses to lie in them will reduce the opportunities for conflict. Apparently paradoxically, inviting a dog to jump up onto a sofa for a reward can facilitate success in asking him to get off again. By allowing access instead of prohibiting it, the resource is devalued, which in turn reduces the need to guard and increases willingness to relinquish.

f) Without making any gender assumptions, it is worth asking couples to give non-judgemental opinions as to why one seems more successful in certain areas than others. It is not uncommon to find blame being apportioned for the dog's behaviour as well as varying degrees of guilt and self-criticism. Whatever has happened in the past and however ill-advised, is water under the proverbial bridge as we strive for improvement going forward.

g) Neutering before social maturity may lead to a loss of confidence and an increase in aggression towards other dogs (McGreevy et al. 2018). In the absence of evidence that

human-directed aggression falls into the same category, it is more likely in Benji's case that oversolicitous human behaviour following surgical intervention may lead to condoning of any apparent behavioural change, and a consequent increase in attention-seeking by stealing.

REFERENCES

American Veterinary Society of Animal Behaviour (2008) *Position Statement on the Use of Dominance Theory in Behaviour Modification of Animals.* Available at: https://avsab.org/wp-content/uploads/2018/03/Dominance_Position_Statement_download-10-3-14.pdf.

McGreevy, P.D., Wilson, B., Starling, M.J. & Serpell, J. A. (2018) Behavioural risks in male dogs with minimal lifetime exposure to gonadal hormones may complicate population-control benefits of desexing. *PLoS One* **13**(5):e0196284. doi: 10.1371/journal.pone.0196284.

2.3 Poppy, 12-yo FN DSH: not eating, face different?

a) Clinical parameters used to help assess hydration status are MM colour and moisture, CRT, skin turgor, eye position in the orbit, pulse volume, HR, corneal lustre, and body weight. Mentation and responsiveness are also important criteria.

b) Tables like these are an attempt to give objective criteria. In the end, it is a spectrum and clinical judgement always applies. Patients do vary, but some of the signs commonly seen with the degree of dehydration are shown in Table A2.3. Quoting a percentage range in your clinical notes can be useful.

Table A2.3 **Clinical signs of dehydration. Entries in bold define progression to the next level of clinical severity**

DEGREE OF DEHYDRATION	CLINICAL SIGNS
5–8%	• Tacky to dry MMs • Pale MMs • Skin tenting
8–10%	• Tacky to dry MMs • Pale MMs • Skin tenting • **Globe retraction**
10–12%	• Tacky to dry MMs • Pale MMs • Skin tenting marked • Globe retraction • **Dull cornea**
>12%	• Tacky to dry MMs • Pale MMs • Skin tenting marked • Globe retraction • Dull cornea • **Depression/collapse**

c) Yes, Poppy appears to be in shock as shown by the prolonged CRT, pale MMs, and weak pulses. Cats may show normal or reduced HRs in the early phase of shock, unlike dogs, who are normally tachycardic at this point. In late-phase shock in both dogs and cats, HRs are 'normal' or low. Repeated monitoring is required.

d) The immediate priority is to treat the shock (IV fluids, warmth) and obtain some basic blood work to check for underlying conditions. Regular repeat clinical examinations are needed throughout the morning, both to monitor Poppy's haemodynamic status and to pick up anything missed on the initial exam in the clinic. Temperature should be monitored.

e) Sodium chloride 0.19% and glucose 4% is a hypotonic solution. The glucose in glucose saline does not provide energy; it is metabolised to free water. At this stage, Poppy requires a physiological replacement fluid such as Lactated Ringer's (Hartmann's solution), which will help correct acidosis, not a hypotonic fluid. Due to her critical state (her shock could worsen quickly), Poppy should be prioritised over other cases, e.g. animals receiving maintenance or intra-operative fluids, who can safely receive normal (physiological) saline (0.9%). If 0.9% saline was the only fluid in the practice, it could also be given to Poppy on the basis that any fluid is better than none at all (within reason), but hypotonic fluids can lead to dangerous hyponatraemia in hypovolaemic patients (Pardo et al. 2024).

f) Possible conditions include chronic renal failure, hyperthyroidism, thoracic or abdominal neoplasia (in cats, lymphoma is common), triaditis, or cholangiohepatitis. Poisoning/toxicity would appear unlikely as Poppy is an indoor cat with no exposure history.

g) Poppy's face may look different because of globe retraction due to loss of retrobulbar fat caused by weight loss while her owner was in hospital. Her face may appear 'pinched in' due to the dehydration. Another potential cause is pain. In fact, the Feline Grimace Scale can be used by veterinary team members and cat owners to assess acute pain in cats (Monteiro et al. 2023). Owners can be very sensitive to changed facial expression in their animals, so it is worth paying attention when they mention it. In this case, it was the main presenting problem from the owner's point of view, so should be discussed. Other conditions might also be recognised by a change in facial expression, e.g. 'the tragic expression of hypothyroidism' in dogs, facial nerve paralysis, dental abscess, Horner's syndrome, anisocoria, masticatory muscle myositis. See also Case 3.14.

h) Poppy weighs 3.2 kg and is 10% dehydrated. Her dehydration is to be corrected over 24 hours.

   Her fluid **deficit** is as follows: 10% of 3.2 kg = 0.32 kg = 0.32 L = 320 mL.

   Her **maintenance** is as follows: 50 mL/kg/24 hours = (50 × 3.2) mL/24 hours = 160 mL/24 hours.

   Total fluid requirement over 24 hours = 320 + 160 = 480 mL/24 hours.

   Fluid rate per hour = 480/24 = 20 mL/hour.

It is important to try to work out fluids accurately because there is a tendency to underperfuse large animals and overperfuse small animals if you attempt to do it any other way. Animals on fluids should receive regular exams to check on hydration status and clinical parameters including heart and respiratory rates, lung auscultation, CRT, and MM tackiness.

REFERENCES

Pardo, M., Spencer, E., Odunayo, A. et al. (2024) AAHA fluid therapy guidelines for dogs and cats. *Journal of the American Animal Hospital Association* **60**(4):131–163. doi: 10.5326/JAAHA-MS-7444. PMID: 38885492.

Monteiro, B. P., Lee, N. H. Y. & Steagall, P. V. (2023) Can cat caregivers reliably assess acute pain in cats using the Feline Grimace Scale? A large bilingual global survey. *Journal of Feline Medicine and Surgery* **25**(1). doi: 10.1177/1098612X221145499.

2.4 Rocco, 5-yo MN Cocker Spaniel: red eye

a) 'Red eye' is a common, non-specific sign of ocular inflammation. It can involve conjunctival hyperaemia (typically associated with extraocular disease such as conjunctivitis), subconjunctival haemorrhage (usually associated with trauma, clotting disorders, or excessive restraint/strangulation), episcleral injection (congestion of deep, straight, episcleral vessels, usually indicative of intraocular disease such as glaucoma or uveitis), corneal neovascularisation (superficial or deep), and hyphaema (bleeding in the anterior chamber, usually associated with clotting disorders, blunt trauma, uveitis, or systemic hypertension). A red eye usually involves a disorder of the anterior segment of the eye, i.e. a structure or structures anterior to the vitreous humour. This includes the following:
- Anterior uveitis
- Corneal injury, e.g. corneal ulcer and non-ulcerative keratitis
- Glaucoma
- Conjunctivitis
- Blepharitis
- Diseases of the orbit, e.g. cellulitis, neoplasia

Note that ocular abnormalities can be secondary, e.g. uveitis secondary to corneal ulceration, so it is important to try to establish the root cause of ocular disease if you can.

b) The following are the top three that could pose a threat to the dog's vision:

1. **Glaucoma** – primary glaucoma is a medical emergency in dogs, potentially causing blindness within 24 hours
2. **Melting corneal ulcers** – rapidly progressing ulcers
3. **Anterior uveitis** – painful inflammation of the anterior segment of the eye

However, without appropriate treatment, any ocular disease that threatens the integrity of the globe can ultimately lead to blindness.

c) Breed predisposition is very important in ophthalmology. Cocker Spaniels are predisposed to entropion (turning in of the eyelids), distichiasis (eyelash[es] arising from an abnormal part of the eyelid), and keratoconjunctivitis sicca (KCS) (dry eye; inadequate production of the aqueous portion of the tear film by the lacrimal gland), all of which can cause corneal irritation and damage. They are also predisposed to primary glaucoma, meaning that if glaucoma occurs in one eye, it is likely to occur in the other eye as well at some stage.

d) A complete ophthalmic examination should be performed, including ophthalmic reflex testing and ophthalmoscopy and, if possible, tonometry. A Schirmer tear test (STT) and fluorescein stain must be performed in any red eye (Figure A2.4).

e) The order is as follows:
1. **Schirmer tear test**: this should be performed first, before anything else

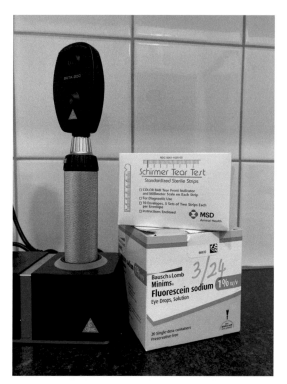

Figure A2.4 An STT and a fluorescein stain are simple and essential tests in eye examination. Fluorescein uptake may be more visible in a darkened room, viewed under ultraviolet light.

is introduced into the eye, to obtain an accurate reading of tear production

2. **Fluorescein staining**: crucial for detection of corneal ulceration, but note that particularly deep corneal ulcers may not stain

3. **Tonometry**: to rule out glaucoma

Use of local anaesthetic (after the STT and fluorescein staining) may permit more thorough examination of the eye and adnexa. The pupillary light reflex (direct and consensual in both eyes) is also important, particularly in a breed predisposed to glaucoma. Eye pain is often associated with miosis (constriction, seen in anterior uveitis especially). However, in the presence of glaucoma, increased intraocular pressure

(IOP) usually results in mydriasis (dilation) and sluggish pupillary light reflexes in the affected eye.

f) If it has been possible to do tonometry and glaucoma can be eliminated, i.e. IOP is within the normal range, reported as 12–24 mmHg (mean 16.3 ± 2.1 mmHg) using a Schiøtz tonometer and 11–25 mmHg (mean 18.1 ± 3.8 mmHg) using a Tono-Pen Vet tonometer (Wrześniewska et al. 2018), conservative management could be undertaken. However, it is important to consider that certain signs may be missed without more specialised equipment. For example, a slit lamp may be needed to detect aqueous flare, which can be associated with anterior uveitis (noting that anterior uveitis can be secondary to another abnormality, such as corneal ulceration, and/or can itself lead to secondary abnormalities such as glaucoma).

If tonometry is not possible, and the pupil is constricted and/or normally light responsive, conservative management could again be considered. But if there is mydriasis and/or the pupillary light responses are sluggish, glaucoma should be assumed and urgent referral offered. It is important to determine if glaucoma is primary (usually due to poor drainage of aqueous fluid due to a malformed iridocorneal angle) or secondary (to uveitis, cataracts, lens luxation, or neoplasia such as ocular melanoma).

If immediate referral is not an option, in a case such as Rocco's, with suspicious signs, you may consider empirical treatment for acute primary glaucoma given that Cocker Spaniels are predisposed to this. You could admit Rocco and administer one drop of latanoprost eye drops (50 µg/mL) (note that this is off label), which increase aqueous outflow. As this causes miosis, lens luxation needs to be ruled out first. Systemic anti-inflammatories (NSAIDs or corticosteroids) may help reduce inflammation, improve aqueous outflow, and improve patient comfort. Tonometry should be repeated in 90 minutes to determine if Rocco has responded. If this fails, systemic medications such as mannitol and furosemide may be required, but specialist advice is recommended. Primary glaucoma is a bilateral condition, so you should advise the owner that Rocco's unaffected eye may develop overt glaucoma in the future (Plummer et al. 2021).

Diagnosis of a red eye is greatly facilitated by the availability of tonometry in general practice. Establishing the primary cause is important. Early referral, if available, is the best option if equipment and expertise are not available in-house, as diagnosis can be challenging if, for example, glaucoma is secondary to uveitis. The eye can quickly deteriorate and does not tolerate sustained inflammation. It is important to become familiar with the acute presentations of anterior uveitis and glaucoma (Table A2.4).

Table A2.4 Differentiating acute anterior uveitis from glaucoma in cases of 'red eye'

	ACUTE ANTERIOR UVEITIS	GLAUCOMA
Redness	Intense reddening of visible parts of eye	Redness due to episcleral injection
Pain	Marked pain with photophobia, blepharospasm, epiphora	Variable levels of pain; may be evident as altered activity/demeanour/appetite
IOP	Low (eye is 'soft') without raised IOP on tonometry	High (eye is 'hard') with IOP raised on tonometry
Pupil	Miosis and/or resistance to dilation via tropicamide	Mydriasis (DO NOT attempt to dilate pupil as this can further increase pressure)
Vision	Vision usually present but may be reduced	No obvious vision loss in early stages; vision loss at >24 hours
Cornea	Corneal changes can include oedema (blue eye), deep vascularisation	Corneal oedema (blue eye)
Anterior chamber	Changes can include hypopyon, aqueous flare, hyphaema, keratic precipitates	Changes may indicate glaucoma is secondary
Iris	Changes can include altered colour, swelling, hyperaemia	Changes may indicate glaucoma is secondary
Initial treatment objective(s)	Immediate management of pain and inflammation to avoid adverse sequelae (including glaucoma): *topical mydriatics and steroids are first-line treatments in many uncomplicated cases.* Refer to the literature	Urgent reduction of IOP to prevent optic nerve damage and loss of vision: *topical latanoprost*
Other considerations	Important to investigate and manage underlying cause	Important to distinguish between primary and secondary glaucoma • If primary, important to monitor other eye • If secondary, manage underlying cause

REFERENCES

Allbaugh, R. A. (2019) Managing uveitis in dogs and cats. *Today's Veterinary Practice* March/April 2019. Available at: https://todaysveterinarypractice.com/ophthalmology/managing-uveitis-in-dogs-and-cats/.

Plummer, C. E., Bras, D., Grozdanic, S. et al. (2021) Prophylactic anti-glaucoma therapy in dogs with primary glaucoma: a practitioner survey of current medical protocols. *Veterinary Ophthalmology* **24**(1):96–108: doi: 10.1111/vop.12820.

Wrześniewska, K., Madany, J. & Winiarczyk, D. (2018) Comparison of intraocular pressure measurement with Schiotz tonometer and Tono-Pen Vet Tonometer in healthy dogs. *Journal of Veterinary Research* **62**(2):243–247. doi: 10.2478/jvetres-2018-0018.

2.5 Carlos, 8-mo MN guinea pig: had a fit

a) Given the clinical presentation and degree of pruritus, the most likely differential diagnoses are ectoparasites:
- Mites, e.g. *Chirodiscoides caviae*, *Trixacarus caviae*, *Demodex caviae*
- Lice
- Dermatophytes, e.g. *Trichophyton mentagrophytes*, *Trichophyton benhamiae*, *Microsporum canis*, although this is less likely than mites or lice given Carlos's clinical presentation.

There may also be secondary bacterial/fungal infections. In a large UK study, dermatophytosis was the second most prevalent primary disorder (following overgrown nails) in guinea pigs registered with veterinarians (O'Neill et al. 2024). Other potential causes of Carlos's signs include allergic reaction to bedding material, infections due to poor sanitation or husbandry, and endocrine alopecia.

b) Direct microscopy of a sticky tape prep or skin scrape allows visualisation of ectoparasites. Fungal cultures may be required to identify dermatophytes. In this case, you identify *Trixacarus caviae* (Figure A2.5).

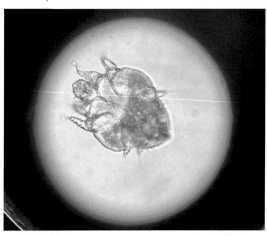

Figure A2.5 *Trixacarus caviae*, **the cause of the 'fits' Carlos experienced.**

c) The goals of treatment are to eliminate the underlying parasitic infestation while providing analgesia and nutritional support. For *T. caviae*, you could treat with ivermectin, 0.4 mg/kg SC q10–14 days for four treatments, or selamectin, 15 mg/kg topically, which may require repeat dosing every 14 days until clinical signs resolve. For analgesia, you could use a non-steroidal anti-inflammatory agent such as meloxicam (0.5 mg/kg PO q12h). Antihistamines can be administered, e.g. diphenhydramine, 1–5 mg/kg PO/SC q12h. If a secondary infection is present, topical antibiotics could be used, e.g. silver sulfadiazine cream, or systemic antibiotics may be required, e.g. trimethoprim sulfamethoxazole, 25 mg/kg PO q12h. Carlos's nails should be trimmed in the meantime to reduce further self-trauma. As guinea pigs are prone to vitamin C deficiency, supplementation with vitamin C (30–50 mg/kg PO q24h) is recommended. It may also be helpful to administer omega-3 and -6 fatty acids, and vitamin A and E, to promote skin barrier function. In severe cases, or if the owner is unable to provide care, euthanasia may be the most humane option. Euthanasia should also be considered in animals with severe secondary infections, or serious concurrent disease including dental disease, or in cases refractory to treatment, which may indicate underlying immunosuppression.

d) It is important to review Carlos's husbandry. Many common disorders are related to husbandry (O'Neill et al. 2024). The cage and environment should be regularly cleaned to reduce the likelihood of reinfestation. Items that cannot be properly washed or cleaned (such as wooden chew toys or bedding) should be discarded and replaced. Adequate nutrition, including access to good-quality grass or hay, high-quality pellets with stabilised vitamin C, and fresh vegetables, should be provided. All guinea pigs in the household should be treated at the same time even if asymptomatic. Owners should be advised that *T. caviae* can transiently infest humans, leading to pruritus.

REFERENCES

Carpenter, J. W. & Marion, C. J. (2018) *Exotic Animal Formulary*, 5th edition. Philadelphia, PA: W.B. Saunders.

O'Neill, D. G., Taffinder, J. L., Brodbelt, D. C. & Baldrey, V. (2024) Demography, commonly diagnosed disorders and mortality of guinea pigs under primary veterinary care in the UK in 2019 – a VetCompass study. *PLoS One* **19**:e0299464. doi: 10.1371/journal.pone.0299464.

Quesenberry, K. E., Orcutt, C. J., Mans, C. & Carpenter, J. W. (2021) *Ferrets, Rabbits and Rodents: Clinical Medicine and Surgery*. St Louis, MO: Elsevier.

2.6 Joey, 18-mo ME Cross-breed: ear flush

a) There are four simple checks in the clinic for normal anatomical dental occlusion (Figure A2.6a). They should form part of every examination of puppies and young dogs.
  1. The upper incisors should sit just rostral to the lower incisors, with the lower incisors resting on the cingulum (groove) of the caudal aspect of the upper incisors. This is 'normal scissor bite'.
  2. The lower canine should sit rostral to the upper canine and evenly occupy the space between the upper canine and the third incisor.
  3. The premolars should interdigitate in a 'pinking shears' fashion (not sit directly above and below each other).
  4. The upper caudal cheek teeth should sit lateral (i.e. buccal) to the lower caudal cheek teeth.

b) Joey's upper incisors are rostral to the lower incisors, but they are too far rostral, producing a marked discrepancy in jaw length (mandibular brachygnathism – 'short mandible'). His lower canines are sitting medial to the upper canines and are not centred in the space between the upper canines and the upper third incisors. The

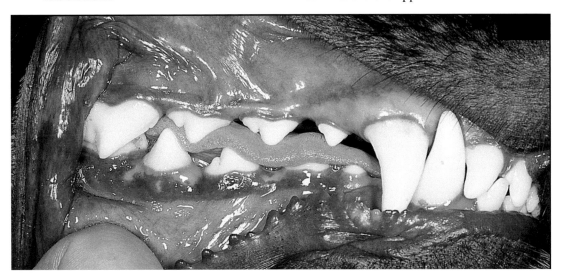

Figure A2.6a Normal anatomical dental occlusion in the dog.

premolars and molars are not visible. There are pits on the hard palate caused by Joey's medially or lingually displaced mandibular canines (also known as linguoverted or 'base narrow' canines).

c) If a medially displaced lower canine touches the hard palate or another structure of the maxilla, the mandible will stop growing rostrally. However, the growth still has to 'go somewhere' so the elongating mandibular body bows ventrally, creating a caudal malocclusion. Thus, Joey's malocclusion can rapidly worsen.

d) This is a common malocclusion in dogs (Berman et al. 2023). Note, however, that not all puppies in a litter may be affected. Puppies with a developing oronasal fistula caused by this problem often appear quiet and may not eat as well as their littermates. Joey should not be bred from as the condition is inherited.

e) (i) Puppies should always be checked for malocclusion at every visit as problems can rapidly develop as they grow. Treatment options include techniques to divert the medially displaced canines laterally (using an inclined bite plane, a distractor device, or, in milder cases, a therapeutic ball of the correct dimensions; Figure A2.6b). (ii) In older dogs, coronal (crown) reduction of the mandibular canines (with root canal treatment) or mandibular canine extraction may be needed, depending on expertise and ability to refer. Joey was referred for bilateral coronal reduction and root canal treatment. Shortly afterwards, his owner

reported a 'new lease of life', suggesting Joey had been in considerable pain before the procedures.

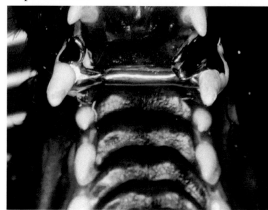

Figure A2.6b Use of an inclined plane to deviate medially displaced lower canines is often a successful technique, but usually requires referral.

REFERENCES

Berman, M., Soltero-Rivera M. & Scanlan, A. J. F. (2023) Prevalence of dental and skeletal malocclusions in mesaticephalic and dolichocephalic dogs – a retrospective study (2015–2018). *Journal of Veterinary Dentistry* **40**(2):143–153. doi: 10.1177/08987564221141826.

Niemiec, B.A. (2012) Pathology in the Pediatric Patient. In: Niemiec, B.A. (ed.) *A Colour Handbook of Small Animal Dental, Oral & Maxillofacial Disease*. Boca Raton, FL: CRC Press, pp. 102–103.

Verstraete, F. J. M. & Tsugawa, A. J. (2016) *Self-Assessment Color Review of Veterinary Dentistry*, 2nd edition. Boca Raton, FL: CRC Press, p. 17.

2.7 Tabitha, 5-mo FE DSH: flank cat spay

a) The tissue layers are as follows:
- Skin
- Subcutaneous layer with fat (it can be useful to remove a small block of fat in

many cats and there may be a small blood vessel to clamp and 'pull')
- External abdominal oblique muscle (fibres run caudoventrally)

- Internal abdominal oblique muscle (fibres run cranioventrally)
- Transverse abdominis (fibres run dorsoventrally)
- Peritoneum

The peritoneum is often penetrated upon incising the transverse abdominis muscle. Many surgeons will tent up the flank muscles individually with fine, rat-toothed forceps and make a small stab incision (using scalpel or point-of-scissor snip), which is then extended with fine Metzenbaum scissors, before moving on to the next layer. Alternatively, the muscles can be separated along the direction of their fibres using a fine forceps opening technique, rather than cut, to create an operative window that 'seals' closed afterwards.

b) Table A2.7 lists the advantages and disadvantages.

Table A2.7 **Advantages and disadvantages of the flank approach to ovariohysterectomy and ovariectomy in companion animals**

ADVANTAGES OF FLANK APPROACH	DISADVANTAGES OF FLANK APPROACH
• Wound easily visible post-operatively (can be important in feral cat projects) • Can be quick surgery once the approach is mastered and refined • Reduced likelihood of major herniation in the case of wound breakdown	• Limited surgical visibility and access; difficult to extend the wound in the case of complication during surgery (may need to convert to midline approach) • Hair may grow back darker in colourpoint breeds, e.g. Siamese, so owners must be warned • More tension applied to tissues to expose ovaries and (especially) elevate right uterine horn. See also answer to part g) below • Cuts through muscle so potentially more post-operative inflammation and associated discomfort

c) Form an equilateral triangle with the fingers of your right hand: the middle finger sits on the greater trochanter of the femur,

the index finger sits on the cranial edge of the wing of the ilium, and then the thumb adopts a position to make an equilateral triangle, and in doing so indicates the point of skin incision. (You can do a similar thing with your left hand!)

d) A useful tip is to place your plain (atraumatic) tissue forceps in between the ventral mesenteric fat (white and lacy) and the more dorsal sublumbar fat (yellowish and more solid). Frequently, you will immediately locate the left uterine horn, which is easily elevated. This relies on your skin incision being in the correct place, but even if the skin incision is slightly 'off', the junction of the two fat colours and textures is a reliable guide for locating the uterine horn and it can usually be found. The uterine horn can look a bit like intestine (or even like ureter in very small patients), so it is vital you identify the correct structure before placing any ligatures or cutting. The flank approach offers a far more limited view; therefore, it is important to identify tissues and organs accurately, and to knot carefully and securely because when you let the pedicle go you will not be able to find it again easily.

Distinguishing the uterine horn from intestine or other structure (e.g. ureter):
- The uterine horn is usually regular and tubular in shape, compared with the intestine, which is flatter and ribbon-like
- The uterine horn can be traced to an ovary cranially and the uterine body caudally (although the uterine body can sometimes be difficult to locate using the flank approach in cats)

e) Midline coeliotomy might be expected to cause less pain than flank laparotomy since abdominal entry is through the fibrous, avascular linea alba. Better exposure could also mean less tension during surgery.

However, studies have so far failed to determine if one approach is superior to the other (Merritt & Collinson 2020). Probably the most significant factors are the skill of the surgeon and their adherence to Halsted's principles (see Case 1.11). Ultimately, you should use the technique that you are most comfortable with.

f) Cats are seasonally polyoestrous (dependent on photoperiod). During a breeding season, cats will enter oestrus approximately every 3 weeks. Rescheduling a cat spay because of oestrus could inadvertently coincide with the next oestrus phase unless you are careful. Many owners will not be fully observant of their cat's behaviour and there are few physical signs of oestrus in cats, compared with dogs. This does mean that you will be likely to occasionally end up spaying a cat while she is in oestrus. However, the behavioural signs of oestrus in some cats can be so marked that it may prompt an emergency call about a cat 'going mad'.

g) This is a situation where the flank spay is disadvantageous. The uterine tissues will be haemorrhagic and friable and liable to disintegrate under minimal tension. If you have the choice, the midline approach will be easier. Sometimes you have already started flank surgery when it becomes apparent that the cat is in oestrus. The following are some tips:

- Use an especially gentle technique and be careful when using instruments on the tissues, e.g. routine clamping of a uterine horn may completely bisect it. Consider a more gentle clamping technique (e.g. using small Doyen forceps) and tying ligatures extra carefully, avoiding over-tightening, which could cause cheese-wiring of tissue.
- Extend the incision if it means less traction to elevate the uterine horn.
- Tie the uterine horns off more cranially. As long as the ovaries are completely removed, the procedure will be successful. Pulling the horn to find the uterine body could result in it coming away in your hand (this also applies to non-oestrus flank spays).

h) No, it does not have to be the left flank. Right flank is also possible, as are (though rarely indicated) bilateral flank incisions. If problems are encountered, conversion to a midline approach will always be the safest option.

REFERENCE

Merritt, B. & Collinson, A. (2020) Midline versus flank approach for spaying cats – is one less painful than the other? *Veterinary Record* **186**(17):565–567. doi: 10.1136/vr.m2008.

2.8 Gemima, 10-mo FN Springer Spaniel: spay wound burst

a) The linea alba ('white line') is the fibrous band running along the ventral midline between the paired rectus abdominis muscles. It is composed of the aponeuroses of the right and left abdominal wall muscles. The blended aponeuroses from the abdominal wall muscles form the external and internal sheaths of the rectus abdominis muscle. The rectus sheath is a reliably strong holding layer for coeliotomy closure, and muscle need not generally be included in midline coeliotomy closure. Incorporating large bites of muscle could result in post-operative pain and swelling, which might lead to self-trauma and wound breakdown. Having said this, paramedian abdominal approaches necessarily incorporate abdominal muscle, as do flank laparotomies. In the cranial two-thirds of the abdominal wall, full-thickness bites of the linea alba are used for closure. In the caudal third, only the external sheath of the rectus sheath is used (Figure A2.8). If this structure is not clearly identified and incorporated into the coeliotomy closure, dehiscence is a real possibility.

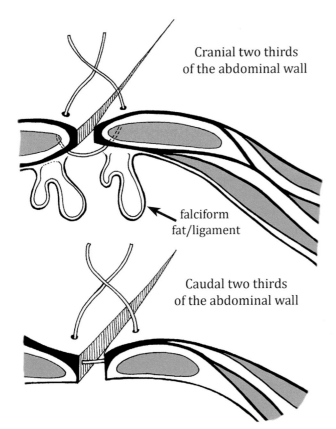

Figure A2.8 **Anatomy of coeliotomy closure using the rectus sheath. In the caudal third of a long incision, only the external leaf is used in closure.**

b) Long-lasting, synthetic, monofilament absorbable suture material should be used whenever possible. Simple interrupted and simple continuous patterns are suitable (Baines 2012, Hunt 2012, Roberts 2017). With the latter, 6–8 knot throws should be present at each end of the suture line. If you are in a situation where your preferred or most familiar suture choice is not available, simple interrupted closure will be prudent.

c) Failing to incorporate the rectus sheath can lead to dehiscence. Suturing subcutis instead of fascia will seriously compromise the closure. Correct tissue identification is important and may be difficult in obese patients. Dissection to properly expose and visualise the linea alba will help. Too much dissection and undermining can lead to increased risk of seroma, but this is less serious than dehiscence. Other risk factors for herniation or evisceration include the following (from de Rooster 2016):

- Inappropriate suture choice, poor knotting, or damaging the suture material by clamping or entanglement in instruments
- Metabolic disease (e.g. diabetes, Cushing's disease, hypoproteinaemia)

- Unrestricted activity after surgery
- Obesity
- Post-operative self-trauma

d) Gemima should be given IV fluids, broad-spectrum IV antibiotics and analgesics. She should be kept warm, anaesthetised, and prepared for surgery, avoiding the use of detergents and alcohol solutions on exposed viscera. The exposed viscera should be lavaged with warm saline (litres) outside the abdomen. The abdomen should be explored, lavaged extensively with warm saline, and any devitalised tissues resected. Lavage fluids must be removed with suction due to the large volumes necessary. The original suture remnants should all be removed. After a change of instruments, drapes, and gloves, the rectus fascia should be closed with long-lasting absorbable suture material. The rest of the closure is routine. Gemima should be hospitalised until eating and outside immediate danger of peritonitis (24–48 hours).

e) It is always challenging when unforeseen complications occur, incurring further expense for the owner. Generally, complications are charged according to individual practice policy, often taking account of specific context. In cases like Gemima's, having a sound clinical protocol for routine abdominal closure will help reassure both vets and owners that good practice has always been followed. In the unfortunate event of complication, this makes context-appropriate charging appear fair and reasonable.

REFERENCES

Baines, S. J. (2012) Suture Materials. In: Baines, S. J., Lipscomb, V. & Hutchinson, T. (eds) *BSAVA Manual of Canine and Feline Surgical Principles: A Foundation Manual*. Quedgeley: BSAVA Publications, pp. 39–47.

Hunt, G. B. (2012) Principles of Operative Technique. In: Baines, S. J., Lipscomb, V. & Hutchinson, T. (eds) *BSAVA Manual of Canine and Feline Surgical Principles: A Foundation Manual*. Quedgeley: BSAVA Publications, pp. 264–276.

de Rooster, H. (2016) Celiotomy. In: Griffon, D. & Hamaise, A. (eds) *Complications in Small Animal Surgery*. Oxford: John Wiley & Sons, pp. 355–361.

Roberts, C. (2017) Choice of suture pattern for linea alba closure. *Veterinary Evidence* **2**(3). doi: 10.18849/ve.v2i3.99.

2.9 Rikki, 4-mo ME Golden Retriever: ?stung on face

a) Bees and wasps belong to Hymenoptera, a group comprising bees (Apoidea), wasps (Vespoidea), and ants (Formicidae). Unlike wasps and ants, which can sting multiple times, bees lose their barbed stinger and venom sac in the stung tissues of the victim and die shortly thereafter (Flores & Thawley 2019). Bee venom contains a range of peptides responsible for signs. Melittin, a detergent that compromises cell membrane integrity, causes pain and acts with phospholipase A2 to lyse RBCs, platelets, WBCs, and vascular endothelial cells. Bee venom also contains mast cell degranulating factor, leading to the release of vasoactive amines such as histamine, dopamine, and noradrenaline, causing angioedema, urticaria, pruritus, and erythema at the site of envenomation (Fitzgerald & Flood 2006). The venom also contains hyaluronidase, which disrupts collagen and facilitates the spread of venom to adjacent tissues (Fitzgerald & Flood 2006). Bee stings most frequently cause local hypersensitivity reactions. Without treatment, signs may resolve within

24 hours, though there is a risk that pruritic dogs will traumatise themselves. Some dogs have regional reactions, involving erythema and oedema of an entire extremity, which may be mistaken for cellulitis. This can take 24–48 hours to develop following a bee sting (Fitzgerald & Flood 2006).

b) It is preferable, but not essential, to remove the sting. While all the contents of the venom sac have usually been delivered during the sting (Fitzgerald & Flood 2006), it can act as an irritating foreign body. Depending on the site, applying ice or cold compresses to the site of the sting can provide relief (Flores & Thawley 2019). In addition, treatment for a localised reaction to bee envenomation typically consists of an antihistamine (e.g. chlorpheniramine, 0.5 mg/kg SC, or diphenhydramine, 1–4 mg/kg PO or IM) to antagonise histamine in the venom and that released with mast cell degranulation. Steroids (e.g. dexamethasone sodium phosphate at 0.1 mg/kg IV) have historically been given for anti-inflammatory action and to stabilise cell membranes, but a study has shown that they offer no advantage over antihistamine treatment alone (Helgeson et al. 2021). Animals presenting with localised signs like these should be monitored for a short period (usually for at least 1 hour after the sting) to ensure that their signs do not progress.

c) While uncommon, bee stings can cause life-threatening anaphylaxis in dogs. In most cases, this occurs within 15–30 minutes of the dog being stung (Fitzgerald & Flood 2006). Anaphylaxis is associated with immunoglobulin E-mediated release of large amounts of chemical mediators, predominantly histamine, from mast cells and basophils (Flores & Thawley 2019). Clinically, this is characterised by cutaneous, gastrointestinal, cardiovascular, or respiratory signs (Hoehne & Hopper 2019). Cutaneous signs are similar to those mentioned previously. Gastrointestinal signs include nausea, ptyalism, vomiting, and diarrhoea (which may or may not include blood) (Flores & Thawley 2019). In the dog, histamine released from the GIT leads to sinusoidal and hepatic venous congestion, which can progress to hepatic haemorrhage and hepatocellular necrosis. This, as well as increased vascular permeability, in turn leads to distributive shock (Hoehne & Hopper 2019). This manifests in cardiovascular signs, including collapse, pallor, poor tissue perfusion (evidenced by increased CRT), and hypotension (secondary to vasodilation and increased vascular permeability). Affected dogs may be tachycardic or, rarely, bradycardic. Aggressive fluid resuscitation is required. BP of patients should be monitored to ensure that normotension is restored and maintained. The use of adrenaline as a first-line treatment for canine anaphylaxis is controversial (Hoehne & Hopper 2019). Respiratory signs are less common, and may include tachypnoea and increased respiratory effort associated with pulmonary congestion and haemorrhage, stridor due to oedema of the larynx or pharynx, and coughing due to increased mucus production and bronchoconstriction (Flores & Thawley 2019). Bronchodilators such as albuterol and terbutaline, and oxygen supplementation, may be required. In the longer term, rush venom immunotherapy has been used to prevent further severe adverse reactions in dogs with known Hymenoptera hypersensitivity (Moore et al. 2023).

REFERENCES

Fitzgerald, K. T. & Flood, A. A. (2006) Hymenoptera stings. *Clinical Techniques in Small Animal Practice* **21**(4):194–204. doi: 10.1053/j.ctsap.2006.10.002.

Flores, R. & Thawley, V. J. (2019) Hymenoptera Envenomation. In: Drobatz, K. J., Hopper, K.,

Rozanski, E. & Silverstein, D. C. (eds) *Textbook of Small Animal Emergency Medicine*. Hoboken, NJ: John Wiley & Sons, pp. 930–934.

Helgeson, M. E., Pigott, A. M. & Kierski, K. R. (2021) Retrospective review of diphenhydramine versus diphenhydramine plus glucocorticoid for treatment of uncomplicated allergic reaction in dogs. *Journal of Veterinary Emergency and Critical Care* **31**:380–386. doi: 10.1111/vec.13054.

Hoehne, S. N. & Hopper, K. (2019) Hypersensitivity and Anaphylaxis. In: Drobatz, K. J., Hopper, K., Rozanski, E. & Silverstein, D. C. (eds) *Textbook of Small Animal Emergency Medicine*. Hoboken, NJ: John Wiley & Sons, pp. 936–941.

Moore, A., Burrows, A. K., Rosenkrantz, W. S. et al. (2023) Modified rush venom immunotherapy in dogs with Hymenoptera hypersensitivity. *Veterinary Dermatology* **34**(6):532–542. doi: 10.1111/vde.13189.

2.10 Dotty, 4-yo MN DSH: dental prophy

a) Given Dotty's age, and that there were no abnormalities on the clinical examination or the history, blood work in this case is unlikely to reveal any abnormalities that are clinically significant (Alef et al. 2008). One study showed that over 90% of pre-anaesthetic blood results would not have changed the anaesthetic plan (Davies & Kawaguchi 2014). A complicating factor with cats, in particular, is that they can become very stressed with the manual handling required for blood collection, which can impact physical examination and laboratory findings (e.g. cats are prone to situational hypertension and tachycardia, and stress-associated hyperglycaemia). Agents used for sedation and chemical restraint may also impact results (Robertson et al. 2018).

b) An Ayres T-piece is the most appropriate breathing system; however, a Mini Lack could be used as an alternative.

c) Assuming a T-piece is used, the fresh gas flow is 2–3 × the minute volume.

$$\text{Minute volume (MV)} = \text{tidal volume (V}_t\text{)} \times \text{respiratory rate (RR)}$$

For dogs and cats, we usually use V_t of 10 mL/kg and RR of 20 breaths per minute; therefore:

$$\text{MV} = V_t \times \text{RR} = 10 \text{ mL/kg} \times 20 \text{ bpm}$$
$$= 200 \text{ mL/kg/min}$$

For our 4.6-kg cat that means:

$$\text{MV} = 200 \text{ mL/kg/min} \times 4.6 \text{ kg} = 920 \text{ mL/min}$$

So the fresh gas flow of 2–3 × MV is:

$$2\text{–}3 \times 920 \text{ mL/min} = 1840\text{–}2760 \text{ mL/min}$$
$$= 1.8\text{–}2.7 \text{ L/min}$$

d) Induction agents, especially when given quickly as a bolus, can cause apnoea. In most cases, this is self-limiting and will resolve spontaneously. Delivering manual breaths to the patient will only increase the time they remain apnoeic as the levels of CO_2 in the blood (the trigger to breathe) remain low. Attaching a pulse oximeter to monitor for hypoxaemia and giving 1 manual breath every 30 seconds should supply enough oxygen without suppressing the normal stimulus to breathe for too long.

REFERENCES

Alef, M., Von Praun, F. & Oechtering, G. (2008) Is routine pre-anaesthetic haematological and biochemical screening justified in dogs? *Veterinary Anaesthesia and Analgesia* **35**(2):132–140. doi: 10.1111/j.1467-2995.2007.00364.x.

Davies, M. & Kawaguchi, S. (2014) Pregeneral anaesthetic blood screening of dogs and cats attending a UK practice. *Veterinary Record* **174**(20):506. doi: 10.1136/vr.102211.

Robertson, S. A., Gogolski, S. M., Pascoe, P. et al. (2018) AAFP Feline anesthesia guidelines. *Journal of Feline Medicine and Surgery* **20**(7):602–634. doi: 10.1177/1098612X18781391.

2.11 Chuck, 17-yo MN DSH: 'gone downhill'

a) Aside from questions about Chuck's physical status (including recent appetite, water intake, toileting, vomiting, demeanour, and activity levels), it is also important to assess Chuck's QOL. For example, you might ask the following:

- Is Chuck able to enjoy his usual routine and daily activities?
- Is he experiencing any level of anxiety or distress, or changes in sleeping pattern?
- Has his personality changed?
- Is he engaging with you or is he hiding?
- Would you say Chuck is happy?

There are validated QOL scoring tools (such as *www.vetmetrica.com*) and unvalidated scoring sheets (such as 'How Will I Know? Assessing Quality of Life and Making Difficult Decisions for Your Pet' from the Ohio State University Veterinary Medical Center [*https://vmc.vet.osu.edu/sites/default/files/documents/how-will-i-know_rev_mar2024ms_0.pdf*]) that may be used to aid this discussion. Asking about how the owners are coping can also be helpful. The following are some approaches you could use:

- How are you coping with all of this?
- What are you most worried about?
- How are you getting on with giving his medications/treatments? Is it stressful?

Asking these questions of the owner allows them to discuss the burden of Chuck's care, and allows you insight into their capabilities and willingness to continue treating him.

b) We know Chuck has CKD, so it is helpful to check his blood work (CBC, urea, creatinine, electrolytes) and USG to determine his current hydration and to guide fluid therapy, if that is decided upon, or this may help the owner regarding a euthanasia decision if returned results are very bad. We need to keep an open mind as to other comorbidities – including urinary tract infection (UTI), hypertension, hyperthyroidism, heart disease, or neoplasia – that may exacerbate CKD causing an 'acute on chronic' crisis. Adjunctive tests including BP measurement, comprehensive blood work including T4, urinalysis, and thoracic radiographs may be indicated. However, Chuck is a very unwell cat, and we should be minimising handling and stress. Diagnostics should be run only if they are going to change the treatment plan.

c) Discussing ending the life of someone's companion animal is a delicate subject, but bringing QOL and euthanasia into the conversation is a professional responsibility. The owners may have drawn their own conclusions about Chuck's QOL – they will have noticed his change in routine and current decline. Your job is to help them understand the extent of Chuck's suffering. Cats are very good at hiding pain – they tend to just 'do less' and will often withdraw from the family. Start by discussing your concerns about Chuck's QOL, using relatable human terms such as exhausted, nauseated, constantly thirsty, disorientated, etc. where appropriate. State clearly that these signs are indicators of severe compromise, and compassionately express that they make you concerned about his QOL. You may use pain scoring tools (e.g. the Feline Grimace Scale for acute pain), QOL scoring tools, and your own clinical findings to support your concerns.

d) After discussing Chuck's poor QOL, it is important to present options to improve this, such as diagnostics and treatment. Highlight the limitations of such treatment to improve Chuck's condition, and invite the owners to weigh up the benefits versus costs to Chuck, as well as financial considerations and medium- and long-term prognoses. Present euthanasia as one option alongside treatment. Bringing this topic into the conversation invites owners to consider it. Make it clear that euthanasia allows us to spare animals from protracted dying and prevents further unnecessary pain and discomfort. In the past, they may have opted for you to provide fluid therapy and hospitalisation and seen marked improvement in Chuck. If you do not believe treatment other than euthanasia to be in Chuck's best interest, you need to explain this to the owners. If the owners are adamant that they are not ready to euthanase, a palliative plan can be discussed. It is important to be clear to the owners that Chuck may not pull through 'like he did last time'. Organ failure is a rollercoaster of ups and downs, but ultimately it is a downward trajectory. The owners may need a little more time or may ask for the advice of a 'senior' or favourite vet. Try not to take this personally, and support them however you can, reassuring them that you understand how difficult this decision is and inviting them to talk things through. Make sure you allow them privacy to discuss with each other without you present. If they need more time to make their decision, stress to the owners that Chuck must be kept comfortable, and send them home with a clear plan, including pain relief and treatment for nausea, assuming Chuck is fit for this.

e) To minimise any discomfort, fear, and anxiety for Chuck, whom we know finds veterinary visits stressful, sedation or even anaesthesia should be used prior to performing euthanasia. Some common agents used to sedate cats in this context are listed in Table A2.11.

Table A2.11 **Some drug combinations to sedate cats prior to euthanasia**			
DRUG	**BUTORPHANOL (10 mg/mL)**	**ACEPROMAZINE (10 mg/mL)**	**TILETAMINE/ZOLAZEPAM* (100 mg/mL)**
Bright, aggressive/anxious, or young cats (heavy sedation)	0.4 mg/kg SC	2 mg/kg SC	If deeper sedation is needed, add 6 mg/kg SC
Elderly, weak/debilitated cats (heavy sedation)	0.2 mg/kg SC	0.6 mg/kg SC	6 mg/kg SC

* To achieve anaesthesia, tiletamine/zolazepam (Figure A2.11) can be given at 6 mg/kg SC. This can be given in combination with butorphanol and acepromazine (combined in the one syringe) or administered 5–10 minutes after to avoid reaction as it can sting. Tiletamine/zolazepam combination is not available in all countries (see alternatives below).

Alternatives to tiletamine/zolazepam

You can use alfaxalone CD (2–3 mg/kg IM) to achieve anaesthesia, however this is a large volume and can cause discomfort. Alternatively, you can combine medetomidine (0.04–0.06 mg/kg), butorphanol (0.4–0.6 mg/kg), and ketamine (7 mg/kg) and administer SC for reliable deep sedation/anaesthesia. Dexmedetomidine at the appropriate dose can be substituted for medetomidine.

Once the patient is fully anaesthetised, pentobarbital can be administered via an IV or intraorgan route, including intrarenal, intrahepatic, intraperitoneal, or intracardiac. Anaesthetic depth must be checked before administering pentobarbital intraorgan to avoid pain. If the patient is not fully anaesthetised, the IV route is the only appropriate option.

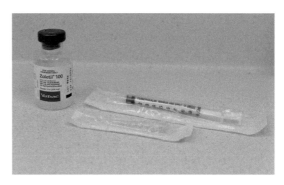

Figure A2.11 Zoletil is a ready mixture of tiletamine and zolazepam.

2.12 Busy, 4-yo MN DSH: rash on chin

a) Feline chin acne is an idiopathic condition affecting follicular keratinisation (Jazic et al. 2006). It generally causes mild signs and tends to be more noticeable in white and light-coloured cats. Sebaceous material plugs hair follicles, forming comedones and hair casts. Where it occurs, secondary infection presents as erythema, papules, pustules, draining tracts, swelling of the region, and pain in the area (Scott and Miller 2010). No single cause has been identified, though potential triggers include alterations in the hair-growth cycle, dysfunction of sebum production, immunosuppression (including that induced by stress), underlying viral diseases including feline herpesvirus and feline calicivirus, or allergies including contact dermatitis, food allergies, and atopic dermatitis (Jazic et al. 2006, Scott and Miller 2010). Poor grooming, or contact dermatitis associated with plastic food and water bowls, have also been suggested as risk factors. In Busy's case, the stress of relocating from a familiar to an unfamiliar environment, coupled with the introduction to other animals, may have triggered the development of feline acne. Alternatively, it is possible that he has had this condition for some time and the previous owners did not notice.

b) As Busy does not have visible papules, pustules, erythema, draining tracts, or other signs of bacterial infection, conservative management is appropriate. It may be useful to clean the area with an antiseptic such as chlorhexidine, and physically remove the comedones (some veterinary team members and animal carers really enjoy this process!). The caudal lesion in Figure 2.12 in the question text is a little different, characterised predominantly by scale and alopecia. Ideally, it would be helpful to rule out dermatophytosis. In addition, it is important to manage Busy's stress. Replacing plastic bowls, if used, with ceramic bowls may also help and certainly won't harm Busy.

c) It is important to rule out concurrent bacterial infection. In one study, all cats with pruritic chin acne had evidence of bacterial pyoderma, with coagulase-positive staphylococci and alpha-haemolytic streptococci the most common agents identified (Jazic et al. 2006), although *Pasteurella multocida* has also been implicated (Scott and Miller 2010). Antibiotic selection should be based on cytology at a minimum, and ideally C&S. Malassezia and dermatophytes have also been reported concurrently with feline acne (Jazic et al. 2006). There is currently insufficient evidence of differing efficacy when comparing topical versus systemic treatment of moderate to severe feline acne with secondary folliculitis and furunculosis (Jazic et al. 2006). It may be prudent to commence treatment with a topical antibacterial agent such as 2% mupirocin ointment, applied twice daily for 3 weeks, in cases where infection is diagnosed. Systemic therapy should be reserved for deep or severe bacterial infections.

REFERENCES

Jazic, E., Coyner, K. S., Loeffler, D. G. & Lewis, T. P. (2006) An evaluation of the clinical, cytological, infectious and histopathological features of feline acne. *Veterinary Dermatology* **17**(2):134–40. doi: 10.1111/j.1365-3164.2006.00507.x.

Scott, D. W. & Miller, W. H. (2010) Feline acne: a retrospective study of 74 cases (1988–2003). *Japanese Journal of Veterinary Dermatology* **16**:203–209. doi: 10.2736/jjvd.16.203.

2.13 Benji, 5-yo MN Cockerpoo: check, seen OOH

a) There are multiple puncture wounds with extensive bruising and areas of blackened skin, indicative of devascularisation and necrosis. Other areas are erythematous. The true extent of the necrosis is probably not yet evident and may result in a large area of skin sloughing from the tail base towards the ilium and down to the mid-femur level over the biceps femoris. Due to the questionable viability of this tissue, surgical management of the wound should be delayed, and the wound should be re-evaluated in another 24 hours.

b) Management of Benji's pain and preventing infection are the immediate priorities. His degree of pain can be assessed subjectively or objectively using a pain score (e.g. Glasgow Pain Score), and appropriate analgesia selected. Multimodal analgesia is appropriate. Continuation of meloxicam as the non-steroidal anti-inflammatory is warranted and the addition of an opioid (e.g. buprenorphine) and/or paracetamol can be considered.

While antibiotics are frequently administered in cases of dog-to-dog bite wounds (Kalnins et al. 2022), the decision to use antibiotics should be made carefully. Given the cause of the injury and speed of veterinary intervention (wound <6–8 hours old at initial presentation), the wound in this case is classified as contaminated, not dirty. Evidence shows a significant correlation between delayed veterinary intervention and wound infection. While C&S would ideally be performed to determine if antibiotics are needed, at this stage there is no reason to suspect infection. An alternative approach would be to administer an antibiotic of lower importance pending C&S, and adjusting treatment as required (Kalnins et al. 2022).

c) When communicating medical concepts to clients, it is essential to use appropriate language to ensure understanding and build rapport. This will vary between clients, e.g. some clients may work in healthcare settings and have a higher baseline understanding than others. Establishing the client's level of medical knowledge can be achieved by directly asking them, e.g. 'How much experience do you have with wound management?'

Once this is achieved, the response should be tailored appropriately. For clients with minimal medical understanding, formal terminology can still be used, but would need to be followed or preceded immediately by an explanation of the term. An example of how to use this approach in this case is detailed below.

'Unfortunately, when Benji was bitten, the damage caused devascularisation, which means the blood supply to the skin in this area was stopped. Without a blood supply, the cells in the skin haven't been able to get everything they need to survive, for example oxygen and nutrients, and they are dying. As the skin cells die, they turn black, like you can see here. This black, necrotic, dead skin cannot be saved and if we leave it, it will drop off, leaving a large open wound.'

d) **Step 1**
With the patient in sternal recumbency, fill the exposed edges of the wound with a sterile lubricant/gel before clipping the surgical site (Figure A2.13a). Despite the wound being classified as contaminated already, we need to minimise the potential for further contamination during preparation. Placing sterile lubricant over the exposed wounds enables clipped hair to be captured without adhering to the surgical site. Sterile lubricant should be used rather than an opened communal lubricant, in order to prevent cross-contamination. Note the edges of the wound do not need to be clipped perfectly (Figure A2.13b); this can be addressed later.

Step 2
Remove the necrotic flap of tissue by peeling back the edge and using a sterile surgical blade as necessary to free any remaining attachments (Figure A2.13c). Removal of this non-viable tissue outside theatre enables the underlying wound to be prepared appropriately for surgery and any contaminants to be moved away from the surgical field.

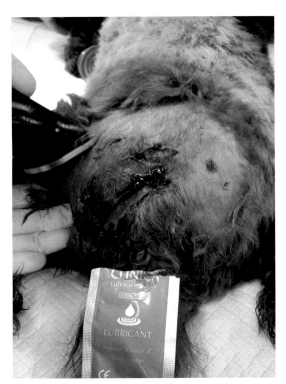

Figure A2.13a Sterile lubricant placed in wounds prior to clipping of fur.

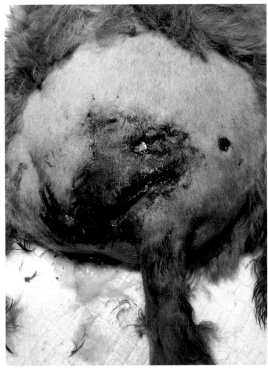

Figure A2.13b Wound clipped with an appropriate surgical perimeter for a contaminated wound.

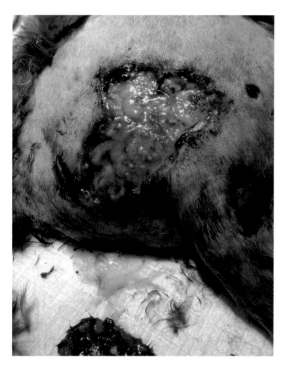

Figure A2.13c Wound after removal of necrotic tissue.

Step 3

Using a sterile surgical blade, debride any areas of contamination on the wound bed. This step should be repeated until evidence of healthy tissue with superficial bleeding is apparent (Figure A2.13d).

Effective lavage of contaminated wounds is best achieved at a pressure of 300 mmHg, which, in the absence of an accurate measuring system, can be achieved with a 35-mL syringe and 19-G needle being depressed at maximum speed. Excessive pressure (e.g. due to using smaller syringes) can drive debris deeper into the wound, thereby inhibiting the desired effect. Sterile Hartmann's is recommended as it has minimal toxic effects on healing tissues, despite having no antiseptic properties. A towel or equivalent should be placed below the wound to soak up the flush used and catch contaminants.

Preparing the surgical field outside the theatre is best practice for any surgery to minimise contamination of a 'clean room'. In this instance, aerosolised droplets would be generated during flushing that cannot be captured, in addition to gravitational run-off. Use of a towel to absorb run-off has the additional advantage of keeping the patient as dry as possible. Wet patients can have an increased risk of becoming hypothermic under anaesthesia, which has been proven to prolong recovery and wound healing post-operatively. Standard aseptic surgical solutions are toxic to healing wounds and should not be used; however, they can be made suitable by diluting in an isotonic solution, e.g. to create 0.05% chlorhexidine or 1% povidone-iodine for flushing.

e) A plan for wound closure should be made prior to anaesthetising the patient whenever possible, to ensure any necessary equipment can be gathered and to guide the surgical preparation of the patient. For example, if grafts or axial pattern flaps are to be used, then multiple areas on the patient would

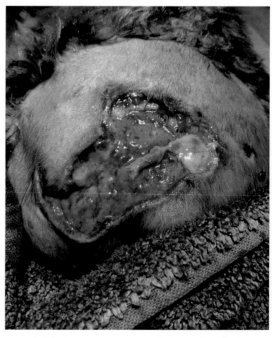

Figure A2.13d Wound after sharp debridement and lavage.

need to be prepped. In this case, the skin around the wound should be handled prior to debridement to assess which planes may allow for primary closure without creating tension at the wound edge. With any large, wide wound, there is a risk of dead space following primary closure, which could result in seroma formation. Consideration of how to manage this should be anticipated and the necessary equipment ordered and sterilised, e.g. a drain if required. While primary closure is the goal, consideration and discussion of how to manage healing by second intention is sensible in order to manage client expectations.

f) **Step 1**

After draping the surgical area, excise the edge of the entire wound to create a fresh surface free of hair and debris. The margin taken should be wide enough to ensure healthy clean edges, but narrow enough to minimise impact on wound closure. Debride the surface of the entire wound until micro-bleeding is evident (see Figure A2.13e). Both actions aid healing. Presence of micro-bleeding demonstrates adequate blood supply, essential to the survival of cells, and promotes chemotaxis, which attracts leukocytes to aid the healing process and fight any potential infection. Fresh edges promote faster healing where direct tissue apposition is achieved and healing by primary intention can occur.

Step 2

Evaluate which areas of the wound can be closed with primary intention without creating wound tension. Close these areas using a suitable suture material and pattern. In this case, a 2/0 (3 metric), absorbable, monofilament (e.g. poliglecaprone 25) and intradermal pattern were used to achieve primary closure of the dorsal and lateral aspects of the wound (Figure A2.13f). The smallest suture possible that ensures adequate mechanical resistance is advised in all surgical circumstances. For canine skin, 4/0–2/0 USP (1.5–3.0 metric) is recommended.

The choice of suture pattern is determined by surgeon preference. In this case, intradermal sutures were used. Bear in mind the need to avoid excess suture material in healing wounds.

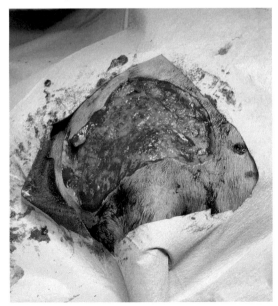

Figure A2.13e Wound with fresh edges and micro-bleeding after excision and debridement.

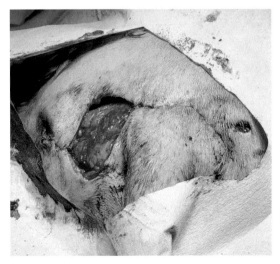

Figure A2.13f Partial wound closure with an intradermal suture pattern.

Step 3

Primary closure of the central aspect of the wound cannot be achieved without creating tension. Tension-relieving sutures such as horizontal or vertical mattress patterns can be used to 'walk' the skin edges as close together as possible while minimising dead space (Figure A2.13g). In this case, interrupted horizontal mattress sutures were placed to balance the need to prevent tension while minimising the wound surface area for healing by second intention. Tension-relieving sutures should ideally be placed at least 0.5 cm from the edge of a wound to avoid being pulled through the delicate/damaged tissue edges. Dead space was not considered to be a concern and no surgical drain was needed in this case. To achieve primary closure of this wound, an alternative option would have been to make tension releasing incisions over the left dorso-lateral pelvis region. However, when this was discussed with the client pre-operatively, it was decided to manage the wound by second intention.

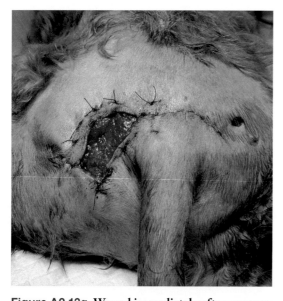

Figure A2.13g Wound immediately after surgery, demonstrating a mixed closure approach.

Step 4

Post-operative management of the wound will involve the use of dressings to balance moisture and promote epithelialisation. A highly absorbent dressing is indicated to begin with; this should be changed to a foam dressing as exudate declines and epithelialisation commences. A hydrogel sheet (with or without Manuka honey) can be used to balance the wound moisture and prevent the dressing sticking to the wound. This is essential during epithelialisation as the cells are fragile and easily damaged, delaying wound healing. Frequency of dressing changes is variable and in the early stages will depend on the degree of exudate production. Aiming to review the wound every 2–5 days is sensible and can be adjusted as appropriate, depending on progress and occurrence of any complications. When clients become familiar with the process, it is also possible and often practical to train them to perform dressing changes and send photograph updates. In areas where it is awkward to apply conventional dressings, suture loops can be placed to allow a tie-over dressing to be applied.

In addition to dressings, the patient should also be monitored for pain, and analgesia prescribed as needed. If there is a concern of wound interference, then measures such as an Elizabethan collar or pet bodysuit would be appropriate, depending on wound location and preference of pet and client.

REFERENCES

Balsa, I. M. & Culp, W. T. N (2015) Wound care. *Veterinary Clinics of North America: Small Animal Practice* **45**(5):1049–1065. doi: 10.1016/j.cvsm.2015.04.009.

Findji, L. & Dupré, G. (2005) *Handbook of Ligatures and Sutures in Veterinary Surgery*. Lure: Vetóquinol.

Kalnins, N. J., Gibson, J. S., Stewart, A. J. et al. (2022) Antimicrobials in dog-to-dog bite wounds: a retrospective study of 1526 dog bite events (1999–2019). *Journal of Veterinary Internal Medicine* **36**(6):2028–2041. doi: 10.1111/jvim.16574.

2.14 Henry, 6-yo MN CKCS: dental, *murmur*

a) The stages of MMVD are outlined in Table A2.14.

Table A2.14 Staging system for MMVD (adapted from Keene et al. 2019)

STAGE	A	B1	B2	C	D
Characteristics	Dogs at high risk of developing heart disease with no currently identifiable cardiac structural disorder, e.g. at-risk breeds such as Cavalier King Charles Spaniel without a murmur	Asymptomatic dogs with a murmur, but with no radiographic or echocardiographic evidence of remodelling of the heart; these dogs have never developed clinical heart failure	Asymptomatic dogs with a murmur, with radiographic and echocardiographic evidence of remodelling of the heart; these dogs have never developed clinical heart failure	Dogs with current or previous clinical heart failure caused by MMVD	Dogs with refractory MMVD where clinical heart failure is refractory to treatment
Key recommendations (note: please refer to guidelines for comprehensive recommendations)	No treatment recommended; avoid breeding from dogs if a murmur is identified	Thoracic radiography, echocardiography, BP measurement; no treatment recommended but repeat echo in 6–12 months (more often in larger dogs)	Pimobendan ± angiotensin-converting enzyme (ACE) inhibitor and mild dietary sodium restriction; frequency of monitoring depends on clinical progression	Varies with acute versus chronic; for chronic, pimobendan + furosemide + ACE inhibitor ± spironolactone with monitoring of renal parameters; frequency of monitoring depends on clinical progression	See guidelines (Keene et al. 2019)

b) Clinically, Henry's heart disease appears stable. Cardiologist recommendations would generally be to re-evaluate B2 MMVD with echocardiography, radiography, and BP measurement every 4–6 months; therefore, this may be an opportunity to re-evaluate Henry's heart disease if the owner is amenable to cardiology referral (Pinkos & Stauthammer 2021). Otherwise, informed consent could be obtained after suitable discussion of the nature of Henry's heart problems and the clinical need for anaesthesia and dentistry. Although routine pre-anaesthetic blood testing is not generally indicated in healthy non-geriatric animals, Henry's cardiovascular disease may predispose him to other organ damage (e.g. kidney); therefore, biochemistry and/or urinalysis could be considered (Ferreira 2020).

c) Pimobendan can be administered on the day of anaesthesia; however, ACE inhibitors (and angiotensin receptor antagonists) may predispose to difficult-to-manage hypotension. It has been recommended that they are discontinued 24 hours prior to anaesthesia (Congdon 2022).

d) Regurgitation of blood through the incompetent mitral valve limits cardiac output, which is generally compensated for by an increase in heart rate. Drugs associated with significant heart rate reductions may therefore limit cardiac output. In addition, increasing afterload (vasoconstriction) will cause an increased regurgitant fraction. For these reasons, alpha-2 adrenoceptor agonists are generally avoided, being associated with both vasoconstriction and bradycardia. Induction of general anaesthesia with slow administration of propofol or alfaxalone (both associated with vasodilation) or ketamine/midazolam is generally well tolerated. Volatile anaesthetics are associated with vasodilation and negative inotropy may be associated with hypotension, so use of anaesthetic-sparing drugs, including opioids and local anaesthetics, to minimise doses of maintenance volatile agents is recommended. Positive pressure ventilation, by its effect of reducing preload, may decrease stroke volume and further limit cardiac output (Yartsev 2023). In Henry's case, a suitable approach would be premedication with an opioid followed by midazolam (0.2–0.3 mg/kg IV) as a co-induction agent, administered once the patient is lightly anaesthetised from the slow administration of propofol IV. Note that administration of midazolam prior to the induction agent has been shown to increase the dose of induction agent required to achieve full anaesthesia (Sánchez et al. 2013, Zapata et al. 2018).

e) Opioids are likely to form the mainstay of background analgesia. Pure μ agonists such as methadone could be supplemented with potent agonists such as fentanyl administered by infusion intraoperatively, although this may be associated with hypoventilation and require ventilatory support, and so may be less practicable in general practice. Local anaesthetic techniques can provide intraoperative and early post-operative analgesia; however, bilateral mandibular block is not recommended due to loss of sensation of the tongue, which can result in self-trauma (bilateral maxillary or infra-orbital block is generally well tolerated). Caution is warranted with the administration of NSAIDs in dogs with heart disease; hypotension, through a combination of vasodilatory anaesthetic drugs and limited capability to increase cardiac output, may predispose the patient to renal injury if prostaglandin E2 and I2 production is inhibited by NSAIDs. Prescription of NSAIDs post-anaesthetic recovery could be considered on a risk/benefit basis. Paracetamol could be considered in dogs, as it appears less associated with prostaglandin inhibition and may pose less risk of nephrotoxicity. Ketamine could be considered as an analgesic/anti-hyperalgesic, in addition to its potential use as an anaesthetic induction agent.

f) The considerations outlined in answer d) still apply; however, profound chemical restraint of the patient may be necessary to protect the health and safety of veterinary staff, and to reduce arousal and negative emotional states in patients. Alfaxalone

(4 mg/kg) administered IM (unlicensed in dogs) can provide useful sedation with limited cardiovascular effects in healthy dogs, but large volumes need to be injected (Cruz-Benedetti et al. 2018), which may be challenging. Lower doses of alfaxalone (2 mg/kg) combined with an opioid (e.g. methadone, 0.2 mg/kg), ketamine (3–5 mg/kg), and preservative-free midazolam (0.3 mg/kg) can achieve profound sedation in agitated patients; however, studies evaluating cardiovascular effects associated with this combination in dogs have not been published. For clinical, welfare, and health and safety reasons, sedation is always preferable to struggling with a patient.

REFERENCES

Congdon, J. (2022) Cardiovascular Disease. In: Johnson, R. A., Snyder, L. B. C. & Schroeder, C. A. (eds) *Canine and Feline Anesthesia and Co-Existing Disease*, 2nd edition. New York: John Wiley & Sons. doi: 10.1002/9781118834305.ch1.

Cruz-Benedetti, I. C., Bublot, I., Ribas, T. et al. (2018) Pharmacokinetics of intramuscular alfaxalone and its echocardiographic, cardiopulmonary and sedative effects in healthy dogs. *PLoS One* 13:e0204553. doi: 10.1371/journal.pone.0204553.

Ferreira, J. (2020) Preanaesthetic screening in dogs and cats. *In Practice* 42(4):197–207. doi: 10.1136/inp.m1448.

Keene, B. W., Atkins, C. E., Bonagura, J. D. et al. (2019) ACVIM consensus guidelines for the diagnosis and treatment of myxomatous mitral valve disease in dogs. *Journal of Veterinary Internal Medicine* 33(3):1127–1140. doi: 10.1111/jvim.15488.

Pinkos, A. & Stauthammer, C. (2021) Degenerative valve disease: classification, diagnosis, and treatment of mitral regurgitation. *Today's Veterinary Practice*. September/October 2021. Available at: https://todaysveterinarypractice.com/cardiology/degenerative-valve-disease-classification-diagnosis-and-treatment-of-mitral-regurgitation/.

Sánchez, A., Belda, E., Escobar, M. et al. (2013) Effects of altering the sequence of midazolam and propofol during co-induction of anaesthesia. *Veterinary Anaesthesia and Analgesia* 40(4):359–366. doi: 10.1111/vaa.12038.

Yartsev, A. (2023) 'Effects of positive pressure ventilation on cardiovascular physiology'. Deranged Physiology. Available at: https://derangedphysiology.com/main/cicm-primary-exam/required-reading/respiratory-system/Chapter%20523/effects-positive-pressure-ventilation-cardiovascular-physiology.

Zapata, A., Laredo, F. G., Escobar, M. et al. (2018) Effects of midazolam before or after alfaxalone for co-induction of anaesthesia in healthy dogs. *Veterinary Anaesthesia and Analgesia* 45(5):609–617. doi: 10.1016/j.vaa.2018.04.002.

2.15 Smithers, 13-yo MN DSH: recheck throat

a) In the region of the right palatoglossal arch in the caudal oral cavity/fauces area, there is a swollen and slightly erythematous mass. It does not seem to be associated with the caudal teeth.

b) Inflammatory lesion, neoplasia, dental-associated lesion, foreign body, or trauma would be some of the most likely diagnoses here. The most common inflammatory diseases of the feline oral cavity are feline chronic gingivostomatitis, followed by eosinophilic granuloma complex (EGC) (Falcão et al. 2020). Neoplastic disease can be characterised as odontogenic (arising from structures associated with dentition) or non-odontogenic. The latter are more common in cats, with the majority of these comprising SCC (60–80% of feline oral tumours) or fibrosarcoma (up to 20% of feline oral tumours). The most common odontogenic tumours in cats are peripheral odontogenic fibromas (Falcão et al. 2020). Because SCC and EGC can be clinically indistinguishable, but treatment is different, cytology or, ideally, histopathology is required to differentiate them.

c) Smithers appears recovered but does have a history of weight loss, which should be monitored. While it is true that older cats tend to lose body mass, if weight loss continues, it may indicate concurrent or underlying disease, including neoplasia. It is possible that Smithers had an inflammatory lesion that has completely resolved, or else the treatment given is working in a palliative fashion and reducing the symptoms. The fact that Smithers's teeth look okay suggests that it is not an odontogenic tumour or dental lesion. His mandibular lymph nodes are not enlarged. Options for treatment would be as follows:

- Do nothing but alert the owner for return of symptoms and monitor Smithers's weight. This could be done at home using Smithers's carrier and bathroom scales.
- Repeat the previous treatment, as per the owner's request. This assumes a palliative effect when there may be none needed (i.e. the problem has indeed resolved), but is inconsistent with principles of antimicrobial stewardship.
- Modify the previous treatment, e.g. do not repeat the antibiotics but put Smithers on a tapering oral dose of prednisolone and observe. This is assuming some palliative anti-inflammatory effect. If Smithers cannot be dosed orally, another long-acting steroid injection at reduced dose before stopping is a possibility.

Which option is chosen should be informed by discussion, but note that repeating an antibiotic such as a long-acting cephalosporin is contrary to good prescribing practice. Giving steroids unnecessarily could compromise Smithers's immune system. The owner should certainly be informed of the possibility of a developing malignant lesion (e.g. tonsillar carcinoma), but that a period of 'watchful waiting' is acceptable given the aforementioned constraints, as long as Smithers appears comfortable. Palliative anti-inflammatories could then be restarted on an ongoing basis, if needed. The main thing in cases like these is to ensure that the owner is fully informed about the potential risks of an approach that does not allow a second view of the lesion to monitor it. Such discussions should be recorded in the clinical notes. Assuming no major deterioration, rechecks initially at 1-2 weeks and then monthly would seem appropriate here.

d) It should not be necessary to ask the owner to sign a release form that states that they are 'going against veterinary advice' since the options listed above comprise professional veterinary advice, informed by the context (owners' economic constraints). The plan should be recorded in the clinical record as a contemporaneous note. This is a good example of contextualised care.

REFERENCE

Falcão, F., Faísca, P., Viegas, I. et al. (2020) Feline oral cavity lesions diagnosed by histopathology: a 6-year retrospective study in Portugal. *Journal of Feline Medicine and Surgery* **22**(10):977–983. doi: 10.1177/1098612X19900033.

2.16 Maggie, 6-yo FN Doberman Pinscher: freq urination

a) The signalment, history, and presentation are sufficient to presumptively diagnose cystitis with a probable bacterial component. C&S testing on a cystocentesis sample remains the gold standard in confirming a UTI. If cystocentesis is not feasible at this point, it may be preferable to omit C&S. The voided sample is certainly adequate for urinalysis (dipstick, USG, and cytological examination of the sediment), which is recommended by the International Society for Companion Animal Infectious Diseases (ISCAID) in all cases to provide supporting evidence and detect potential comorbidities (e.g. as inidicated by glucosuria, crystalluria) (Weese et al. 2019).

b) While veterinarians have historically tended to select broad-spectrum, medium-importance amoxycillin–clavulanate for cystitis, the Australian (University of Melbourne) guidelines (University of Melbourne 2019) and international (ISCAID) guidelines (Weese et al. 2019) suggest low-importance amoxycillin or a trimethoprim sulfonamide (TMS) for empirical treatment (Weese et al. 2019). Furthermore, an analysis of C&S results from more than 6000 Australian dog and cat urinary isolates showed that selecting the drug based on bacterial morphology improves expected success. Rods should be treated with TMS (15 mg/kg q12h); cocci with amoxycillin (11–15 mg/kg q8–12h). If a mixture of rods and cocci are seen, or cytology is not possible, use TMS.

c) Unless contraindicated, always prescribe NSAIDs to reduce discomfort. Although evidence in animals is not available, in some human trials, cyclooxygenase (COX)-2 inhibitors alone have been found to be as effective as antimicrobials for resolving uncomplicated cystitis. Encouraging high fluid consumption, e.g. offering unsalted meat broth, would also be expected to assist clearance of bacteria from the bladder. The vulval inflammation should clear with resolution of the infection and administration of NSAIDs, but the owner should be instructed to clean the area. Topical cortisone cream applied to the vulva to reduce inflammation could be added if appropriate.

d) Recommended antimicrobial treatment duration is 3–5 days only. This might be shorter than you are used to; there is increasing evidence in human and animal trials that shorter durations of antimicrobial therapy often work just as well as longer durations. Remember that the goal of antimicrobial therapy is to temporarily suppress bacterial growth so that the animal's immune system can clear the infection. In immunocompetent dogs, 3 days is likely to be sufficient. For immunocompromised dogs, treating for 5 days is preferable. It is wise to forewarn the owner that, in the unlikely event that this empirical treatment is not successful, you will need to collect a cystocentesis sample for laboratory testing.

Note: if significant clinical improvement is not seen within 48 hours of commencing TMS or amoxycillin, the treatment is unlikely to be effective. The antimicrobial should be discontinued (while pain relief continues) and a cystocentesis sample collected for C&S. If available, perform ultrasonography-guided cystocentesis so that you can simultaneously assess the bladder for uroliths or masses. If the urine sample cannot be processed immediately, refrigerate and ensure culture begins within 24 hours of collection. Continue pain relief while awaiting C&S results. Then select an antimicrobial with the lowest importance rating to which the bacteria are susceptible. Check the traffic-light poster for dog and cat antimicrobials on the University of Melbourne Australian Veterinary Prescribing Guidelines website if you are unsure of the importance ratings (University of Melbourne 2020).

e) Using the shortest effective duration reduces adverse effects, dysbiosis, and antimicrobial resistance, and also makes it easier and cheaper for the client. Using TMS for only 3–5 days greatly reduces – and might effectively eliminate – the risk of serious adverse effects, including dry eye and hepatopathy, even in breeds at reportedly higher risk, such as the Doberman Pinscher. (All serious adverse effects reported in the veterinary literature have been in animals given TMS for >7 days.)

f) The infection is resolved when clinical signs have resolved. Repeat urinalysis or C&S is not required in the absence of clinical signs. The presence of bacteria does not equal infection and subclinical bacteriuria does not require treatment with antimicrobials.

g) An additional episode of cystitis within 1 month strongly suggests an underlying problem. Common underlying problems include uroliths, bladder wall masses, reduced immunity due to endocrinopathy such as diabetes mellitus, or anatomical abnormalities that increase the chance of faecal or skin bacteria entering the bladder,

such as a recessed vulva. Dogs with urethral sphincter mechanism incompetence (USMI) may experience recurrent UTI due to ascending infections. After performing a complete physical examination, repeat urinalysis and perform ultrasonography-guided cystocentesis. Send urine for C&S. While awaiting the results, provide analgesia such as NSAIDs and encourage increased fluid consumption. Investigations for underlying conditions include imaging of the urinary tract and blood work.

REFERENCES

University of Melbourne (2019) *Australian Veterinary Prescribing Guidelines – Resources*. Melbourne, VIC: University of Melbourne. Available at: https://vetantibiotics.science. unimelb.edu.au/about/resources/.

University of Melbourne (2020) *Australian Veterinary Prescribing Guidelines – Dog and Cat Antimicrobial Traffic Light Card, Version 2*. Melbourne, VIC: University of Melbourne. Available at: https:// drive.google.com/file/d/1tpgHtE7-W8TFhBHwS9QMtUgeZvZlc98s/view.

Weese, J. S., Blondeav, J., Boothe, D. et al. (2019) International Society for Companion Animal Infectious Diseases (ISCAID) guidelines for the diagnosis and management of bacterial urinary tract infections in dogs and cats. *Veterinary Journal* 247:8–25. doi: 10.1016/j. tvjl.2019.02.008.

2.17 Spaghetti, 9-mo ME rat: bleeding nose & eyes

a) Chromodacryorrhoea (porphyrin-pigmented tears) are usually seen as a response to stress or underlying disease. Porphyrin will fluoresce under a Wood's lamp, so can be differentiated from blood.

b) This condition most likely indicates underlying respiratory disease and is the most common presenting complaint in

rats. It is often caused by an infectious agent (*Mycoplasma pulmonis* being the most common, but also *Streptococcus pneumoniae* and *Corynebacterium kutscheri*) and concurrent infections with other respiratory pathogens. Coinfection with Sendai virus, mice pneumonia virus, *Pneumocystis carinii*, and *Haemophilus* species can all increase the severity of disease. Rat respiratory disease is a multifactorial syndrome of chronic respiratory disease combined with bacterial pneumonia. The disease usually causes bronchitis and secondary infection due to inflammation and damage to the respiratory epithelium. Respiratory disease can be exacerbated by environmental, husbandry, or nutritional factors. Rats with chronic respiratory disease can have a good QOL and may live to their full lifespan with the disease (2–3 years) as long as they are well managed.

c) Possible diagnostic tests include cytology of nasal discharge. The presence of Gram-positive diplococci facilitates a tentative diagnosis of *S. pneumoniae*. A respiratory pathogen panel, plus C&S, can be performed on respiratory secretions. Thoracic radiography necessitates general anaesthesia for diagnostic-quality images due to a high movement artefact in conscious rats, but rats are difficult to intubate and those with respiratory disease are at increased risk of anaesthetic complications, including death. Radiographic findings may not reflect the severity of disease. While CT is more accurate, this also requires anaesthesia and is not routinely available in general practice. Empirical treatment is not unreasonable.

d) The mainstays of treatment are husbandry changes, antibiotics, and anti-inflammatories. Patients with mild clinical signs will often improve with husbandry changes and anti-inflammatories. Ideally a C&S test would be performed and appropriate antibiotics would be used. If a culture is not possible, first-line antibiotic treatment usually consists of doxycycline (5–10 mg/kg PO q12h for 28 days), which is the treatment of choice for the most common pathogen *M. pulmonis*. In the case of severe infection, enrofloxacin (5–20 mg/kg PO q12h) may be administered concurrently. The treatment of choice for *S. pneumoniae* is amoxycillin–clavulanic acid (20 mg/kg PO q12h). Meloxicam may be administered at a dose of 1–2 mg/kg PO q12–24h. In more severe cases, a mucolytic such as bromhexine (0.5 mg/kg PO q12–24h) may be administered. Rats can be nebulised with saline, hypertonic saline, diluted F10, or diluted bromhexine for periods of 15 minutes every 12 hours. Bronchodilators such as theophylline (10–20 mg/kg PO q8-12h) can be administered.

e) Given that rat respiratory disease tends to be chronic and is a result of multifactorial causes, good husbandry is crucial in managing the disease. Mycoplasma multiplies more rapidly where environmental ammonia levels are higher (50–100 ppm). Ensure that Spaghetti's cage is appropriately large, well ventilated, easy to clean, and spot cleaned daily. It should be completely cleaned once per week using an agent such as F10. As a general rule, if you can smell anything other than fresh bedding, the cage needs to be cleaned. The substrate should generate minimal dust, e.g. recycled paper kitty litter, paper-based bedding and fabric pieces (must be laundered frequently). Avoid sawdust/wood shavings as these produce a lot of dust, which can irritate airways. Bedding should be easily washable, e.g. cloth hammocks, or easily disposable, e.g. clean cardboard boxes. Rats should be offered a diet of good-quality rat pellets in restricted portions, fresh vegetables or salad daily, with small amounts of fruit, invertebrates, and seeds as treats. They require mental stimulation and benefit from a complex environment incorporating hides, tunnels, toys, a nesting area, and opportunities outside their enclosure interacting with people. Rat enclosures should also be away from predatory pets (such as cats and dogs) to minimise stress levels, which may flare up respiratory disease.

REFERENCES

Carpenter, J. W. & Marion, C. J. (2018) *Exotic Animal Formulary*, 5th edition. Philadelphia, PA: W.B. Saunders.

Quesenberry, K. E., Orcutt, C. J., Mans, C. & Carpenter, J. W. (2021) *Ferrets, Rabbits and Rodents: Clinical Medicine and Surgery*. St Louis, MO: Elsevier.

2.18 Pat, 7-yo MN Shetland Sheepdog: licking bottom ++

a) Externally, you can evaluate perianal masses and the perianal skin. You can assess anal tone and perineal reflex. To test the latter, you can lightly tap the perineum with a thermometer or similar on both the right and the left sides. This should stimulate contraction of the anal sphincter and flexion of the tail, if present. Weakness or absence of this reflex occurs with lesions impacting the pudendal nerve or spine at S1–3. Laterally, there may be masses associated with the anal sacs (located at approximately 4 and 8 o'clock). These may be neoplastic, inflammatory, or granulomatous. Within the rectum, you can assess the presence, texture, and consistency of stool, and intraluminal masses in the terminal rectum. You may be able to palpate urethral masses or uroliths in the pelvic urethra through the ventral rectal wall. Depending on the patient size, you may be able to palpate the prostate and evaluate its size and symmetry. The normal prostate should be symmetrical, with a median sulcus, and should not be painful on palpation. It can help to palpate the abdomen simultaneously with your free hand, and gently direct the prostate caudally. Dorsally, you may be able to palpate enlarged sublumbar lymph nodes or elicit the presence of lumbosacral pain. Relative to the anus, the sacral lymph nodes are positioned orally, at approximately 11 and 1 o'clock. Sedation or anaesthesia may be required to perform a complete (360°) rectal examination, as this can cause discomfort to the dog (and the veterinarian, if the dog is moving or tense).

b) Non-neoplastic anal gland disease is classified as impaction (characterised by full, sometimes difficult to express anal glands), anal sacculitis (characterised by inflammation of the anal sac, with or without infection), or anal sac abscessation (characterised by infection of the anal sac walls, local cellulitis, and, ultimately, draining tracts) (Lundberg et al. 2022). It can be difficult to differentiate the last two. Other possibilities include neoplastic disease (perianal adenoma or adenocarcinoma, or other cutaneous neoplasia such as SCC, malignant melanoma, mast cell tumour, or haemangiosarcoma) and perianal fistula. Rectal or abdominal palpation may reveal sublumbar lymphadenomegaly in dogs with anal sac adenocarcinomas. Given the acute onset, the nature of the mass, and the absence of other findings on physical examination, anal sac abscessation is most likely with Pat.

c) Risk factors associated with non-neoplastic anal sac disease include diarrhoea, dietary change, obesity, skin disease (particularly atopic dermatitis), and breed, with Labradors, German Shepherds, and small-breed dogs at increased risk (Corbee et al. 2021).

d) The mainstays of treatment for anal sac abscessation are drainage, antibiotic treatment, and analgesia. Sedation may be required to facilitate expression of an abscessed anal gland. This can also facilitate gentle flushing of the affected anal sac using a tom cat catheter and saline, and instillation of a topical antibiotic

(Lundberg et al. 2022). Local treatment has been argued to be better antimicrobial stewardship (Lundberg et al. 2022), but the need for sedation may increase the costs to owners. Alternatively, systemic antibiotics may be administered. Selection of analgesia should be based on an assessment of the patient, and may include NSAIDs. It is also critical to treat concurrent skin disease. In many cases, increasing the fibre content of the diet may reduce the risk of future anal sac impaction. Because anal sac abscessation tends to be a clinical diagnosis, it is critical to repeat the anal and rectal examination around 1 week later to check that the mass is reduced in size or resolved, and to express anal residual material in the gland (if required).

e) The problem may not resolve if the infection is associated with antibiotic-resistant organisms or neoplastic disease. Most anal sac tumours are malignant. A detailed history and complete physical examination should be repeated. Dogs with neoplastic anal sac disease may have other signs, including tenesmus, abnormally shaped stool, urinary incontinence, stranguria, bleeding from the rectum or anus, reduced appetite, weakness, or weight loss. In addition, affected dogs may have PU/PD due to hypercalcaemia of malignancy, which is reported to occur in 27–53% of dogs with anal sac adenocarcinoma (Repasy et al. 2022). This occurs due to the release of parathyroid-related protein from the tumour, leading to hypercalcaemia, which inhibits antidiuretic hormone. In cases not resolving as expected, a complete 360° rectal examination should be performed (with sedation if required). If, based on history and thorough physical examination, infection is still the leading differential, it is important to collect material from the anal sacs for C&S to guide ongoing antimicrobial therapy. If treated locally, the anal sacs may need to be flushed multiple times before infection resolves.

If there are signs of systemic illness, a CBC, serum biochemistry profile, and ionised calcium should be performed. If neoplasia is suspected, abdominal and thoracic radiography are recommended to screen for metastatic disease. Perianal masses should be aspirated using a fine needle (22–25 G) through the skin, which can aid cytological diagnosis.

REFERENCES

Corbee, R. J., Woldring, H. H., Van den Eijnde, L. M. & Wouters, E. G. H. (2021) A cross-sectional study on canine and feline anal sac disease. *Animals (Basel)* **12**(1). doi: 10.3390/ani12010095.

Lundberg, A., Koch, S. N. & Torres, S. M. F. (2022) Local treatment for canine anal sacculitis: a retrospective study of 33 dogs. *Veterinary Dermatology* **33**(5):426–434. doi: 10.1111/vde.13102.

Repasy, A. B., Selmic, L. E. & Kisseberth, W. C. (2022) Canine apocrine gland anal sac adenocarcinoma: a review. *Topics in Companion Animal Medicine* **50**:100682. doi: 10.1016/j.tcam.2022.100682.

2.19 Spot, 5-yo FN Lagotto: ate fishing line

a) A single lateral radiograph incorporating the oesophagus and stomach may be adequate in an emergency when screening for a recently ingested metallic foreign body, but this dog has ingested at least one non-metallic foreign body (fishing line) and potentially others, such as plastic lures, which may be revealed in high-quality radiographs. As thoracic and abdominal radiography in the dog require different exposures, it would be ideal to perform at least a single thoracic view to visualise the oesophagus, and both a lateral and VD view of the abdomen to visualise and help localise the foreign body in the stomach. Heavier sedation or general anaesthesia can minimise movement artefact.

b) Potential approaches for managing the foreign body/bodies are outlined in Table A2.19.

Table A2.19 **Potential approaches for managing gastric foreign bodies (adapted from Zersen et al. 2020)**

APPROACH	POTENTIAL ADVANTAGES	POTENTIAL COMPLICATIONS
Monitor until foreign body is passed	• Inexpensive if foreign body is passed • Can repeat radiography to determine whether foreign body is passing/has passed	• Contraindicated with sharp objects due to risk of perforation of the GIT, or pain as the material progresses through the GIT (Figure A2.19a,b) • Risk of intestinal plication and perforation with a linear foreign body if anchored under the tongue, the pylorus, or via the hook in Spot's case; this may require surgery to resolve
Induce emesis	• Relatively inexpensive • Does not require anaesthesia or surgery • No risk of surgical-site dehiscence	• Contraindicated with sedated patients (will need to reverse sedation prior to administering) • Contraindicated if ingested foreign body is sharp, as may lead to tissue perforation (e.g. in oesophagus) • Plication if the linear foreign body is anchored • Incomplete elimination of foreign body via emesis may necessitate endoscopic or surgical intervention (thoracotomy or laparotomy) • Aspiration of gastric contents or foreign body • Aspiration pneumonia • Vasovagal response • Oesophagitis • Where apomorphine is used, emesis may not be induced initially in up to one-fifth of cases (Fischer et al. 2021), necessitating a follow-up dose • Potential adverse effects of apomorphine include sedation, respiratory depression, hypotension, tachyarrythmias, and protracted vomiting (Fischer et al. 2021)
Endoscopy	• No risk of surgical-site dehiscence if foreign body retrieved endoscopically • Can convert to gastrotomy if foreign body cannot be removed	• Cost • Requires general anaesthesia and attendant risks • May be difficult to locate and retrieve the foreign body with a full stomach (may require extended anaesthetic time) • Perforation of stomach or oesphagus and associated structures with sharp foreign body, e.g. fish hook • Regurgitation and aspiration or stricture formation • Pneumothorax • Pleural effusion • Respiratory arrest
Gastrotomy	• In Spot's case, can retrieve hook and line and any other foreign bodies • Higher success rate than inducing emesis, allows direct visualisation of foreign body, and facilitates cutting of hook in Spot's case	• Cost • Requires general anaesthesia and associated risks • Post-operative morbidity (pyrexia, anorexia, vomiting, surgical-site infection, development of seroma, wound dehiscence) • Aspiration pneumonia

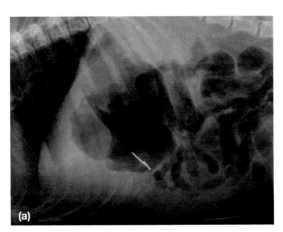
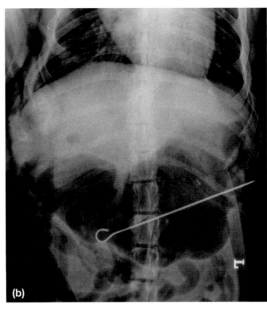

Figure A2.19a,b Lateral (a) and VD (b) abdominal radiographs of a canine patient with a sharp, metallic foreign body in the stomach. Induction of emesis would be contraindicated due to a high likelihood of gastric or oesophageal perforation. The benefit of taking two views is reinforced when these images are compared.

REFERENCES

Fischer, C., Drobatz, K. J., & Thawley, V. J. (2021) Evaluation of subcutaneous versus intravenous administration of apomorphine for induction of emesis in dogs. *Journal of the American Veterinary Medical Association* **259**:283–287. doi: 10.2460/javma.259.3.283.

Peterson, M. E. (2013) Toxicologic Decontamination. In: Peterson, M. E. & Talcott, P. A. (eds) *Small Animal Toxicology*, 3rd edition. Saint Louis, MO; W.B. Saunders, pp. 73–83. doi: 10.1016/B978-1-4557-0717-1.00010-7.

Zersen, K. M., Peterson, N. & Bergman, P. J. (2020) Retrospective evaluation of the induction of emesis with apomorphine as treatment for gastric foreign bodies in dogs (2010–2014): 61 cases. *Journal of Veterinary Emergency and Critical Care* **30**:209–212. doi: 10.1111/vec.12942.

2.20 Confidential meeting with T

PART 1

a) The GIBOR outlines 12 fundamental rights of trans and gender-diverse people in veterinary workplaces. These 12 fundamental rights can be broken down into three broad categories.

Rights of affirmation
- Right to identity
- Right to names
- Right to pronouns

Rights of self-determination
- Right to privacy
- Freedom of gender expression
- Freedom from gender affirmation timelines

Rights of protection
- Right to advocacy
- Right to safety
- Freedom from explanation
- Protection from co-worker discrimination/harassment
- Protection from client discrimination/harassment
- Right to correct information

The complete GIBOR with an expanded explanation of these rights can be found online (*https://pridevmc.org/global-gibor/*).

b) It is critical that T is a part of the decision-making process regarding their coming out at work. Trans and gender-diverse people almost always have control of their lives and their bodies taken from them by media, family, medical services, and society generally. While well-intentioned, the planning and execution of the email campaign would disempower T and remove their right to freedom from gender affirmation timelines. The best course of action is to talk to T, listen to their needs, and give them the primary role in the decision-making processes around their transition and coming out at work.

Practical options to help with T's transition at work include changing T's name on the clinic website if they wish this, and for everyone at the clinic to have pronouns added to their clinic name badges and on clinic profiles. In addition, setting up a regular schedule of get-togethers where you can discuss how things are going would be very helpful.

PART 2

a) These 'offhand comments' are often called microaggressions. Microaggressions are subtle and sometimes unintentional comments, actions, or situations that negatively target a marginalised person or group. Microaggressions are often seen as harmless or inconsequential by both the transgressor and the target person; however, cumulatively, they can have a marked negative impact on the targeted individual and on team culture. The key to addressing microaggressions is education. Education programmes that comprehensively address awareness, impact, and removing microaggressions from the workplace are a vital part of any diversity and inclusion programme and help to create a psychologically safe workplace for everyone, not just marginalised people.

PART 3

a) This client has clearly breached T's right to protection from client discrimination/harassment. Regardless of the financial value of the client, they need to know that you will support the rights of T and of your team first. Any compromise of this will send the message to your team that they are not valued and respected and will put at risk the psychological safety of your team at work. An email reply should express this clearly and concisely. In particular the email should make the following clear:

1. That you support your staff member in their calling-out of the client and you will not ask them to apologise for this
2. That you expect all clients to treat T with respect and dignity
3. That if the client repeats the above comments or behaviour, then they will be declined service and asked to seek the services of a different veterinary practice

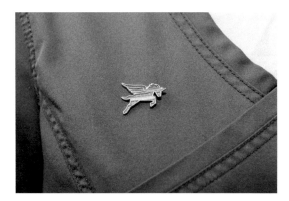

Figure A2.20 **Pin badge of the Australian Rainbow Vets and Allies on a scrub top.**

TODAY'S CASE LIST

3.1 Spot, 5-yo FN Lagotto: emergency from last night

3.2 Jason, 12-yo MN Golden Retriever: not himself

3.3 Flora, 6-yo FE Cross-breed: in labour *CARE*

3.4 Ned, 16-wo ME Miniature Poodle Cross: vomiting ++

3.5 Nigel, 10-yo MN DSH: nail trim

3.6 Donald, 2-yo MN Old English Bulldog: routine vacc

3.7 Gladys, 6-yo FN Australian Shepherd: new dog check-up

3.8 Padme, 10-yo FN Chihuahua: post-op check, not doing well

3.9 Evie, 1-yo FE Border Collie: lap spay admit

3.10 Phil, 10-yo MN Maltese Chihuahua: lame HLs

3.11 Franco, 6-yo MN Poodle: still not right

3.12 Jeremy, 3-yo ME Cocker Spaniel: routine castration

3.13 Thumper, 4-yo MN Dwarf Lop: not eating or moving

3.14 Sarah, 10-wo FE Labrador Cross: vacc

3.15 Pearl, 6-mo FE DSH: health check

3.16 Benny, 4-yo MN Miniature Dachshund: bloody faeces

3.17 Tracy, 12-yo FN SBT: O noticed lump

3.18 Fella, 12-yo MN DSH: left for euthanasia

3.19 Tully, 12-mo FE Lab: post-op wound check

3.20 Womble, 6-yo MN English Bull Terrier: seizures

3.21 Rex, 8-yo ME Rottweiler: dental (extractions)

Recipes: Two soups

DOI: 10.1201/9781003278306-3

3.1 Spot, 5-yo FN Lagotto: emergency from last night

You saw Spot last night after she swallowed fishing line with an attached hook. After taking X-rays, which showed a barbed hook in her stomach, you sent her to an emergency clinic for ongoing treatment (see Case 2.19).

This morning, you receive an email from the emergency facility enclosing Spot's records. The records indicate that, upon admission, emesis was induced using apomorphine (0.03 mg/kg SC) (Figure 3.1). The hook and line were found in the vomitus, and Spot was discharged home within an hour.

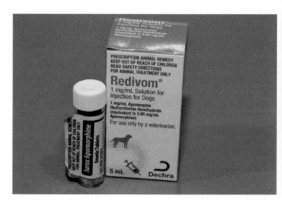

Figure 3.1 Two apomorphine formulations for use in dogs.

a) What are the risks and benefits of emesis as used by the emergency clinic in Spot's case? Would this be different in a general practice context?
b) How might you therefore respond if Spot's owner asks why you didn't just induce emesis at the time of initial presentation, thereby saving the owner money?
c) In general, and in more routine cases, which route of administration (SC or IV) for apomorphine is most effective for inducing emesis?
d) How would you manage any adverse effects associated with apomorphine?
e) Can apomorphine be used to induce emesis in cats?
f) What is a safe product to advise owners for inducing emesis in dogs at home, e.g. after ingestion of common intoxicants?

3.2 Jason, 12-yo MN Golden Retriever: not himself

Jason presents with a 24- to 48-hour history of 'not being himself'. Jason has a poor appetite, is lethargic, and is sleeping much more than usual. He walks slowly into your clinic from the waiting room and immediately lies down. Jason is not on any medication. He has no known exposure to trauma or toxins and Jason is not a scavenger. Jason is not insured and his owner makes it clear he has no budget for comprehensive diagnostics or treatment.

You perform a clinical exam and find:

- Mentation: dull, depressed
- RR: 45 breaths per minute, no audible crackles or wheezes; no cough
- HR: 110 bpm without a murmur; matching, bounding pulses

- Temp: 37.2 °C
- Pale MMs
- CRT – hard to assess due to pallor
- Abdominal palpation: distended, slightly painful abdomen with a fluid wave detected
- Jason's extremities are cool to the touch

Jason lies down immediately you have finished examining him.

You take a small blood sample for PCV and TP (Table 3.2).

Table 3.2 **Jason's PCV and TP results**		
PARAMETER	**RESULT**	**REFERENCE RANGE**
PCV	0.25	0.35–0.50
TP	5.1 g/dL	6.0–7.5

A blood smear shows no evidence of regeneration, and no evidence of platelet clumping.

The ultrasound machine happens to be in the room. You place a probe at the costophrenic location and obtain an image (Figure 3.2).

a) The owner asks for a prognosis. Outline possible causes and outcomes based on the information you currently have.

b) What do you do next?

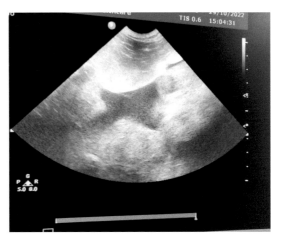

Figure 3.2 **The image obtained at the costophrenic location on Jason.**

3.3 Flora, 6-yo FE Cross-breed: in labour *CARE*

Flora, an otherwise healthy dog who has a history of prior pelvic fracture (Figure 3.3), is presented in stage 2 labour. One puppy in posterior presentation was delivered at home by the owner. You examine this puppy in the clinic and find him dead with traumatic injuries to the head. You suspect these injuries were incurred during delivery. Flora has now been in stage 2 labour with her next puppy for 40 minutes and is increasingly distressed. On vaginal examination, you detect a puppy's head at the pelvic inlet. You judge attempted manual delivery unsafe, so obtain consent to perform a caesarean section. Once hospitalised, Flora shows fear aggression and becomes extremely difficult to handle. It is not possible to insert an IV cannula without sedation/premedication.

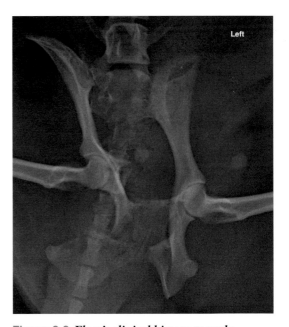

Figure 3.3 **Flora's clinical history records a previous pelvic fracture. Pelvic fracture, especially if managed conservatively, is a risk factor for obstructive dystocia.**

a) What are the advantages and disadvantages of premedication before caesarean section?

b) Which drugs are best avoided?

c) Outline key principles of general anaesthesia for caesarean section.

d) How can you assess neonates immediately after birth to guide resuscitation?

3.4 Ned, 16-wo ME Miniature Poodle Cross: vomiting ++

Ned has had vomiting, depression, and apparent pain overnight. Prior to this, he had been a normal, healthy, and active puppy.

On a physical exam, Ned has pain in the caudal abdomen, with a palpable mobile mass approximately the size of a thumb present. Palpation of this mass produced a marked pain response. The rest of the physical exam was within normal limits. Abdominal radiographs were taken (Figure 3.4a).

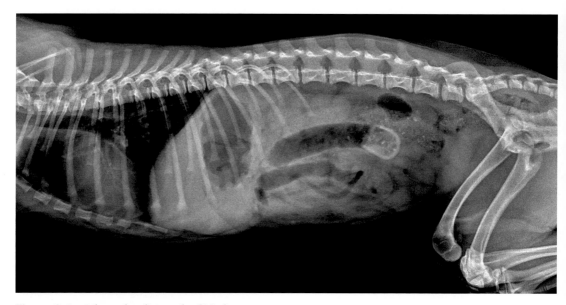

Figure 3.4a **A lateral radiograph of Ned.**

a) Describe the radiographic findings. What is your diagnosis and recommended treatment?
b) You determine that Ned requires surgery (Figure 3.4b). Describe the procedure, giving step-by-step details of surgical approach, assessment of abdominal organs, treatment of the problem found in Ned, and closure of the surgical sites.
c) Outline peri- and post-operative medications and care that can improve Ned's recovery.

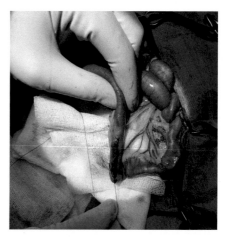

Figure 3.4b **Intraoperative view during Ned's surgery.**

3.5 Nigel, 10-yo MN DSH: nail trim

Nigel was brought in to the clinic for a nail trim. The nail on the third digit of Nigel's right hind paw is ingrown (Figure 3.5a). A nurse manages to clip the nail, but is concerned that Nigel may require antibiotics (Figure 3.5b). They ask if you can fit Nigel in for a consultation.

a) What underlying condition(s) may lead to ingrown nails in cats?

b) As well as clipping the nail, how would you treat this condition?

c) How might you assess the effectiveness of treatment?

d) Nigel's owner has limited funds. How might you proceed?

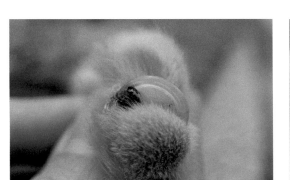

Figure 3.5a The nail of the third digit of Nigel's right hind paw, photographed from the medial aspect. The dorsal surface of the paw is on the right side of the image.

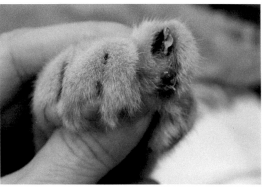

Figure 3.5b View of the paw immediately following clipping of the toenail, prior to cleaning with antiseptic. There is purulent discharge from the site of nail penetration of the digital pad.

3.6 Donald, 2-yo MN Old English Bulldog: routine vacc

Donald presents for a routine vaccination, during which his owners mention that they are having problems with Donald humping them and showing aggressive behaviour when interrupted. He can be resting on the floor and then suddenly lunge towards the owners for no apparent reason and start humping an arm or leg. This tends to happen for a few days every 2–3 weeks. He is also becoming increasingly sensitive to certain noises and will bark excessively at the window when vehicles go past. Some days he can ignore these noises, but other days he seems on edge and hypervigilant.

a) What are the differentials for humping behaviour in a neutered dog?

b) Is there anything in Donald's history that would make you suspicious of a physical cause for his behaviour problems?

On examination, you note that Donald is reluctant to fully extend his hips. The clients mention that he can sometimes have problems jumping onto furniture, but otherwise exercises normally.

c) You suspect that musculoskeletal pain may be contributing to Donald's behaviour problems, but the clients are reluctant to opt for radiographs of his hindlimbs without further evidence of this. What would be a reasonable way of confirming your suspicions?

d) What first-aid advice would you give to Donald's owners to keep them safe and prevent escalation of Donald's behaviour problems?

3.7 Gladys, 6-yo FN Australian Shepherd: new dog check-up

Gladys has been recently acquired by the owners from relatives who have relocated overseas. On examination, you note that her irises are distinctly different colours (Figure 3.7). Gladys has normal menace responses, direct and consensual pupillary reflexes, palpebral responses, and pupillary light reflexes in both eyes.

You perform some eye diagnostics:

- A Schirmer tear test reveals 22 mm/minute in her right eye, and 19 mm/minute in her left eye
- IOP, as measured by tonometry, is 16 mmHg in the right eye and 18 mmHg in the left eye
- Fluorescein staining is negative when visualised under a blue light

a) Which of the above components of the examination tested Gladys's vision? What other tests might you perform if you suspected that Gladys had vision loss?

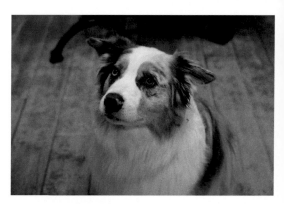

Figure 3.7 Gladys's eyes showing different-coloured irises.

b) What do the ophthalmic abbreviations OD, OS, and OU stand for?
c) What is the normal IOP for a dog?
d) What is the most likely cause of Gladys's condition?
e) What condition(s) could this be associated with?

3.8 Padme, 10-yo FN Chihuahua: post-op check, not doing well

Padme has presented 10 days after exploratory laparotomy and surgical excision of a benign hepatocellular adenoma. Padme was under anaesthetic for approximately 2 hours. The histopathology report confirms clear margins. The owners report that Padme has yet to return to her normal self. They feel that she is moving tentatively, her appetite is significantly reduced (she is refusing to eat anything unless hand-fed warmed chicken), and she seems generally unhappy.

Several days after surgery, they noted a small, red spot appear over her left shoulder. They had 'spoken to someone in the practice' who suggested that the spot corresponded to the site of a pain-relief injection, and that it would soon clear up. However, they feel the redness has spread. Concerningly, similar red spots have appeared around Padme's tail base.

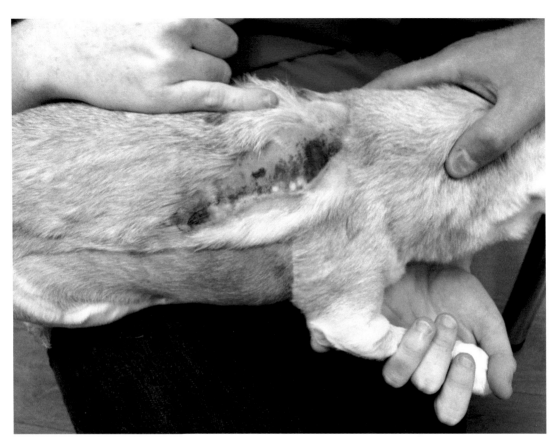

Figure 3.8a The area around the right shoulder has a mottled appearance, is oedematous, and blanches when touched gently.

Physical findings:

- BCS: 4/5
- Weight: 4.0 kg (she was 4.9 kg on the day of her surgery)
- Demeanour: quiet, alert, responsive; Padme trembles during the examination
- MMs pink, CRT <2 s
- Temp: 38.3 °C
- HR: 120 bpm (no murmurs)
- RR: 26 breaths per minute, with no increased effort
- The fur over the areas of concern is matted

There is patchy alopecia over the tail base, with the skin having a mottled red to black, erythematous, blistered appearance. It blanches when light pressure is applied, and feels both moist and oedematous. In addition, over the

right shoulder, there is a ridge of skin that feels quite leathery.

You clip away some fur, revealing what seems to be a well-circumscribed, darker area of skin. It has a red to waxy white appearance around the edges, and has a mottled red to black erythematous appearance. The area dorsal to the ridge is profoundly oedematous and blanches when light pressure is applied (Figure 3.8a).

You clip more fur and realise that the spots you have seen occur at the edge of a large, oval-shaped lesion covering Padme's entire dorsum (Figure 3.8b). You are concerned that this is a delayed presentation of thermal burn, secondary to exposure to a heat pad during surgery.

a) Supplemental heating methods are used to prevent hypothermia (just under 98 °F, or 36.5 °C) in veterinary patients. What adverse effects are associated with hypothermia in veterinary patients?
b) Why are heat pads contraindicated?
c) What is the safest way to reduce the risk of hypothermia in small animal patients?
d) What other differentials for Padme's skin lesion might you consider?
e) Assuming this is an iatrogenic burn, what should you do next?

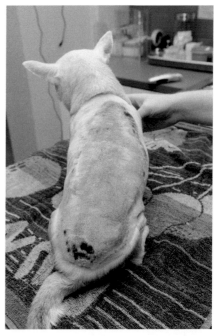

Figure 3.8b A more extensive clip reveals a large, oval-shaped area encompassing Padme's dorsum.

3.9 Evie, 1-yo FE Border Collie: lap spay admit

Evie (Figure 3.9a) is a fit and lively dog with no pre-existing conditions, presenting for a laparoscopic spay. She had one season 4 months ago that was uneventful. Her recent history and clinical exam are unremarkable. Today she has no mammary development or milk production and her vulva is small. Evie's owner, a retired vet who stopped working before laparoscopic spays were introduced, has some questions for you.

a) What are the main differences between a laparoscopic spay and a 'normal' spay?
b) What are the advantages and disadvantages of a laparoscopic spay?
c) The vet asks you to talk through the two-port procedure step by step.
d) What are the possible complications?
e) What post-operative care is needed?

Your nurse today is a new colleague and asks you to check the equipment table (Figure 3.9b).

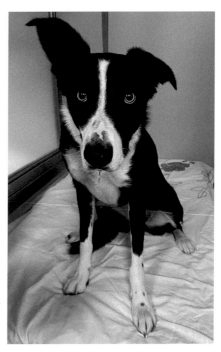

Figure 3.9a Evie on admission for her laparoscopic spay.

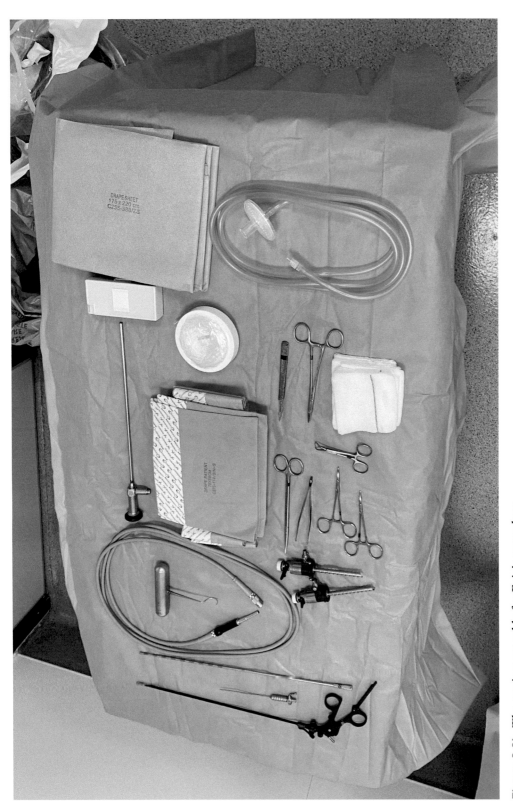

Figure 3.9b The equipment table for Evie's procedure.

f) List all the items needed for a laparoscopic spay (they are mostly shown in Figure 3.9b).

Is there anything missing in Figure 3.9b?

3.10 Phil, 10-yo MN Maltese Chihuahua: lame HLs

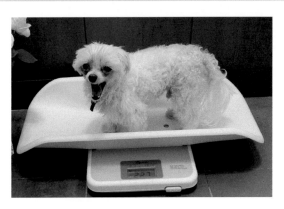

Figure 3.10 **Phil on the scales.**

Phil (Figure 3.10) is presented with a history of intermittent hindlimb lameness. He also occasionally 'skips' with one or other hindlimbs when he runs quickly. His appointment today was prompted by several occasions during which Phil fell over and held one hindlimb extended in what the owner called a 'weird position'. Phil was agitated and, at first, the owner thought he was 'having a fit', but the problem resolved when the owner 'massaged' the offending leg. Phil then stood up normally.

Phil was recently adopted from a rescue organisation. To the owner's knowledge, Phil has no previous history of trauma or surgery, but the rescue could not supply a full history.

Examination findings:

- BCS: 2.7/5
- Weight: 2.27 kg
- Upright hindlimb gait, with occasional 'skipping' lameness of the hindlimbs when running
- On physical examination, both patellas can be luxated medially and remain luxated until the stifle is extended, when they can be replaced
- The patellas do not re-luxate spontaneously. You do not elicit a drawer sign. You do not palpate an effusion in either stifle joint
- The rest of the physical exam is normal

a) What is the pathogenesis of medial patellar luxation?
b) What grade (I–IV) of patellar luxation does Phil have?
c) What happened when the owner massaged Phil's leg after he collapsed?
d) Would you perform diagnostic tests? If so, what tests?
e) What treatment would you recommend?

3.11 Franco, 6-yo MN Poodle: still not right

This is Franco's second visit to the clinic. At the previous visit, which was a vaccination appointment 3 weeks ago, the owner reported to your colleague that the otherwise healthy, active Franco was drinking more, possibly urinating more frequently and maybe – though the owner really wasn't sure – jumping a bit less than he had been. Franco's urine was moderately concentrated (USG 1.022), but there were no other abnormalities on urinalysis. One of your colleague's differentials was Cushing's syndrome. A CBC, biochemistry panel, and T4 were sent off. The results are given in Table 3.11.

Table 3.11 **Franco's blood count, biochemistry panel, and total T4 results. Abnormalities are highlighted in red**

PARAMETER	RESULT	REFERENCE RANGE
Haematocrit	0.44	0.38–0.57
RBC count	6.2×10^{12}/L	$5.7–8.3 \times 10^{12}$/L
Haemoglobin	165 g/L	129–201 g/L
Reticulocyte-Hb equivalent	26.1×10^{12}/L	$21.3–28.1 \times 10^{12}$/L
MCV	72 fL	63–75 fL
MCH	27 pg	22–27 pg
MCHC	372 g/L	328–378 g/L
WBC count	10.8×10^9/L	$4.7–12.8 \times 10^9$/L
Neutrophils	8.7×10^9/L	$3.1–9.0 \times 10^9$/L
Lymphocytes	1.2×10^9/L	$1.0–3.5 \times 10^9$/L
Monocytes	0.9×10^9/L	$0.2–1.0 \times 10^9$/L
Eosinophils	0.001×10^9/L	$0.1–1.0 \times 10^9$/L
Basophils	0.01×10^9/L	$<0.2 \times 10^9$/L
Platelets	215	$150–539 \times 10^9$/L
Plasma glucose	3.6 mmol/L	3.6–6.2 mmol/L
Serum glucose	1.4 mmol/L	3.6–6.2 mmol/L
Creatinine	62 µmol/L	50–127 µmol/L
Urea	5.9 mmol/L	3.0–9.8 mmol/L
Phosphate	1.66 mmol/L	0.80–1.7 mmol/L
Calcium	2.43 mmol/L	1.87–2.83 mmol/L
Sodium	151 mmol/L	145–152 mmol/L
Potassium	4.8 mmol/L	4.3–5.9 mmol/L
Chloride	107 mmol/L	100–120 mmol/L
Bicarbonate	23 mmol/L	16–25 mmol/L
Anion gap	26 mmol/L	16–29 mmol/L
TP	60 g/L	53–72 g/L
Albumin	42 g/L	28–44 g/L
Globulin	18 g/L	18–37 g/L
Albumin:globulin ratio	2.3	0.8–2.3
Creatinine kinase	230 U/L	89–467 U/L
ALT	150	18–89 U/L
Aspartate aminotransferase (AST)	50 U/L	21–52 U/L
ALP	52 U/L	11–129 U/L
GGT	18 U/L	<7 U/L
Bilirubin – total	1 µmol/L	<6 µmol/L
Cholesterol	9.0 mmol/L	3.6–10 mmol/L
Triglyceride	2.1 mmol/L	0.2–1.7 mmol/L
Total T4	19 nmol/L	13–47 nmol/L

At the initial visit, Franco's owner felt that their dog had a strain or sprain. After discussion with the owner, your colleague dispensed a course of NSAIDs, but told the client to monitor for signs of Cushing's syndrome.

When seen by you today, Franco is much the same as before. You manage to catch your colleague for a quick word in the prep room. They feel that Franco 'probably has an endocrinopathy', but are uncertain about the case and want you to take over.

a) Take a few minutes to think about possible sources of uncertainty in veterinary general practice. What sorts of things create uncertainty in decision-making in the general practice context?

b) Studies in human healthcare suggest that clinicians vary significantly in their tolerance to uncertainty. What are the potential negative impacts of intolerance to uncertainty on clinicians (including veterinarians)?

c) Individual clinician responses to uncertainty may be maladaptive, or adaptive. List potential strategies for diagnosing and managing uncertainty.

3.12 Jeremy, 3-yo ME Cocker Spaniel: routine castration

Jeremy is being prepared for surgery when you are called to examine the electrocardiogram (ECG) due to concerns over the HR (Figure 3.12). He was premedicated with 2 µg/kg of dexmedetomidine and 0.2 mg/kg of methadone IV 15 minutes ago.

a) What is the ECG abnormality displayed in Figure 3.12?

b) Would you treat this abnormality? If yes, how?

c) Would your actions change in a non-anaesthetised dog?

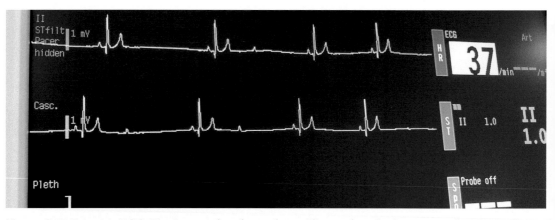

Figure 3.12 Jeremy's ECG 15 minutes after dexmedetomidine and methadone were administered.

3.13 Thumper, 4-yo MN Dwarf Lop: not eating or moving

Thumper presents with a history of lethargy since this morning. His owner reports that he is not interested in his greens or favourite treats (Figure 3.13). Thumper's litter tray has also been empty overnight.

Key physical findings:

- Demeanour: quiet, flat
- HR 160 bpm
- Temp: 36.7 °C
- RR: rapid panting
- Abdominal palpation: uncomfortable in cranial abdomen with a large non-compressible stomach, and painful on palpation
- Moderately delayed skin tent
- Coat: lots of moulting

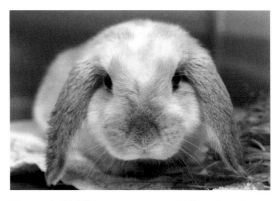

Figure 3.13 **Thumper presents lethargic and anorexic with no faeces passed overnight.**

a) What is the most likely cause of Thumper's clinical signs?
b) What diagnostic tests would you recommend?
c) What are the treatment options for this condition?

d) What is the prognosis and what aftercare is required?

3.14 Sarah, 10-wo FE Labrador Cross: vacc

Sarah is presented for routine vaccination. During the examination, you comment on her unusual facial expression – she seems to be 'smiling' and her ears are held in an abnormal position (Figure 3.14). On further questioning, the owners recall that Sarah's facial expression has indeed changed over the last 24–48 hours. To her owners' knowledge, Sarah has not experienced trauma or been exposed to any toxins.

a) What condition does this puppy have and what is the likely cause?
b) What type of clinical reasoning do experienced clinicians use when they make

a diagnosis based on appearance? What are the advantages and disadvantages of this approach? (You may or may not have been

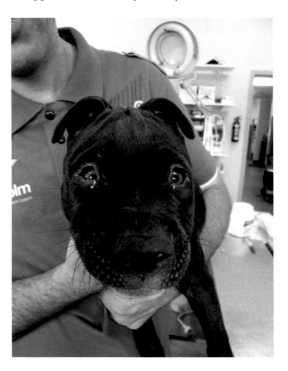

Figure 3.14 **Signs of tetanus include *risus sardonicus* (changed facial expression, a 'sardonic smile' caused by spasm of facial muscles), trismus (contraction of jaw muscles), erect ear carriage, and third eyelid protrusion. Sarah shows two of these.** *This image has been previously published (Fawcett & Irwin 2014a,b) and is reproduced here with permission. Full references in Answers section.*

able to use this approach yourself for Sarah's condition. If not, this question will probably ensure you do in future.)

c) How would this disease present in cats?

d) How would you treat this condition and how does treatment address the underlying pathophysiology?

e) Given the history provided, how might Sarah have contracted this condition?

f) How can this condition be prevented?

3.15 Pearl, 6-mo FE DSH: health check

You are seeing Pearl for a general health check. During your overall preventive medicine discussion, you bring up the topic of gonadectomy (Figure 3.15). The owner responds that they have been doing some reading and found conflicting information. They have questions about timing or even whether to go for this procedure at all.

a) What factors will impact your general recommendations about gonadectomy/neutering in cats?

b) What is your recommendation for the timing of gonadectomy for Pearl?

c) What is your recommendation for the timing of castration for a male cat?

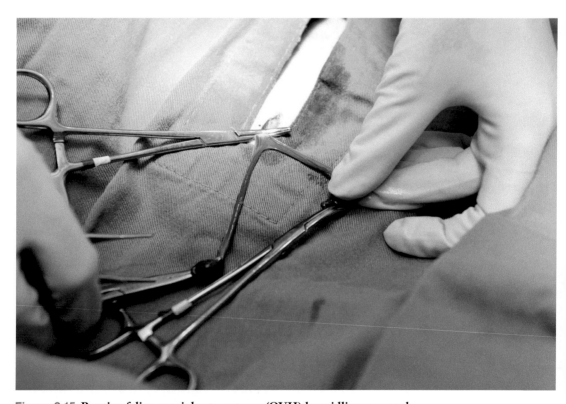

Figure 3.15 Routine feline ovariohysterectomy (OVH) by midline approach.

3.16 Benny, 4-yo MN Miniature Dachshund: bloody faeces

Benny, an 8.0-kg male Miniature Dachshund (Figure 3.16a), has not eaten his breakfast and is slightly subdued in demeanour. His owner is mildly concerned as Benny has a habit of eating garbage, duck faeces, and other foreign material, and normally always eats his breakfast. Benny lives on a rural property with an Australian Cattle Dog. Vaccinations and endoparasite control are up to date. His diet consists of a variety of high-quality wet and dry dog food, with occasional treats and leftovers.

Benny is bright and responsive, normothermic, and has no palpable signs of abdominal pain or discomfort. Shortly after examination, Benny passes a solid faecal motion followed by some bloody, loose, mucous faeces (Figure 3.16b) and a worm (Figure 3.16c).

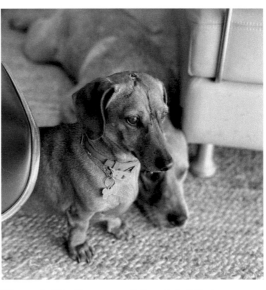

Figure 3.16a **Benny, an 8-kg adult Miniature Dachshund.**

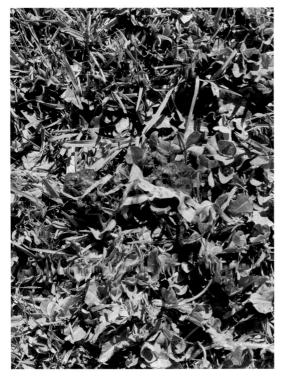

Figure 3.16b **Benny's faeces. Note the presence of blood, mucus, and a parasite.**

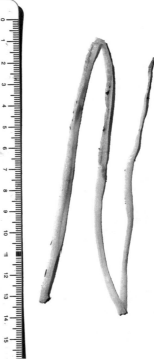

Figure 3.16c **The parasite in Figure 3.16b, identified as *Spirometra erinacei*.**

a) What *type* of worm is shown in Figure 3.16c?
b) How might Benny have become infected?
c) Is it zoonotic?

d) Is this parasite responsible for Benny's clinical signs?
e) Is routine endoparasite treatment effective in the control of this parasite?

3.17 Tracy, 12-yo FN SBT: O noticed lump

Tracy presents with a mammary mass in the caudal left mammary gland measuring approximately 2 × 4 cm. The mass is thought to have appeared over the previous 3 months and the owner now feels it is enlarging quickly. The mass feels relatively mobile and is not fixed to underlying structures.

Tracy also has moderate to severe dental disease (Figure 3.17a). The owner reports that Tracy sometimes exhibits mouth pain, such as crying out when eating a hard biscuit, and that Tracy's breath has had an unpleasant odour for some time.

Tracy seems otherwise healthy. Her water intake is normal. A urine dipstick yields no

issues; USG is 1.028. On a minimum database, PCV, TP, and both BUN and glucose test strips are within normal ranges, and the blood smear is unremarkable.

The owner wishes to proceed with treatment, but funds are limited. The owner declines further blood testing for economic reasons.

It is proposed to admit Tracy for chest radiography, excision of the mammary mass with histopathology, and dental treatment as a single procedure. This would save the owner the cost (and Tracy the stress) of a second anaesthetic.

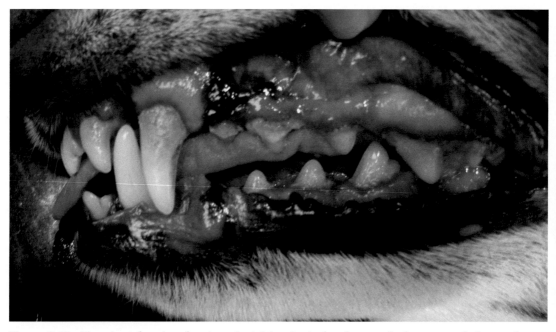

Figure 3.17a **Tracy's oral cavity, showing gingivitis, gingival oedema, calculus accumulation, and possibly pus at the gingival margin of some teeth.**

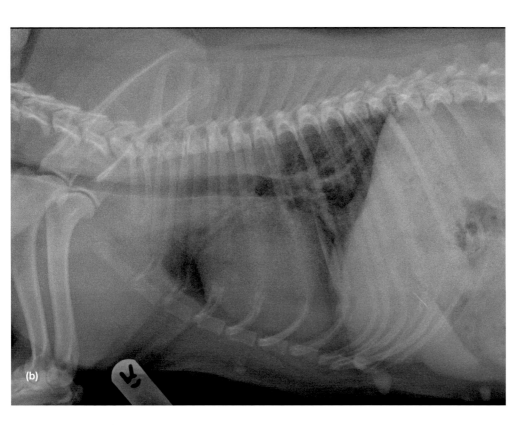

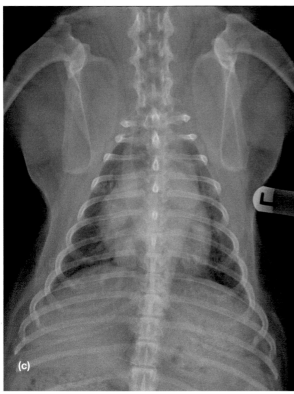

Figure 3.17b,c Two views of Tracy's chest.

a) Comment on the decision to carry out mammary mass removal and dental surgery under the same anaesthetic.

b) Are antibiotics indicated?

c) What other measures could be implemented to guard against wound infection when the combined operation is scheduled?

d) Tracy received three-view chest radiographs. Two views are shown in Figure 3.17b,c. No obvious pulmonary metastases were seen on the X-rays; however, a very subtle incidental finding is noted in the cranial abdomen on both views. Can you spot it?

e) How would you approach this further comorbidity issue with an already financially stretched owner?

f) Tracy's histopathology report arrives 10 days after surgery. The mass is described as a 'canine simple mammary carcinoma, grade 1, complete excision with >2 cm margins'. Tracy's teeth were scaled and polished and six removed. Early furcation exposure (on probing) was noted on 108 and 309, but, in order to reduce total operating time, these teeth were not removed. When discharging Tracy to her owner, what is your plan going forward regarding the following?

i) Mammary tumour

ii) Teeth

iii) Incidental finding, bearing in mind that the owner has limited finances

3.18 Fella, 12-yo MN DSH: left for euthanasia

A drop-off euthanasia was placed in your appointment column. You were tied up with an emergency and could not admit Fella yourself, but a senior nurse talked to the owner. She informs you that the owners were curt, to the point of appearing rude, and insisted that they did not want to be present for the euthanasia (Figure 3.18). They signed the consent forms, paid, and left the premises. You attempt to examine Fella, but he is hissing and backing away from you in his carrier. He has extensive damage to his nose and upper jaw due to what is likely an SCC. The nurse is very upset – she can't believe that Fella's owners 'could be so cruel as to let him live like this and then just dump him at the clinic to be euthanased'.

a) How will you approach Fella's euthanasia in a humane and stress-free way?

b) Would you sedate Fella prior to euthanasia? If so, how?

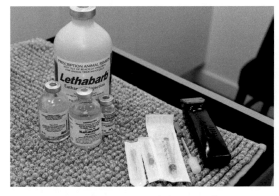

Figure 3.18 Fella's owners did not wish to stay for the euthanasia.

c) How can you administer the pentobarbital?

d) How might you respond to the nurse's distress?

e) Should you contact the owners following euthanasia?

3.19 Tully, 12-mo FE Lab: post-op wound check

Tully presents for a recheck of her abdominal wound 5 days after exploratory laparotomy. The owner reports that Tully has been eating, drinking, and toileting normally, but did not tolerate the hard plastic Elizabethan collar she was wearing when discharged. She appeared subdued and miserable (Figure 3.19). They admit that Tully has been caught licking her wound occasionally, but that she stops when told not to. Tully is not currently on any medication.

Physical examination findings:

- Demeanour: very BAR
- BCS: 3/5
- Weight: 23.2 kg (was 23.5 kg on the day of surgery)
- MMs pink, CRT <2 s
- HR: 160 bpm with no pulse deficits
- RR: panting (you suspect due to excitement)
- Temp: 38.3 °C
- Abdominal palpation: soft, normal
- Wound: there is mild erythema associated with the surgical wound, and a small, fluid-filled swelling cranially. There is no discharge and the skin does not feel warm. Tully does not react when you inspect the site

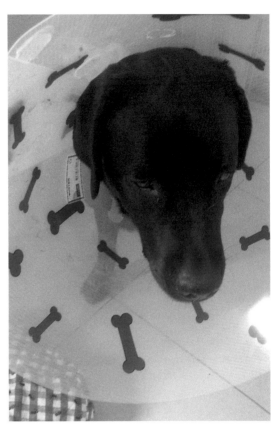

Figure 3.19 Tully was miserable when wearing a hard plastic Elizabethan collar.

a) Apart from an Elizabethan collar, what other steps can be taken to reduce self-trauma in veterinary patients?
b) Should you drain the swelling?
c) Tully's owners ask if she needs antibiotics. What would you advise?

d) Elizabethan collars are one means of protecting surgical sites from self-trauma, yet Tully's owners have not adhered to your advice to keep the collar on. How might you advise clients in relation to Elizabethan collars?

3.20 Womble, 6-yo MN English Bull Terrier: seizures

You saw Womble 3 weeks ago for a vaccination. Aside from mild dental disease (grade 1/4), you found him to be in good health. The owner reports that Womble had been fine on his lead walk around the park this morning. He ate his usual breakfast of tinned food, but 20 minutes later his owner found him seizuring. She rushed him straight down to the clinic and arrives just as you are finishing afternoon clinic. He is still seizuring (Figure 3.20).

a) What are the first steps you would take in managing Womble?

b) One cause of seizures in companion animals is toxins. Can you think of any drugs/toxins/agents that may cause seizures in dogs?

c) Assuming Womble has not been exposed to any agent that causes seizures, and he presents in status epilepticus, how might you attempt to control his seizures?

d) What should you do once Womble's seizures are controlled?

e) Womble's owners have limited funds, but want to know Womble's prognosis. What can you advise?

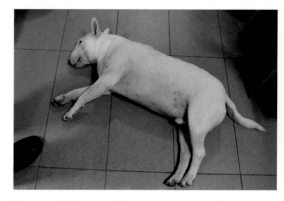

Figure 3.20 **Womble presents in lateral recumbency and seizuring.**

f) In dogs at risk of status epilepticus (e.g. those with idiopathic epilepsy), aside from anti-seizure medication, what veterinarian-supplied at-home treatment could potentially be administered to try to stop seizures and prevent progression to status epilepticus?

3.21 Rex, 8-yo ME Rottweiler: dental (extractions)

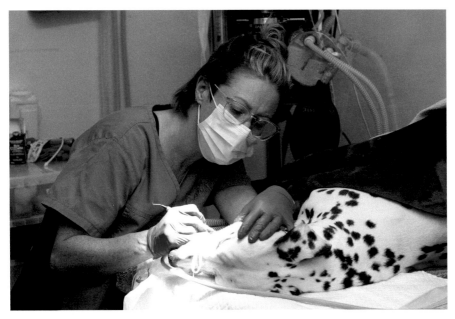

Figure 3.21a **Handling large-breed dogs is associated with health and safety risks during dentistry and other procedures due to their size and weight.**

List at least five possible health and safety hazards associated with a case like Rex, who weighs 55 kg. For each hazard, identify at least one action you can undertake to reduce the risk of a health and safety impact to yourself or your team.

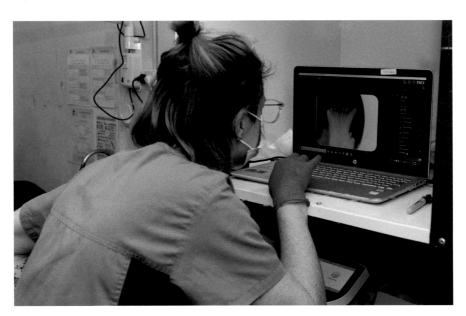

Figure 3.21b **Extraction procedures can be lengthy and involve multiple dental radiographs.**

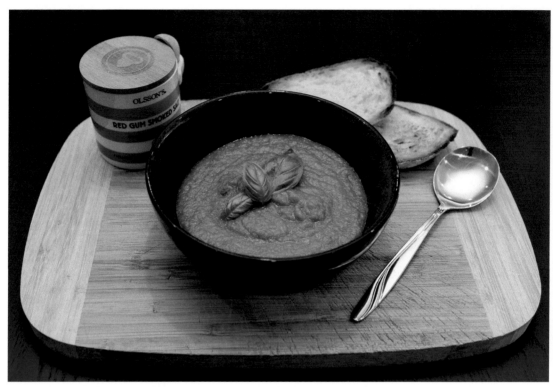

Figure 3.22a **The tomato soup.**

'TWO SOUPS'

With homage to great British comedy actress Julie Walters.

TOMATO SOUP

Ingredients

55 g margarine
115 g onion diced
115 g carrots chopped
115 g leeks chopped
15 g corn flour
570 mL vegetable stock
400 g tin of tomatoes
2 cloves
1 teaspoon sugar
Clove of garlic (crushed)
2 bay leaves
Pinch of marjoram
2 tablespoons tomato puree

Method

1. Melt margarine in soup pan and soften onion, carrot, and leek.
2. Add flour and cook for 2 minutes on medium heat.
3. Add stock.
4. Add rest of ingredients.
5. Simmer gently until carrots are cooked (30 minutes).
6. Can liquidise or serve as is (but beware of cloves!).

PUMPKIN SOUP

Ingredients

Scooped or chopped flesh of 1 medium pumpkin
6 plum tomatoes (halved)
Dash of olive oil
25 g butter or margarine
1 onion, diced
2 cloves garlic (crushed)
700 mL vegetable stock
30 g fresh basil, chopped
Salt and pepper

Method

1. Preheat oven to 180 °C or gas 4.
2. Wash pumpkin flesh until seeds removed – retain seeds.
3. Roast seeds for 30 minutes until crisped.
4. Place tomatoes on a baking sheet and drizzle with olive oil and season. Roast for 15–20 minutes.
5. Add onion, garlic, and pumpkin to the pan with butter/margarine and olive oil. Sautee for 2–3 minutes.
6. Add roasted tomatoes and vegetable stock. Simmer for 20 minutes.
7. Add chopped basil. Simmer for 10 minutes.
8. Liquidise the soup with a stick blender and sieve to remove any pips.
9. Serve garnished with the toasted seeds.

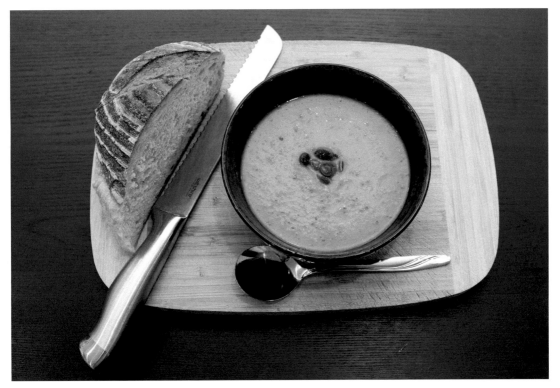

Figure 3.22b **The pumpkin soup.**

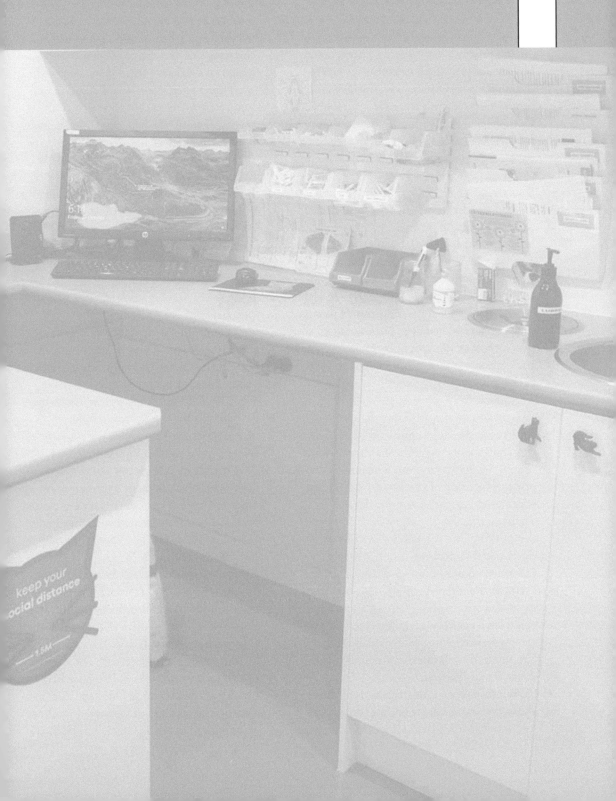

3.1 Spot, 5-yo FN Lagotto: emergency from last night

a) Inducing emesis when the foreign body is a sharp object, such as a fish hook, risks laceration or penetration of tissues during forceful vomiting. The hook could become lodged in the oesophagus, larynx, pharynx, or oral cavity, any of which could produce dangerous and distressing sequelae. Oesophageal foreign bodies can be difficult to retrieve and, in some cases, may require thoracotomy, which has associated risks and potential complications. Benefits of emesis, if successful, as was the case with Spot, include an inexpensive, simple, and quick process requiring no anaesthesia or surgical intervention. In this case, the thinking may have included the observation that the stomach was very full; therefore, the food could potentially act as a protective covering for the vomited fish hook during its passage orally. There is, however, also the possibility that there was a failure of communication, and emesis was induced before the nature of the foreign body was actually realised (or seen on the X-ray). In an emergency referral situation, with immediate access to anaesthesia, endoscopy, and (if needed) surgical support to perform a thoracotomy should the hook cause oesophageal damage, perhaps the risks of emesis may have been considered mitigated to some degree. In a general practice situation, at the end of the working day, the context is different, especially if endoscopy is not available. Informed consent is another aspect. If, for example, any other form of intervention was ruled out on cost grounds, then emesis could have been seen as a treatment of last resort. Nevertheless, there is still the risk of potentially making the situation much worse for the patient.

b) Owner discussion along the lines of the above considerations would be important (see also Table A2.19 in Chapter 2 [Answers section]). This would also be a case in which a phone call to the emergency practice would be in order, to understand their thinking and treatment rationale with Spot, which could then inform your discussion with the owner. This would demonstrate a concerned and caring approach to the owner. If a mistake had indeed been made, e.g. emesis induced before the history and radiographs were reviewed, it would also help future learning.

c) Both SC and IV routes are equally effective, but in a randomised trial of 42 client-owned dogs, emesis was delayed when apomorphine was given via the SC route (median time to emesis of 13.5 minutes), compared with when it was given via the IV route (median time to emesis of 2 minutes) (Fischer et al. 2021). Apomorphine can also be administered via the conjunctiva if diluted with sterile water. The oral route is less reliable owing to a significant 'first pass' effect. In some countries (e.g. Australia, UK), licensed injectable preparations may be available for the SC route only.

d) For respiratory and central nervous system effects, naloxone can be administered (0.01–0.04 mg/kg IV) (Peterson 2013). Following successful production of a foreign body, and when no more are present, ongoing nausea and emesis can be treated with maropitant (1 mg/kg SC or IV) or metoclopramide (0.2–0.4 mg/kg IV or SC).

e) Apomorphine should not be used in cats. In cats, alpha-2 agonists such as xylazine, medetomidine, and dexmedetomidine are the most reliable emetics (Dunayer 2023) (Figure A3.1), though hydromorphone or brimonidine may be used. The dose of dexmedetomidine is 7–10 μg/kg IM or 3.5 μg/kg IV (Lee & Odunayo 2022). Oral administration of dexmedetomidine at 20 μg/kg has been reported to be a safe and effective means of inducing emesis in cats with no known cardiovascular disease (Maxwell et al. 2024). Medetomidine and dexmedetomidine can be reversed with atipamezole. The dose of xylazine is 0.44 mg/kg SC or IM. This can be reversed with yohimbine (Lee & Odunayo 2022) or atipamezole.

f) The safest product for home use, for use in dogs only, is 3% hydrogen peroxide dosed at 2 mL/kg PO (Dunayer 2023). Do not give more than 45 mL in any dog. It can be administered with milk or ice cream and light exercise may stimulate vomiting.

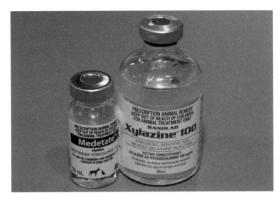

Figure A3.1 Alpha-2 agonists such as medetomidine and xylazine are the most reliable emetics in cats.

Contraindications to use of emetics
- Sharp or barbed gastric foreign bodies
- Corrosive agents or petroleum swallowed
- Seizuring or comatose animal

Note that animals at increased risk of aspiration, including brachycephalics, need careful monitoring.

REFERENCES

Dunayer, E. (2023) Emetics in small animals. *Today's Veterinary Practice*. March/April 2023. Available at: https://todaysveterinarypractice.com/pharmacology/emetics-in-small-animals/.

Fischer, C., Drobatz, K. J. & Thawley, V. J. (2021) Evaluation of subcutaneous versus intravenous administration of apomorphine for induction of emesis in dogs. *Journal of the American Veterinary Medical Association* **259**(3):283–287. doi: 10.2460/javma.259.3.283.

Lee, J. & Odunayo A. (2022) Drugs used for emesis induction in cats. *Clinician's Brief*. Available at: www.cliniciansbrief.com/article/drugs-used-emesis-induction-cats.

Maxwell, K. M., Odunayo, A. & Wissel, C. (2024) Use of orally administered dexmedetomidine to induce emesis in cats. *Journal of Feline Medicine and Surgery* **26**(5). doi: 10.1177/1098612x241248980.

Peterson, M. E. (2013) Chapter 10: Toxicologic Decontamination. In: Peterson, M. E. & Talcott, P. A. (eds) *Small Animal Toxicology*, 3rd edition. St Louis, MO: W.B. Saunders. doi: 10.1016/B978-1-4557-0717-1.00010-7

Zersen, K. M., Peterson, N. & Bergman, P. J. (2020) Retrospective evaluation of the induction of emesis with apomorphine as treatment for gastric foreign bodies in dogs (2010–2014): 61 cases. *Journal of Veterinary Emergency and Critical Care* **30**(2):209–212. doi: 10.1111/vec.12942.

3.2 Jason, 12-yo MN Golden Retriever: not himself

a) The signs of lethargy and increased RR with pale MMs, together with a fluid wave, point towards cardiac or haemorrhagic causes. The low PCV and TP suggest loss of whole blood; the non-regenerative smear suggests acute onset. The ultrasound shows characteristic black triangular shapes indicating fluid separation of liver lobes and liver/diaphragm. Jason probably has a haemoabdomen, most likely due to a bleeding mass in the abdomen. This does not necessarily imply inoperable malignancy, but approximately four out of five cases of non-traumatic haemoabdomen are associated with malignant neoplasia, with two-thirds to three-quarters of these associated with splenic haemangiosarcoma (Pratschke 2020). Furthermore, it has been found that 17% of dogs diagnosed with 'non-malignant' splenic histopathological findings following splenectomy for non-traumatic haemoabdomen died prematurely of a suspected malignancy in the months following surgery (Millar et al. 2022). This suggests that histopathologic signs of malignancy may be missed, and prevalence of malignancy underestimated. Other potential causes of non-traumatic haemoabdomen include coagulopathies, bleeding benign masses, hepatic or splenic torsion, or gastric dilatation and volvulus (GDV) (Pratschke 2020). You cannot provide a definitive prognosis without performing costly major surgery. On the balance of probability, it is more likely than not that Jason – an old, large-breed dog – has a splenic haemangiosarcoma or hepatic tumour. The prognosis is therefore guarded.

b) Exactly what you do next will depend on discussion with the owner. One minimally invasive, inexpensive test is abdominocentesis and measurement of PCV. If the PCV of the abdominal fluid collected is similar to or higher than the PCV from Jason's peripheral blood sample, and it does not clot, this is supportive of a diagnosis of haemoabdomen. Blood clotting suggests accidental organ puncture or venous sampling, as free blood in the abdomen is defibrinated (Pratschke 2020).

Further diagnostics, even if the owner could afford them, are unlikely to give more information. Stabilisation of Jason (e.g. with IV fluid resuscitation, analgesia, oxygen supplementation, potentially exogenous or autologous blood transfusion, and placement of an abdominal wrap) will be required at the outset, though the owner has already stated severe cost constraints. Decision-making may be aided with three-view thoracic radiography once Jason is stable, as the detection of metastatic disease signifies a grave prognosis. Progression to exploratory laparotomy with an option for intraoperative euthanasia would be a rational way forward, but immediate euthanasia at this point is also justified as, unfortunately, the outlook for Jason is likely to be poor. Despite the constraints discussed by the owner at the outset, this is an emotionally charged situation. It is still important to explain the options, costs, and benefits. All things considered, this could be a case for euthanasia without further intervention.

REFERENCES

Millar, S. L., Curley, T. L., Monnet, E. L. & Zersen, K. M. (2022) Premature death in dogs with nontraumatic hemoabdomen and splenectomy with benign histopathologic findings. *Journal of the American Veterinary Medical Association* 260(S1):S9–S14. doi: 10.2460/javma.21.01.0033.

Pratschke, K. (2020) Approach to haemoabdomen in small animal patients. *In Practice* **42**(1):5–19. doi: 10.1136/inp.l6819.

3.3 Flora, 6-yo FE Cross-breed: in labour *CARE*

a) With a patient like Flora, the advantages for sedation/premedication include a compliant, stress-free patient at induction and the fact that less general anaesthetic drugs will be required during the procedure, i.e. the

principles of balanced anaesthesia apply in caesarean section as in other surgeries. Disadvantages theoretically include longer exposure of puppies to depressant drugs. Ultimately, you want the safest induction and maintenance of anaesthesia for the patient, puppies, and staff. Fighting and struggling with a distressed or aggressive dog in stage 2 labour is neither medically nor ethically acceptable, so Flora should be premedicated appropriately.

b) It is best to avoid drugs that cannot be reversed, or to use them in very low doses, but with Flora we do need adequate sedation to ensure that she can be handled safely. Acepromazine should be avoided as it can cause prolonged sedation, and the vasodilation seen with this drug can also exacerbate hypotension, and may exacerbate aggression (Simon et al. 2014). There is also no reversal agent available. Full μ-opioid receptor agonists (methadone, morphine, pethidine) are very good choices as they are reversible with naloxone and have minimal cardiovascular effects. They will provide some sedation when used alone, but in a dog like Flora another drug will probably be required. Benzodiazepines (Figure A3.3a) can be effective with opioids in sick or debilitated animals (and can be reversed with flumazenil), but will be less effective with aggressive dogs like Flora. Medetomidine or dexmedetomidine (avoid xylazine) could be cautiously used at a low dose such as 10–20 μg/kg, in combination with an opioid. In combination with opioids, these drugs can cause profound sedation, but are quickly reversible with atipamezole. If reversing these drugs during the anaesthetic, be aware that the patient may make a rapid return to consciousness if being maintained on low levels of a volatile agent. It is therefore prudent to have more IV induction agent to hand.

c) Use rapid IV induction with propofol or alfaxolone (neither has advantage over the other) after a few minutes of pre-oxygenation. Administer an anti-emetic (e.g. maropitant) with the premedication and beware of regurgitation immediately after

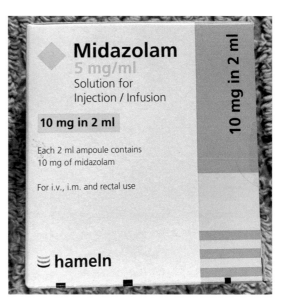

Figure A3.3a The benzodiazepine/opioid combination is a good choice for sick or debilitated animals, but would be unlikely to provide adequate sedation in Flora's case.

induction: use the reverse Trendelenburg position (elevating the head above the pelvic limbs) and intubate with a well-fitting, cuffed endotracheal tube. Local anaesthetic techniques are suitable and anaesthetic-sparing; use low-end doses as these drugs undergo some placental transfer (Grubb & Lobprise 2020). Use the lowest effective levels of volatile agent as high levels may depress the neonatal respiratory system. This volatile-sparing effect is a good argument for opioid premedication in caesarean section. Do not induce by mask. This is likely to result in resistance, intense struggles, and adrenaline release, with risk of regurgitation. Other disadvantages of mask induction include the need to use very high settings on the vaporiser, thereby increasing the risk of exposure of veterinary staff to anaesthetic gases.

d) The appearance, pulse, grimace, activity, respiration (Apgar) scoring system for neonates is useful (Table A3.3).

Table A3.3 **The Apgar scoring system for canine neonates: a combined assessment is made across the five criteria. Scores of <7 are associated with a poorer survival (Veronesi 2016)**

	SCORE OF 0	SCORE OF 1	SCORE OF 2
HR	<180	180–220	>220
RR	<6, silent	6–15, quiet crying	>15, strong vocal
Reflexes	Absent	Present	Vigorous
Movement	None	Some	Active
MMs	Cyanotic	Pale	Pink

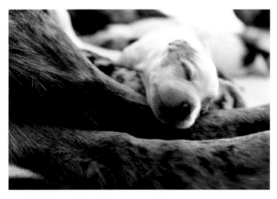

Figure A3.3c The hoped-for result post-caesarean is a comfortable and relaxed dam and litter.

REFERENCES

Grubb, T. & Lobprise, H. (2020) Local and regional anaesthesia in dogs and cats: descriptions of specific local and regional techniques (Part 2). *Veterinary Medicine and Science* **6**(2):218–234. doi: 10.1002/vms3.218.

Simon, B. T., Scallan, E. M., Siracusa, C. et al. (2014) Effects of acepromazine or methadone on midazolam-induced behavioral reactions in dogs. *Canadian Veterinary Journal* **55**(9):875–885.

Veronesi, M. C. (2016) Assessment of canine neonatal viability – the Apgar score. *Reproduction in Domesticated Animals* **51**(Suppl. 1):46–50. doi: 10.1111/rda.12787.

Resuscitation techniques for puppies

- Clear airway (head down, mild suction with bulb syringe)
- Gentle rubbing of puppies with warm towels simulates licking by the mother
- Insert and rotate an orange or insulin needle in the nasal philtrum acupuncture point GV26 (Renzhong point) at the base of the nose. Insert until bone is felt (Figure A3.3b)

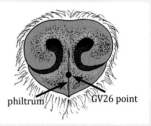
philtrum   GV26 point

Figure A3.3b The GV26 Renzhong acupuncture point.

- Administer naloxone (one drop, sublingually) to depressed neonates if opioids have been given to the mother
- 1 drop of 1:10,000 adrenaline sublingually may be administered to neonates for cardiovascular stimulation
- Provide flow-by oxygen or brief intubation
- Provide forced warm air blanket or heat pad
- Place puppies back with the dam as soon as possible (Figure A3.3c)

Remember to explain to owners that no anaesthetic drugs are specifically licensed for use in caesarean section, to ensure fully informed consent.

3.4 Ned, 16-wo ME Miniature Poodle Cross: vomiting ++

a) A lateral radiograph including the thoracic and abdominal cavities is shown. There is gas in the stomach and three discrete gas accumulations in the small intestines. One of these gas shadows terminates at a U-shaped radiopaque mass. The intestines appear generally thickened; there are normal-appearing faeces in the large intestine. The thoracic cavity appears normal and no abnormalities of the musculoskeletal system are observable. Based on the history and radiographic findings, a diagnosis of GIT obstruction with a foreign body is made. Recommended treatment is exploratory laparotomy to remove the foreign body.

b) A ventral midline coeliotomy is the standard approach for exploratory laparotomy in small animals. The process is as follows:

1. An incision is made through the skin from the umbilicus to approximately 2–3 cm cranial to the pubic rim. The linea alba is identified and incised along a similar length. The incision may be extended cranially to approximately 2 cm caudal to the xiphoid and caudally almost to the pubis, if required. In male animals, the skin incision deviates laterally to avoid the prepuce and the preputial blood vessel is ligated. The reflected penis and prepuce allows caudal extension of the linea alba incision on the midline. The use of self-retaining retractors or a second surgeon to assist with retraction facilitates visibility and isolation of structures.

2. The entire GIT from the stomach to rectum should be checked for obstructions. This can be done by gentle palpation and running the intestines between the thumb and forefinger. The intestines should also be observed for discolouration and peristaltic motility.

3. Obstructed intestine is exteriorised from the abdomen and packed off with moistened large, laparotomy sponges. Any spillage can thus be safely contained. The obstructed section is observed closely for viability based on assessment of perfusion and motility. There are no set rules on viability; however, intestine that is non-motile on palpation and red-brown to purple in colour has a poor prognosis for viability.

4. Provided the intestinal segment is assessed to be viable, then an enterotomy can be performed to remove the foreign body. A linear incision is made through the intestinal wall opposite the mesenteric attachment (an 'anti-mesenteric' incision). The incision should be made just distal to the obstruction such that it is in viable, healthy intestine to aid rapid healing. The incision should be long enough to enable the obstruction to be removed without too much pressure. The obstruction is gently massaged out of the incision.

5. The intestine should be lavaged with sterile saline and reassessed for viability. As a general rule, intestine that was questionable will often look much more viable once the obstruction is removed, so do not rush this stage and allow the tissue time to recover.

6. If the intestine is assessed to be non-viable, then the non-viable segment should be excised and an end-to-end anastomosis performed. In Ned's case, an enterotomy was all that was required.

7. Using gentle digital pressure, or suitably guarded atraumatic forceps, the intestinal lumen is gently occluded proximal and distal to the enterotomy. 3/0 or 4/0 synthetic absorbable suture material is suitable for performing the

closure. A simple continuous closure is performed with full thickness bites of the intestine wall no further than 3 mm apart. The closed intestine is lavaged again with warm sterile saline. An omental patch can be placed by mobilising some of the greater omentum, wrapping the repaired intestine, and loosely tacking the omentum with suture material (Figure A3.4).

8. The intestine can now be returned to the abdomen. If suction is available, then the abdomen can be flushed with warm saline. Abdominal flush should be removed as much as possible with suction.

9. The abdomen is closed routinely using simple continuous or simple interrupted sutures in the linea alba using a synthetic, absorbable, monofilament suture of suitable duration of effectiveness for this closure, e.g. polydioxanone (PDS). The SC and skin layers are closed routinely.

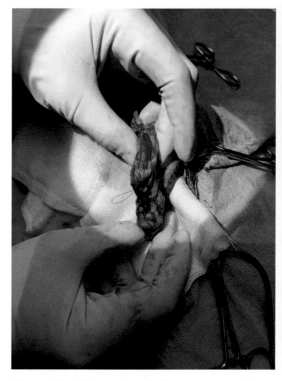

Figure A3.4 A loosely tacked omentum patch applied to the enterotomy incision.

c) Ned has undergone major abdominal surgery and will require regular monitoring. He should be contained/rested appropriately at home and given lead exercise only. The wound should be checked by the owner at least twice daily and a clinic recheck scheduled for 2–3 days after discharge.

- **Antibiotic usage**. Enterotomy is a clean-contaminated procedure. The use of a broad-spectrum perioperative antibiotic such as an augmented penicillin is appropriate for perioperative use. Provided there is no gross contamination during surgery, then there is no indication for post-operative antibiotics.

- **Pain relief**. Appropriate analgesia with opiate medications should occur intraoperatively and post-operatively. Maropitant (1 mg/kg SC or IV) may provide some degree of visceral analgesia in both dogs and cats. In dogs, paracetamol can be used safely at 10–15 mg/kg IV q8h as a post-operative analgesic following surgery (Hernández-Avalos et al. 2020). Depending on the patient, judicious NSAID use may be considered.

- **Nausea** can be a common cause of post-operative morbidity following GIT surgery. Ondansetron can be used in addition to maropitant. If post-operative ileus is suspected (usually confirmed on abdominal ultrasound), metoclopramide may be administered as a constant rate infusion (CRI).

- **Omeprazole** can be helpful to reduce GIT acidity, reflux, and ulceration.

- **Fluid therapy** and **feeding** post-operatively: oral food and water can and should be offered as soon as possible post-operatively to promote gut healing and prevent ileus. IV fluids should be continued at maintenance fluid rates until oral water consumption is observed and urination is normal. Vomiting, abdominal pain, malaise, dehydration despite fluids, or any signs of shock should prompt immediate re-examination and review, as these can be signs of post-operative peritonitis (DePompeo et al. 2018).

REFERENCES

DePompeo, C. M., Bond, L., George, Y. E. et al. (2018) Intra-abdominal complications following intestinal anastomoses by suture and staple techniques in dogs. *Journal of the American Veterinary Medical Association* **253**(4):437–443. doi:10.2460/javma.253.4.437.

Hernández-Avalos, I., Valverde, A., Ibancovichi-Camarillo, J. A. et al. (2020) Clinical evaluation of postoperative analgesia, cardiorespiratory parameters and changes in liver and renal function tests of paracetamol compared to meloxicam and carprofen in dogs undergoing ovariohysterectomy. *PLoS One* **15**:e0223697. doi: 10.1371/journal.pone.0223697.

3.5 Nigel, 10-yo MN DSH: nail trim

a) Chronic musculoskeletal pain, such as that caused by degenerative joint disease, trauma, or injury, may reduce normal wear and scratching behaviour by which cats normally regulate the length of their nails. This can lead to thickening of nails, or even ingrown nails (Ray et al. 2021).

b) Once the nail has been clipped and the component penetrating the digital pad removed, antibiotics are generally not indicated. The wound can be cleaned with an antiseptic such as dilute povidone-iodine. It is important to assess Nigel by taking a history from his owner and performing a complete physical examination. The owner may have noted that Nigel has been less active, or behaving differently (e.g. avoiding jumping or not using his scratching post). All nails should be checked, as multiple ingrown nails are not uncommon in older cats. As chronic pain can be difficult to detect in cats, orthopaedic examination under sedation and survey radiographs may be helpful. If suitable, analgesia can be dispensed. For musculoskeletal pain, analgesics may include NSAIDs, gabapentin or pregabalin, or monoclonal antibodies targeting nerve growth factor. If Nigel is overweight, weight reduction should be instituted (Gruen et al. 2022). In addition, Nigel's nails should be monitored and trimmed regularly. Environmental modification, such as provision of horizontal scratching surfaces, may be beneficial.

c) Aside from monitoring Nigel's nails, assessing his pain prior to and during treatment can be useful in determining the impact of analgesia and guiding future treatment. Owners can complete the Feline Musculoskeletal Pain Index online (see the supplementary material of Enomoto et al. 2022).

d) If Nigel's owner has limited funds, you might consider proceeding with a treatment trial with an NSAID, as long as Nigel is systemically well, has no history of PU/PD, and has a good appetite. It would be helpful to assess Nigel's urea, creatinine, and USG to screen for CKD prior to commencing a treatment trial, but if this is not possible, the client should be counselled about the potential risks of exacerbating existing kidney disease by administering an NSAID. Nigel's pain can be scored by the client at home, and the client can also commence weight reduction and regular weighing of Nigel. Nigel's home environment can be modified to improve his mobility (e.g. placement of non-slip rugs, ramps, or stairs to access resting spots and ensure easy access to food and litter trays). Depending on Nigel's temperament and the owner's capabilities, they may be able to learn to trim Nigel's nails at home. However, if Nigel is receiving ongoing analgesia for chronic pain (e.g. that associated with degenerative joint disease), he will require regular veterinary check-ups.

REFERENCES

Enomoto, M., Lascelles, B. D. X., Robertson, J. B. & Gruen, M. E. (2022) Refinement of the feline musculoskeletal pain index (FMPI) and development of the short-form FMPI. *Journal of Feline Medicine and Surgery* **24**(2):142–151. doi: 10.1177/1098612X211011984.

Gruen, M. E., Lascelles, B. D. X., Colleran, E. et al. (2022) 2022 AAHA Pain Management Guidelines for Dogs and Cats. *Journal of the American Animal Hospital Association* **58**(2):55–76. doi: 10.5326/jaaha-ms-7292.

Ray, M., Carney, H. C., Boynton, B. et al. (2021) 2021 AAFP Feline Senior Care Guidelines. *Journal of Feline Medicine and Surgery* **23**(10):613–638. doi: 10.1177/1098612X211021538.

3.6 Donald, 2-yo MN Old English Bulldog: routine vacc

a) If this behaviour has been inadvertently reinforced, then it could be attention-seeking in nature. Humping is also considered to be a displacement behaviour that is displayed when a dog is feeling uncertain or conflicted during a social interaction. It can also be displayed when a dog is suffering from abdominal pain or musculoskeletal discomfort.

b) The fluctuations in the frequency of the humping behaviour and inconsistency of the noise sensitivity suggest that these are being impacted by a physical problem. The fact that the humping behaviour can occur from rest without any apparent external trigger is also suspicious of a physical cause. If an animal is suffering from a physical problem, e.g. musculoskeletal pain, then they are likely to be more sensitive to any triggers within their environment. Chronic pain can vary with a dog's level of exercise or other factors. This in turn will have an impact on the frequency/intensity of problem behaviours that are either a direct result of the pain or to which the pain is contributing.

c) It would be appropriate to consider an analgesic trial for Donald. Usually this would consist of 2–4 weeks on an NSAID as a first-line treatment if appropriate. It is essential that the client keeps a diary of the frequency and intensity of problem behaviours during this time, as well as noting the presence of any musculoskeletal signs, e.g. when jumping onto furniture. Reduction or elimination of the behaviour with NSAID administration is supportive of physical pain as a trigger. Not all pain responds to NSAIDs (e.g. neuropathic pain or bone pain due to malignancy can be very refractory), so a lack of response does not rule out pain and a multimodal analgesic trial may be required.

d) Any triggers for the humping behaviour should be identified and minimised. The clients could also cover their windows with frosted film and play white noise/music to help to reduce the frequency of the barking at the window. The clients should be advised not to punish Donald's humping behaviour but to turn/move slowly away from him without saying anything. It may be necessary to use a houseline to help to facilitate this, i.e. Donald's harness is left on and attached to a long light lead that can then be used to help to move him behind a barrier such as a door or baby gate without confrontation when the problem behaviour occurs.

REFERENCES

Ackerman, L. J. & Landsberg, G. M. (2023) Chapter 2, Developmental, Social and Communicative Behaviour. In: Ackerman, L. J. & Landsberg, G. M. (eds) *Behavior Problems of the Dog and Cat*, 4th edition. Philadelphia, PA: Saunders.

Lopes Fagundes, A. L., Hewison, L., McPeake, K. J. et al. (2018) Noise sensitivities in dogs: an exploration of signs in dogs with and without musculoskeletal pain using qualitative content analysis. *Frontiers in Veterinary Science* 5:17. doi: 10.3389/fvets.2018.00017.

Mills, D. S., Demontigny-Bédard, I., Gruen, M. et al. (2020) Pain and problem behavior in cats and dogs. *Animals* 10(2):318. doi: 10.3390/ani10020318.

3.7 Gladys, 6-yo FN Australian Shepherd: new dog check-up

a) The menace response tests vision, as this requires the central and peripheral visual pathways, visual cortex, and both the optic nerve (cranial nerve II) and the facial nerve (cranial nerve VII) to be intact. The pupillary light reflex can be normal in cortically blind animals, and therefore does not rule out blindness. The menace response should be assessed independently in each eye, by covering the other eye. It is performed by making a rapid movement towards the eye, taking care not to cause air movement or contact eyelashes or fur, as this can result in a false-positive response. False-negative responses can occur in cases where the facial nerve is paralysed, hence it is important to assess the palpebral reflex. Menace may also be absent in animals aged <12 weeks. The presence/absence of vision can also be tested by creating a simple obstacle course in the consulting room, covering one eye with a patch, and encouraging the dog to navigate the course in both light and dark conditions. Alternatively, the visual placing response can be assessed in dogs that can be lifted, by moving the animal towards a table. Dogs with vision will lift their legs to stand on the surface as it approaches, whereas those that cannot see will not move their legs as the table approaches.

b) OD = oculus dexter (right eye), OS = oculus sinister (left eye), and OU = oculus uterque (both eyes).

c) IOP can vary depending on the instrument used for measurement. In one study, healthy dogs had IOP ranging from 12 to 24 mmHg when measured with a Schiøtz tonometer (mean 16.3 ± 2.1 mmHg), and 11–25 mmHg when measured with a Tono-Pen Vet tonometer (mean 18.1 ± 3.8 mmHg) (Wrześniewska et al. 2018).

d) Heterochromia iridium, or variation in colour between two eyes, is typically a congenital condition, arising from the incomplete maturation or absence of pigment granules in the iris stroma or anterior pigmented layer of the iris (Miller 2008).

e) In some dog breeds, e.g. Dalmatians, Australian Cattle Dogs, Australian Shepherds, English Setters, Boston Terriers, Old English Sheepdogs and Bulldogs, it is associated with congenital deafness (Miller 2008).

REFERENCES

Miller, P. E. 2008. Uvea. In: Maggs, D. J., Miller, P. E. & Ofri, R. (eds) *Slatter's Fundamentals of Veterinary Ophthalmology*, 4th edition. St Louis, MO: Saunders.

Wrześniewska K., Madany, J. & Winiarczyk, D. (2018) Comparison of intraocular pressure measurement with Schiotz tonometer and Tono-Pen Vet Tonometer in healthy dogs. *Journal of Veterinary Research* **62**(2):243–247. doi: 10.2478/jvetres-2018-0018.

3.8 Padme, 10-yo FN Chihuahua: post-op check, not doing well

a) Delayed drug metabolism, cerebral depression (both of which can prolong anaesthetic recovery), cardiovascular dysfunction, impaired perfusion, respiratory compromise, and increased incidence of wound infection are all adverse effects of hypothermia in the anaesthetised and surgical patient (Grubb et al. 2020).

b) Heat pads, electric mats, electric blankets, wheat packs, and hot water bottles (including those improvised from gloves) have all been associated with burns in veterinary patients (Dunlop et al. 1989). Anaesthetised patients are not able to adjust their position to move away from a static heat source that is causing tissue damage. Wet animals are at an increased risk of being burned as water conducts heat.

c) Convective or forced-air warm blanket systems (such as Bair Huggers) or circulating warm water blankets are currently the most effective patient heating methods (Grubb et al. 2020). Supplemental methods include warming IV fluids, using a fluid-line warmer, and insulating the patient's extremities using bubble wrap and/or baby socks (Grubb et al. 2020). As sedation and premedication cause heat loss via depression of the hypothalamus, it is important to keep patients in a warm environment in the perioperative period. It should feel noticeably warm to humans in scrub suits.

d) The shape of the lesion and the development of an eschar are highly suggestive of a thermal burn. Other differentials to consider include toxic epidermal necrolysis, erythema multiforme, ischaemic dermatopathies, pressure necrosis, or an autoimmune blistering disease such as pemphigus vulgaris or bullous pemphigoid (Gomes 2019). You would need to perform biopsies to rule out these conditions, but in Padme's case, the history of a recent long operation is highly suggestive. It is critical to establish what heating source(s) were used during surgery on Padme.

e) Padme requires significant treatment. A large area of her body is affected, and burns tend to progress. Several weeks later, the lesion appeared as pictured in Figure A3.8. The central concern is Padme's immediate welfare. She has lost a significant amount of weight (18.4% of her body weight), is likely to be suffering from significant pain, and may develop infection and scarring. It is important to evaluate her systemic health (a CBC/multiple biochemical analysis [MBA] and urinalysis are recommended) and prioritise treatment of systemic disease. You will also need to develop an analgesia plan. It would be helpful to talk to the practice management team, insurers, and specialists, and discuss the plan with the owners. Adverse events like this can be discussed confidentially in morbidity and mortality meetings. Padme's treatment may require surgical excision of eschar and scar tissue, wound management, antimicrobial treatment, and supportive care. In addition to a treatment plan, it is essential to establish a communication plan so that both Padme's owners and the veterinary team know who will be communicating, how that communication will take place (e.g. hospital visits, telephone, email, or a combination), and how frequently it will occur. The owners should be informed of the outcome of the internal investigation regarding the source of heat, and any changes made to protocols based on the findings of that investigation.

REFERENCES

Dunlop, C. I., Daunt, D. A. & Haskins, S. C. (1989) Thermal burns in four dogs during anesthesia. *Veterinary Surgery* **18**(3):242–246. doi: 10.1111/j.1532-950x.1989.tb01079.x.

Gomes, P. (2019) Burns. *Clinician's Brief*. Available at: www.cliniciansbrief.com/article/burns.

Grubb, T., Sager, J., Gaynor, J. S. et al. (2020) 2020 AAHA Anesthesia and Monitoring Guidelines for Dogs and Cats. *Journal of the American Animal Hospital Association* **56**(2):59–82. doi: 10.5326/jaaha-ms-7055.

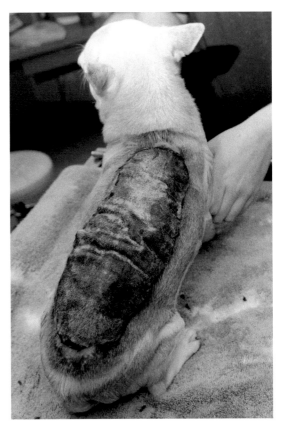

Figure A3.8 Progression of the burn several weeks later. The dramatic and distressing appearance is typical of severe burns.

3.9 Evie, 1-yo FE Border Collie: lap spay admit

a) Traditional OVH involves making a midline incision and removing the ovaries and the uterus. Ligatures are placed to control haemorrhage. Laparoscopic ovariectomy involves creating two or three small incisions and, using a camera and cautery tool, removing the ovaries only (Figure A3.9).

b) **Advantages**
- Less manipulation of tissue and associated haemorrhage
- Increased visualisation of tissue in situ
- Reduced exposure and contamination of abdominal tissues
- Less post-operative pain (Phypers 2017)
- Faster return to normal activity levels
- Reduced post-operative complications (operator dependent)

Disadvantages
- Increased cost to purchase and maintain equipment
- Establishment of a pneumoperitoneum impacts ventilation (Fernández-Martín et al. 2022)
- Additional surgeon training needed
- Additional anaesthetist training needed
- Larger area of fur clipped

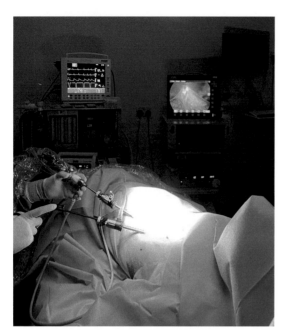

Figure A3.9 Evie's laparoscopic spay underway.

c) The two-port procedure is as follows:
1. Prepare for surgery with a ventral midline clip and chlorhexidine scrub.
2. Insert Veress needle midway between xiphoid process and umbilicus. Insufflate the abdomen to 10–12 mmHg with CO_2.
3. Place caudal port 1 cm caudal to the umbilicus.
4. Remove Veress needle and replace with cranial port – connect to CO_2 insufflation cable. Turn patient onto right lateral recumbency.
5. Place Babcock forceps into caudal port and telescope into cranial port to identify and grasp, with the Babcock's, the left ovarian bursa.
6. Raise the ovary to the ventral body wall with the forceps and isolate it by passing the ovariectomy hook through the left side of body wall and then through the left ovarian bursa. The hook is used to tack the ovarian bursa to the body wall so that the forceps are not needed any more and the caudal port can be used for the ligating tool instead.

7. Remove the forceps and place cautery tool (LigaSure™) into the caudal port. Cauterise and cut below the ovary – through the suspensory ligament and uterus. Check for any haemorrhage.
8. Remove cautery tool and replace with Babcock forceps into caudal port and grasp ovary. Remove ovariectomy hook.
9. Remove ovary and caudal port together – using artery forceps to grasp and manipulate the ovary to remove if needed.
10. Replace caudal port and check entire left ovary removed.
11. Turn patient onto left lateral recumbency and repeat process for right ovary.
12. Return to dorsal recumbency before suturing muscle and SC layers with PDS. The skin can be closed with suture glue or with an intradermal suture such as Monocryl.

d) Possible complications are as follows:
• Gas embolism
• Increased airway resistance (from insufflation of abdomen)
• Iatrogenic trauma to spleen
• Usual abdominal surgery complications – haemorrhage, infection, wound breakdown

e) Post-operative care involves the following:
• Post-operative pain relief (e.g. NSAID) for 3–5 days
• Restricted exercise for 7 days
• Pet medical T-shirt or Elizabethan collar to prevent licking of the wound if needed
• Post-operative check-up 7 days after surgery

f) Equipment needed:
• Carbon dioxide insufflator
• Trocars (5 mm or 10 mm) × 2
• Insufflation cable
• Laparoscopy tower and screen
• Light cable
• Laparoscope – telescope and camera
• Vessel sealing device, e.g. LigaSure™
• Babcock forceps

- Blunt-ended palpation probe
- Veress needle
- Ovariectomy hook
- Camera sheath
- Standard equipment required for surgery – needle holders, Mayo scissors, 2 × artery forceps, scalpel blade (number 11) and holder, rat-tooth forceps, towel clamp
- Surgical drapes
- Suture material – PDS and/or Monocryl
- Suture glue (optional)

Missing items

- Vessel sealing device
- Camera head (cable is in photo)

REFERENCES

Charlesworth, M. & Sanchez, F. (2019) A comparison of the rates of postoperative complications between dogs undergoing laparoscopic and open ovariectomy. *Journal of Small Animal Practice* **60**(4):218–222. doi: 10.1111/jsap.12993.

Devitt, C. M., Cox, R. E. & Hailey, J. J. (2005) Duration, complications, stress and pain of open ovariohysterectomy versus a simple method of laparoscopic-assisted ovariohysterectomy in dogs. *Journal of the American Veterinary Medical Association* **227**(6):921–927. doi: 10.2460/javma.2005.227.921.

Fernández-Martín, S., Valiño-Cultelli, V. & González-Cantalapiedra, A. (2022) Laparoscopic versus open ovariectomy in bitches: changes in cardiorespiratory values, blood parameters, and sevoflurane requirements associated with the surgical technique. *Animals* **12**(11):1438. doi: 10.3390/ani12111438.

Phypers, C. (2017) In cats and dogs does laparoscopic ovariectomy offer advantages over open ovariectomy for postoperative recovery? *Veterinary Evidence* **2**(2). doi: 10.18849/ve.v2i2.59.

Woodlands, C. (2018) Laparoscopic spay. *Veterinary Nursing Journal* **33**(2):56–60. doi: 10.1080/17415349.2017.1395135.

3.10 Phil, 10-yo MN Maltese Chihuahua: lame HLs

a) Patellar luxation is most commonly a developmental disorder (Kowaleski et al. 2017). Most affected patients are small-breed dogs, though patellar luxation does occur in large-breed dogs, in whom patellas may luxate laterally, and occasionally in cats. Medial patellar luxation is the most common form. Malalignment of the quadriceps mechanism can lead to anatomical changes of the distal femur (including the trochlear groove in which the patella usually sits) and proximal tibia, causing patellar instability. Intermittent luxation of the patella can cause wear of the medial trochlear ridge, leading to a shallower and narrower trochlear groove and further increasing the risk of luxation (Kowaleski et al. 2017). Patellar luxation can also be secondary to conditions or treatments that cause laxity of the extensor mechanism of the stifle, including a congenitally decreased angle of the inclination of the femoral neck, hip luxation, or femoral head excision (Vasseur 2003). Less commonly, patellar luxation can occur secondary to trauma to the stifle joint capsule or fascia, causing femoropatellar instability. Acute traumatic patellar luxation can be lateral, medial, or bidirectional, but would be expected to be associated with non-weight-bearing lameness and pain on joint manipulation (Vasseur 2003). It may also occur secondary to surgical treatment of cranial cruciate ligament disease or fractures of the femur or tibia (Di Dona et al. 2018).

b) Phil has grade II patellar luxation. The grading system is outlined in Table A3.10.

c) The owner's rubbing of Phil's leg will have accidentally replaced the luxated patella. It is not unusual for dogs to become agitated in this way when the patella luxates in grade II luxations.

Table A3.10 **Grades of medial patellar luxation in small animals (adapted from Vasseur 2003 and Kowaleski et al. 2017)**

GRADE	DESCRIPTION
I	• This may be an incidental finding • The patella can be manually luxated, but returns to the normal position when released • There is no crepitus and bony deformities are not present
II	• This may cause intermittent lameness of varying severity, often described as a 'skipping lameness' • The patella luxates with internal tibial rotation upon stifle flexion or when the patella is manually pushed over the trochlear ridge • The patella remains luxated until the stifle is extended, or until the patella is manually replaced with stifle joint extension and external rotation • If present, skeletal deformities are mild and may include femoral varus, tibial valgus, and internal tibial rotation at the stifle joint • Bony deformities can progress, leading to more severe lameness or increased grade of patellar luxation • Cranial cruciate ligament rupture may occur
III	• This may be associated with mild, moderate, or severe lameness • The patella is continuously luxated during ambulation • It can be manually replaced, but will re-luxate spontaneously when manual pressure is removed • Skeletal deformities are present, and include femoral varus, tibial valgus, and internal tibial rotation at the stifle joint • Affected dogs may carry the leg in a semi-flexed position or walk with a crouched gait to use the leg in a semi-flexed, internally rotated position
IV	• This is associated with severe lameness • The patella is permanently luxated and cannot be manually replaced • Severe bony deformities are present, including include femoral varus, tibial valgus, and internal tibial rotation at the stifle joint

Varus: limb or part deviated in a medial direction.
Valgus: limb or part deviated in a lateral direction.

d) Survey radiographs of the stifles, and of the hips and hocks, can confirm luxation, and can be used to assess the presence and degree of bony deformities or degenerative changes in the joints of the hindlimbs (Figure A3.10a,b). They may also evidence previous surgical procedures. Views should include the following:
• Lateral stifle: assess position of patella in trochlear groove
• Craniocaudal stifle (including the femur and tibia): screen for varus or valgus deformity of long bones and assess whether patella is medial or lateral to the distal femur.

• A 'skyline' view of the patella in the trochlear groove (to assess trochlear ridges and depth of the trochlea) may be used pre- and post-operatively when surgery is performed, but is not carried out routinely (Kowaleski et al. 2017).

e) While grade I medial patellar luxation does not require surgical treatment, and grade IV often requires surgical treatment, management of grades II and III medial patellar luxation is more dependent on individual patient factors (Kowaleski et al. 2017). Given the lack of pain in Phil, and the small size of the patient, conservative treatment (including NSAIDs or other analgesics, as appropriate), together with exercises designed to strengthen the quadriceps mechanism, may be the most appropriate option. Weight management is not required for Phil, but should be considered if needed on an individual basis

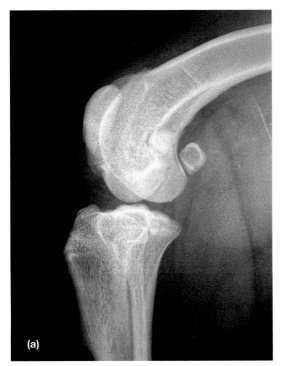

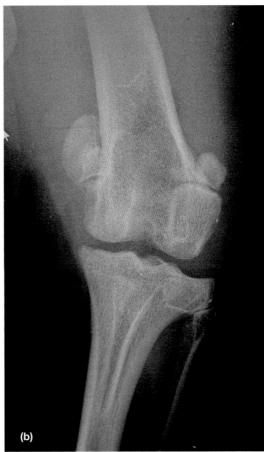

Figure A3.10a,b **Mediolateral and craniocaudal radiographs of the right stifle of a larger dog, demonstrating a medially luxated patella.**

in all patients in order to reduce excess loading of joints. If lameness increases in frequency or the patient's mobility is impaired, surgery should be considered.

The aim of surgery is to restore normal function of the quadriceps mechanism relative to the distal hindlimb, and to stabilise the patella within the trochlear groove of the femur. In growing animals, there is a risk that bony surgical techniques could damage the distal femoral or proximal tibial physes (Kowaleski et al. 2017). In small patients, soft tissue surgery (e.g. lateral imbrication) may be adequate, but in many cases, orthopaedic surgery, such as deepening of the trochlear groove or tibial tuberosity transposition and other procedures, may be required. In bilateral

cases, procedures may be performed concurrently or staged. Post-operatively, the limbs should be bandaged for several days. Activity should be restricted for 6–8 weeks and analgesia administered.

REFERENCES

Di Dona, F., Della Valle, G. & Fatone, G. (2018) Patellar luxation in dogs. *Veterinary Medicine (Auckland)* 9:23–32. doi: 10.2147/vmrr.S142545.

Kowaleski, M. P., Boudrieau, R. J. & Pozzi, A. (2017) Stifle Joint. In: Johnston, S. A. & Tobias, K. M. (eds) *Veterinary Surgery: Small Animal Expert Consult* (e-book). Philadelphia, PA: Elsevier.

Vasseur, P. B. (2003) Stifle Joint. In: Slatter, D. & Holmburg, D. L. (eds) *Textbook of Small Animal Surgery*, 3rd edition. Philadelphia, PA: Saunders.

3.11 Franco, 6-yo MN Poodle: still not right

a) One of the impacts of the 'hidden curriculum' in veterinary training is that it can lead prospective veterinarians to believe that there is always a definitive diagnosis, a 'right' approach to case management, or a 'gold-standard' approach against which other approaches are considered deficient or wanting. Yet there are many potential sources of uncertainty in veterinary general practice. These include decision-making around diagnostic modalities and treatment options when there are multiple options available; managing incidental, unexpected, or ambiguous findings; prognosticating and predicting the effects of both disease and disease management on individual patients (including the probability of certain outcomes); and questions around the best interests of the patient, in particular in the context of the human–animal relationship. Contextual factors that impact our decision-making can increase uncertainty. These include clinician factors (such as fatigue, hunger, physical discomfort, communication skills), client factors (communication skills, expectations and assumptions about veterinary care, finances), factors arising from interpersonal communication (such as misinterpretation, confusion, or conflict), and other factors (such as time constraints, interruptions, and distractions) (Scott et al. 2023).

b) Potential negative impacts of intolerance to uncertainty include poor decision-making, increased vulnerability to cognitive biases, premature referral, inappropriate resource use (e.g. performing unnecessary diagnostic tests or prescribing inappropriate treatment), and avoidance of decision-making (or avoiding cases we feel uncertain about) (Gheihman et al. 2020, Scott et al. 2023). In addition, among healthcare workers, uncertainty is linked to higher levels of distress and burnout, reduced self-compassion, and disengagement from the workplace (Scott et al. 2023).

c) Potential strategies for diagnosing and managing uncertainty in veterinary general practice are listed in Table A3.11.

Table A3.11 **Potential strategies for diagnosing and managing uncertainty in veterinary general practice (adapted from Scott et al. 2023 and Gheihman et al. 2020)**	
STRATEGY	**EXAMPLES**
Consider your emotional or 'gut' reactions to uncertainty	• Reflect on recent cases about which you have felt uncertainty, discomfort, or uneasiness. Which elements of the case do you think contributed to these feelings? Why? • Did you respond maladaptively (e.g. through premature case closure or avoidance) or adaptively (e.g. with curiosity and information-seeking)?
Identify cognitive biases	• Cognitive biases are heuristics, mental shortcuts, or 'rules of thumb' that may be based on false assumptions. • Many cognitive biases have been described, including premature case closure (e.g. finding a single foreign body in the abdomen of a dog, removing it, and closing the site before exploring the remainder of the abdomen), confirmation bias (accepting only information that confirms one's original or favoured diagnosis, and ignoring or rejecting information that might challenge this assessment), and the representativeness heuristic (in which a patient's presentation is compared with a 'typical' case of a condition, without considering atypical presentations). • Ask yourself: What is the basis of my decision? • Is there anything that I have overlooked or dismissed, or that does not quite support my decision-making?

STRATEGY	EXAMPLES
Anticipate and prepare for uncertainty	• Are there types of cases that you avoid or that you would like to avoid (e.g. types of presentations such as musculoskeletal conditions, or types of cases such as endocrinopathies)? Why? • What factors would make you more comfortable with these cases (e.g. additional scientific knowledge, continuing professional development or practical training)? • Could you plan your continuing professional development to address these concerns?
Categorise the type of uncertainty	• Scientific uncertainty (knowledge about diagnosis, treatment, and prognosis) is best addressed using evidence (e.g. knowledge summaries or critically appraised topic summaries, review articles, guidelines if available or subject matter experts such as specialists). • Practical uncertainty (about delivering care) is best addressed by discussing with the client, practice managers, or senior team members. • Interpersonal uncertainty requires a context-specific approach that may involve further discussion, including involvement of other team members, and potentially those within the client's network.
Let go of the need for absolute certainty	• Absolute certainty is rare in clinical practice (e.g. it is rare to definitively diagnose the source of acute gastroenteritis in small animal patients). • Be flexible in the degree of certainty required – it may be enough to rule out certain conditions (through clinical reasoning and diagnostic testing) and be confident about the body systems involved. • Develop the skills to justify, and review, a working hypothesis or presumptive diagnosis.
Triage uncertainty	• Manage those uncertainties that are important to the current presentation, and review others later (e.g. once the patient is stable – this is 'sequential care').
Utilise safety-netting and follow-up	• Management plans should plan for uncertainty and contingencies. For example, what if a test result is negative or inconclusive? What if the patient does not improve with treatment? What if they get worse? • Ask yourself, 'If I am right, what do I expect to happen?' and 'If I am wrong, what might happen and what is the plan?' • Schedule a follow-up visit or phone call within a time frame that enables you to intervene appropriately.
Discuss uncertainty with colleagues	• 'Don't worry alone' – if you are uneasy about a case (e.g. a patient who has a presumptive diagnosis due to gastroenteritis secondary to dietary indiscretion, who has protracted or severe abdominal pain), discuss the case with a colleague. Ask them to examine the animal. • Communicate uncertainty during case handovers. • Discuss uncertainty with a colleague or mentor who has expertise in a particular area. They may be able to give you tips on how to hone your approach and navigate topics you are most uncertain about.
Discuss uncertainty with clients	• Be confident about uncertainty. Uncertainty is common in veterinary practice, as we are dealing with unpredictable biological systems. Definitive diagnosis is far less common than presumptive diagnosis. • Tell the client a diagnosis is presumptive, or a working hypothesis, and let them know the basis of this assessment. For example, it may be that a definitive diagnosis would require diagnostic tests that are beyond the client's financial capacity, or may be considered too invasive to be in the interests of the patient. • Seek the client's involvement in monitoring for any evidence that might challenge assessment (e.g. failure to respond as expected to treatment) and stress the importance of being ready to review the plan.

REFERENCES

Gheihman, G., Johnson, M. & Simpkin, A. L. (2020) Twelve tips for thriving in the face of clinical uncertainty. *Medical Teacher* **42**(5):493–499. doi: 10.1080/0142159x.2019.1579308.

Scott, I. A., Doust, J. A., Keijzers, G. B. & Wallis, K. A. (2023) Coping with uncertainty in clinical practice: a narrative review. *Medical Journal of Australia* **218**:418–425. doi: 10.5694/mja2.51925.

3.12 Jeremy, 3-yo ME Cocker Spaniel: routine castration

a) This ECG shows second-degree Mobitz type 2 atrioventricular (AV) block. AV blocks are described in Table A3.12.

b) In this case, most anaesthetists would not treat the block if the BP was within the normal range, as the block is most likely due to increased vagal tone from the alpha-2 agonist, dexmedetomidine. If the BP was low, atipamezole could be given to antagonise the dexmedetomidine.

c) Second-degree Mobitz type 2 AV block in a non-anaesthetised dog is often a sign of cardiac disease. In such cases, it may progress to third-degree AV block, which would require urgent pacemaker implantation.

Table A3.12 Classification of AV blocks

TYPE OF AV BLOCK	ECG FEATURES
First degree	• Increased PR interval • No skipped beats
Second degree	• Some skipped beats • Conducted beats also present
Second degree, Mobitz type 1	• Gradually increasing PR interval leading to a skipped beat (due to increasing vagal tone)
Second degree, Mobitz type 2	• Intermittent non-conducted P waves without progressive prolongation of the PR interval
Third degree	• Complete AV dissociation with no P waves conducted • Ventricular or junctional escape beats usually seen

3.13 Thumper, 4-yo MN Dwarf Lop: not eating or moving

a) The most likely problem is hypovolaemic shock due to acute gastrointestinal obstruction (also known as bloat), most likely secondary to a compacted hair ball (or possibly other material, such as carpet or cloth fibre, plastic, rubber) causing obstruction. Other differential diagnoses include extraluminal compression of the GIT by neoplasia, post-operative adhesions, or abscesses. Liver lobe torsion is also a possibility.

b) **Abdominal radiographs** are useful to screen for signs of obstruction. Thumper is so unwell that you are able to take a conscious lateral radiograph, which shows a large, fluid-filled stomach with a central gas cap, and a lack of gas in the GIT distal to the stomach. Both lateral and VD/DV views are required for assessment (Figure A3.13a,b).

CBC and biochemistry. Blood work is a useful next step. Hyperglycaemia is common in obstructed rabbits, where blood glucose is often >15 mmol/L. Thumper's blood glucose was 29.6 mmol/L (this may partly be due to stress, but also due to the increase in serum osmolality from sodium loss into the GIT). Obstructed rabbits commonly have increased renal values and can go into acute renal failure (renal values need to be monitored post-treatment). Increased liver values may support a diagnosis of liver lobe torsion, which can be confirmed with abdominal ultrasonography.

c) Medical management may be successful if initiated early. This consists of supportive care (warming the patient, treating hypovolaemic shock, correcting fluid and electrolyte imbalances, and administering analgesia) along with decompression of the stomach to relieve pressure. IV fluids (60–90 mL/kg for the first hour,

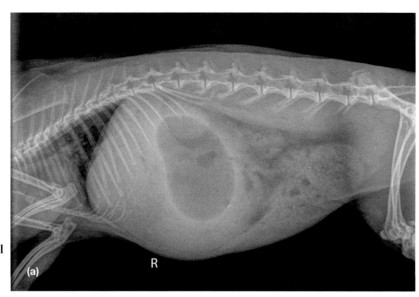

Figure A3.13a,b Lateral and DV radiographs of Thumper.

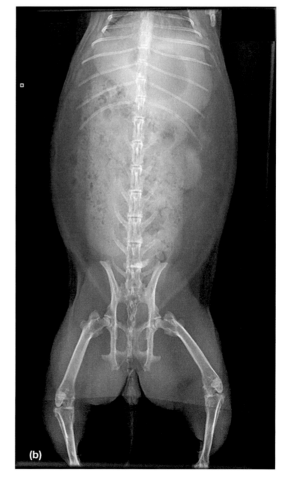

then maintenance of 100–150 mL/kg/day) can be administered via a lateral ear, cephalic, or lateral saphenous vein. For analgesia, a CRI of lignocaine (1.5 mg/kg/h) and fentanyl (0.03 mg/kg/h) can be administered. Alternatively, buprenorphine at 0.03 mg/kg can be administered SC/IM q6–12h. NSAIDs should be avoided unless renal disease is ruled out. Gastric decompression should be performed under sedation ± inhalant anaesthesia. Thumper can be sedated with midazolam, 0.5–1 mg/kg IM, then anaesthetised by administering isoflurane gas in oxygen via a mask over the nose. An 18-Fr (or smaller) red rubber catheter (well-lubricated) may be used for orogastric tubing. Measure the distance from Thumper's nose to his last rib and mark this on the tube. Gently the pass tube from Thumper's mouth into his stomach to release gas and fluid; you may need to pass the tube several times. Following decompression, palpate Thumper's abdomen and assess for pain frequently (usually q1–2h if he is otherwise stable). Most rabbits will begin eating and defaecating within 24 hours of commencing treatment. If Thumper does not improve or bloats again, you will need to repeat decompression. If he bloats repeatedly, exploratory laparotomy may be required. If surgery is performed and an intestinal foreign body identified, it is best to try to manipulate the foreign body into the caecum, or if this is not possible, move the foreign body into the stomach and perform a gastrotomy. This is better tolerated than an enterotomy.

d) Depending on the duration and cause of bloat, Thumper's prognosis may be good to grave. Without treatment, his stomach may rupture, which can lead to shock and death within 6–8 hours. You will need to continue to provide supportive care until Thumper is able to eat and defaecate normally on his own. This can include ongoing pain relief, gastrointestinal motility agents such as metoclopramide, and assisted feeding in small amounts q2–4h.

REFERENCES

Carpenter, J. W. & Marion, C. J. (2018). *Exotic Animal Formulary*, 5th edition. Philadelphia, PA: W.B. Saunders Company.

Quesenberry, K. E., Orcutt, C. J., Mans, C. & Carpenter, J. W. (2021) *Ferrets, Rabbits and Rodents: Clinical Medicine and Surgery*. St Louis, MO: Elsevier.

3.14 Sarah, 10-wo FE Labrador Cross: vacc

a) Sarah has generalised tetanus, caused by tetanospasmin, a neurotoxin produced by the Gram-positive, anaerobic, spore-forming bacteria *Clostridium tetani*. This ubiquitous agent is found in soil, dust, and the GIT and faeces of animals. Once inoculated into a suitable anaerobic environment, such as a penetrating wound, *C. tetani* elaborates the tetanus toxin.

b) Tetanus is generally a clinical diagnosis based on pattern recognition: it produces a distinctive syndrome of generalised extensor muscle rigidity in dogs. Recognition of a disease based on what it looks like, or on the illness script associated with the disease, is called type 1 or system 1 thinking. In conditions such as tetanus, for which there is no reliable clinical diagnostic test, type 1 thinking is rapid and economical. This method of diagnosis is often role-modelled by experienced clinicians. For type 1 thinking to be successful, it requires the practitioner to have previous exposure to the pattern or illness script, which is challenging when it comes to uncommon diseases such as tetanus. Those without experience of this condition will not be able to make a diagnosis based on the type 1 approach. The type 1 approach relies on mental shortcuts ('heuristics'), which are subject to biases.

This contrasts with type 2 or system 2 thinking, an analytical, problem-based approach, which is explicitly taught in veterinary schools. It requires generating a problem list and considering differentials for each problem, ranking the probability of these based on available evidence, and reviewing this ranking in light of new information (such as additional test results). It is slower, more time-consuming, and cognitively demanding, but may be more helpful in assessing uncommon conditions or uncommon presentations of common conditions. By taking a comprehensive approach to problems and requiring the veterinarian to consider all differentials (and thus do some research), it helps the inexperienced clinician consider differential diagnoses, even if they have no former experience with these.

c) In cats, tetanus most commonly presents as spastic paralysis of a single limb ('localised tetanus') (see Figure A3.14a).

d) Tetanus is a progressive disease (Figure A3.14b). Treatment requires removal of the source of the infection and antimicrobial treatment to prevent further toxin elaboration, antitoxin to neutralise any unbound toxin, and supportive care until the effects of bound toxin wear off (Fawcett & Irwin 2014a,b).

Once bound to nerve endings, the toxin prevents the release of inhibitory neurotransmitters, leading to overstimulation of motor neurons and increased muscle tone. As this can worsen with excitement, stimulation (lights, loud noises such as banging of metal cages) should be minimised. Supportive care includes the administration of muscle relaxants, sedatives, analgesics if required, fluid, and nutritional support. A dim and quiet room will help. Supportive care also requires monitoring for and managing autonomic dysfunction, including bradycardia/tachycardia, hypotension, and urine retention, and complications such as laryngospasm, aspiration pneumonia, and respiratory compromise (Dörfelt et al. 2023).

In addition, affected dogs are at risk of complications due to prolonged recumbency and paralysis, such as urinary and respiratory tract infections and decubital ulcers.

e) Sarah is likely to have suffered a deep, penetrating wound contaminated with soil or faeces. Potential routes of infection in puppies include broken or erupting teeth, omphalitis, bite wounds (including snakebite wounds), injections, surgical-site infections, deep penetrating wounds (especially of the digits), and osteomyelitis. In one retrospective study, digital osteomyelitis was frequently identified, thus radiographic examination of the paws was recommended. Because infection with *C. tetani* can originate from a very small puncture wound, such wounds may heal externally and thus not be visible by the time signs of tetanus develop. Therefore, being unable to localise the site of infection does not rule out a diagnosis of tetanus.

f) Appropriate, early wound care, including flushing, debridement, and antimicrobial treatment, is important when wounds can be detected. As dogs and cats are less vulnerable to tetanus than humans and horses, vaccination is currently not listed as

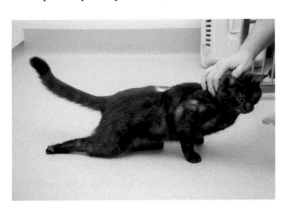

Figure A3.14a Localised tetanus in a feline patient. Note rigid extension of the right hindlimb. *Figure A3.14a has been previously published (Fawcett & Irwin 2014a, 2014b) and is reproduced here with permission.*

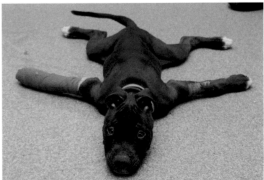

Figure A3.14b Over 24 hours, Sarah developed generalised spastic paralysis with marked extensor muscle rigidity. *Figure A3.14b has been previously published (Fawcett & Irwin 2014a, 2014b) and is reproduced here with permission.*

recommended (Squires et al. 2024). While *C. tetani* is vulnerable to disinfection, the spores are very hardy and resistant to ethanol, phenols, formalin, and boiling water. They can be destroyed if autoclaved at 120 °C for 15–20 minutes.

REFERENCES

Dörfelt, S., Mayer, C., Wolf, G. et al. (2023) Retrospective study of tetanus in 18 dogs: causes, management, complications, and immunological status. *Frontiers in Veterinary Science* **10**:1249833. doi: 10.3389/fvets.2023.1249833.

Fawcett, A. & Irwin, P. (2014a) Diagnosis and treatment of generalised tetanus in dogs. *In Practice* **36**(10):482–493. doi: 10.1136/inp.g6312.

Fawcett, A. & Irwin, P. (2014b) Review of treatment of generalised tetanus in dogs. *Australian Veterinary Practitioner* **44**(1):574–578.

Squires, R. A., Crawford, C., Marcondes, M. & Whitley, N. (2024) 2024 guidelines for the vaccination of dogs and cats – compiled by the Vaccination Guidelines Group (VGG) of the World Small Animal Veterinary Association (WSAVA). *Journal of Small Animal Practice* **65**(5):277–316. doi: 10.1111/jsap.13718.

3.15 Pearl, 6-mo FE DSH: health check

a) Factors that will impact your recommendation include the overall health of the cat and their ability to withstand anaesthesia and surgery, ownership of the cat, and the owner's intentions for the cat. The first is self-explanatory. The second is about ensuring that indiscriminate breeding will not take place. Cats that are being fostered from a humane organisation generally are gonadectomised before adoption. For cats with a dedicated owner, the owner should be included in the decision, bearing in mind that some legislatures mandate desexing by a particular age (e.g. 4 months in New South Wales in Australia).

Those cats that are intended for showing or for eventual breeding obviously should not be spayed or castrated, but some owners will require an explanation of the irreversibility of gonadectomy procedures and of the costs and risks of breeding cats. For those cats intended for companionship only, behavioural concerns should be discussed. Normal reproductive behaviour in female cats is frequent during the breeding season and may be distressing to some owners. Normal reproductive behaviour in intact male cats can be perceived as aggressive and intact male cats also urine mark with a distinctive foul-smelling urine. These behaviours often make intact male cats unsuitable as pets, but are eliminated, or at least minimised, by castration.

b) Most of the research that has been done to date has evaluated OVH as the gonadectomy procedure of choice in cats. OVH decreases the chances of acquiring some disorders, in particular mammary neoplasia and pyometra. Incidence of mammary neoplasia later in life is greatly decreased by spaying earlier in life, with the greatest benefit if spaying is performed before the first oestrus, and decreasing benefit thereafter. Mammary neoplasia in cats is almost invariably malignant adenocarcinoma. Pyometra is common in aged cats and there is obvious benefit in spaying cats before uterine pathology develops. The most common negative effect of OVH in cats is obesity; this can be controlled by diet and encouraging exercise through use of food puzzle balls, playing with the cat, and providing access to the outdoors where allowed (often with supervision). Local legislature may sometimes mandate indoor-only keeping of cats. There are a few reports of increased incidence of feline lower urinary tract disease and diabetes mellitus; the latter may be associated with obesity. Because of the high occurrence and significant morbidity associated with mammary neoplasia, female cats should be spayed prior to puberty, which in most queens will occur around 4–6 months of age during the breeding season.

c) Castration in male cats prevents the behaviours described above and prevents testicular neoplasia. The latter is uncommon and can be treated at the time it develops. Prostate disease, a concern in dogs, is uncommon in cats. The only reported disorder that is more common after castration in male cats is obesity. Because of the negative impact of normal reproductive behaviours in intact male cats that are intended to be companions and the lack of any other negative repercussions of the procedures, male cats should be castrated any time after 8 weeks of age and well before puberty, which, in most

cats, will occur around 4–6 months of age, during the breeding season.

World Small Animal Veterinary Association (WSAVA) reproduction control guidelines are available online (*https://wsava.org/wp-content/uploads/2024/05/J-of-Small-Animal-Practice-2024-Romagnoli-WSAVA-guidelines-for-the-control-of-reproduction-in-dogs-and-cats.pdf*).

REFERENCES

Root Kustritz, M. V. (2007) Determining the optimal age for gonadectomy of dogs and cats. *Journal of the American Veterinary Medical Association* **231**(11):1665–1675. doi: 10.2460/javma.231.11.1665.

Root Kustritz, M. V. (2012) Use of an impact score to guide client decision-making about timing of spay-castration of dogs and cats. *Clinical Theriogenology* **4**(4):481–485.

Root Kustritz, M. V. (2018) Population control in small animals. *Veterinary Clinics of North America Small Animal Practice* **48**(4):721–732. doi: 10.1016/j.cvsm.2018.02.013.

3.16 Benny, 4-yo MN Miniature Dachshund: bloody faeces

a) This is an adult tapeworm. *Spirometra erinacei* is commonly called a zipper worm.

b) Researching a good parasitological textbook (e.g. Lapage 1962, Šlapeta et al. 2018) you would find that *Spirometra erinacei* is a pseudophyllidean cestode that is widely distributed in different species of amphibians, reptiles, and mammals, which serve in most cases as intermediate or paratenic hosts. Following a general pattern seen in many parasites of this type, when released from the definitive host, each egg releases a larva (coracidium), which, when ingested by a copepod (a small aquatic crustacean), develops into a procercoid. After ingestion by a second intermediate host (amphibian, reptile, or mammal), procercoids develop into plerocercoids,

also known as spargana, and can be found throughout the body. When present SC, spargana may result in soft swellings of the body (sparganosis) (Figure A3.16a,b). Oedema and haemorrhage of soft tissues may be associated with this stage. The definitive host is generally a mammalian carnivore (felids, canids).

c) Larval spargana (plerocercoids) and adult Pseudophyllidea may be found in felids, canids, and other animals. Spargana are the causative agents of human larval migration syndromes called sparganosis (spirometrosis), a food- and waterborne zoonotic disease. The disease is endemic in East Asian countries, and has also been reported in populations in Europe, America, Africa, and Australia. Humans acquire

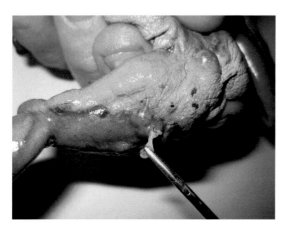

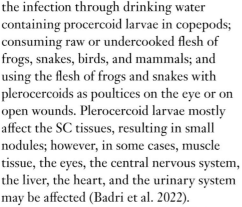

Figure A3.16a Surgical removal of a sparganum (plerocercoid) from a skin nodule of an Australian Green Tree Frog, *Litoria caerulea*.

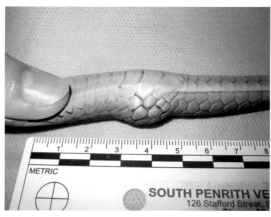

Figure A3.16b Sparganosis in a Common Tree Snake, *Dendrelaphis punctulata*.

the infection through drinking water containing procercoid larvae in copepods; consuming raw or undercooked flesh of frogs, snakes, birds, and mammals; and using the flesh of frogs and snakes with plerocercoids as poultices on the eye or on open wounds. Plerocercoid larvae mostly affect the SC tissues, resulting in small nodules; however, in some cases, muscle tissue, the eyes, the central nervous system, the liver, the heart, and the urinary system may be affected (Badri et al. 2022).

d) Unlike cyclophyllidean cestodes, adults of which are widely regarded as almost non-pathogenic to the dog or cat definitive host, infection with adult *Spirometra* spp. can be associated with gastrointestinal disease in dogs and cats. Clinical signs reported include diarrhoea, weight loss, and vomiting, which usually resolve following appropriate anthelmintic therapy (CAPC 2023). Although, in Benny's case, the diarrhoea was acute, and he had not been seen to vomit, the presence of a cestode in bloody and mucous faeces strongly indicates parasitism as the cause of his condition.

e) No products have been approved for treatment of *Spirometra* spp. infections in dogs and cats. Praziquantel has been used successfully; however, a higher than labelled dose (25 mg/kg PO) and an extended duration of treatment (2 consecutive days) is usually required to eliminate the infection. Treatment of *Spirometra* spp. in dogs and cats must be combined with prevention of ingestion of prey species or reinfection is likely to occur (CAPC 2023). Benny recovered quickly after treatment with praziquantel.

REFERENCES

Badri, M., Olfatifar, M., KarimiPourSaryazdi, A. et al. (2022) The global prevalence of *Spirometra* parasites in snakes, frogs, dogs, and cats: a systematic review and meta-analysis. *Veterinary Medicine and Science* **8**(6):2785–2805. doi: 10.1002/vms3.932.

CAPC (Companion Animal Parasite Council) (2023) *Spirometra* spp. Available at: https://capcvet.org/guidelines/spirometra-spp/.

Lapage, G. (1962) Helminth Parasites. In: Lapage, G. (ed.) *Mönnig's Veterinary Helminthology and Entomology*, 5th edition. London: Baillière, Tindall and Cox, pp. 31–333.

Šlapeta, J., Modrý, D. & Johnson, R. (2018) Reptile Parasitology in Health and Disease. In: Doneley, R., Monks, D., Johnson, R. & Carmel, B. (eds) *Reptile Medicine and Surgery in Clinical Practice*. Oxford: John Wiley & Sons, pp. 425–439.

3.17 Tracy, 12-yo FN SBT: O noticed lump

a) Ideally, these would be separate procedures and the dentistry would be carried out first because this is causing Tracy the most pain and discomfort. However, the owner reports that the mammary mass is growing rapidly, and the owner is both concerned about this and financially challenged. As is so often the case in general practice, context is critical and you are required to manage competing concerns. Many dogs with pre-existing periodontal disease are treated for unrelated conditions with emergency surgery, including orthopaedic surgery with implants, and heal uneventfully without infection disseminating from the mouth. A decision to treat both problems under the one anaesthetic requires owner discussion and informed consent and must be arrived at jointly after considering all factors, including the potential risk of surgical-site infection from bacteraemia or inadvertent aerosol or physical transfer from the oral cavity to the surgical site associated with the dental procedure. Healthy dogs cope well with the transient bacteraemia produced by dental treatment (Blazevich & Miles 2024) and a study in humans showed that bacteraemia induced by dental cleaning without antibiotic prophylaxis was not associated with infection of a central venous catheter in cancer patients (Usmani et al. 2018). Different approaches to this common question in companion animal practice are therefore possible, and rational, and the discussion and decision should be noted in the clinical record. Another approach is to ignore Tracy's dental problems for now. Perhaps the owner could save up for treatment later? This would be an example of a sequential care approach, prioritising the approach to comorbidities to take account of owner finances and other factors.

b) Systemic antimicrobials are not indicated prior to clean surgery (e.g. tumour excision). When performing dentistry in an infected mouth alongside a second clean procedure, many vets will give prophylactic antibiotics. Given Tracey's advanced dental disease, it has been recommended (Bellows et al. 2019) that pre-operative antibiotics may be administered for several days prior to surgery to improve surgical handling of tissues. Antibiotics should also be given prior to surgery on the day of surgery to ensure good tissue levels are present at the time of operation in the mouth and the mammary tissue. Note that the precautions in c) below are at least as important.

c) The clean surgery should take place first in the sterile operating room. Before transfer to the dental room or area, the surgical wound should be covered with a temporary waterproof dressing, and waterproof operating drapes can also cover Tracy's trunk/caudal abdomen to help protect the wound area from aerosolised bacteria. Chlorhexidine rinses should be used in the mouth before and during dental surgery. Dental procedures are notoriously difficult to predict in terms of length and a limit should be set on the total operating time including dental operating time, e.g. 90 minutes. This should be discussed with the owner beforehand, as prolonged operating time is associated with a higher risk of wound infection. This may necessitate performing a 'palliative dental treatment' on Tracy, addressing the worse problems only (sequential care), depending on the state of the mouth. Note that this could mean that Tracy ultimately requires a second anaesthetic at a later date after all, so the owner should not be left assuming that one procedure will definitely fix all of Tracy's problems – it depends what lies underneath the copious calculus in her mouth. This emphasises the need for proper informed consent that has elements of contingency and uncertainty built in (and applies to many procedures, but especially dental surgery).

d) There is a fine straight needle in the liver.

e) The owner should be informed about the needle and asked about any events that could have caused this. (The only explanation was that the owner had done needlework from time to time but stopped several years ago.) The merits of the two approaches to this unexpected finding should be discussed: do nothing or attempt removal (which could be harder than anticipated). However, given financial constraints, adding exploratory coeliotomy to the treatment plan is not feasible. The finding and decision should be prominently marked in the clinical records.

f) i)   The site of mass removal and the mammary area generally should be monitored for recurrence.

ii) Tracy's owner should be shown how to brush Tracy's teeth, focusing especially on the teeth with early furcation exposure. It is probable that these teeth will need to be removed in the future.

iii) The fact that the owner stopped needlework a few years ago suggests that the needle has remained in situ for a long time. This justifies a conservative approach. Repeat imaging could be considered in several months (or at the time of future dental treatment).

REFERENCES

Bellows, J., Berg, M. L., Dennis, S. et al. (2019) AAHA Dental Care Guidelines for Dogs and Cats. *Journal of the American Animal Hospital Association* **55**(2):49–69. doi: 10.5326/jaaha-ms-6933.

Blazevich, M. & Miles, C. (2024) The presence of bacteremia in 13 dogs undergoing oral surgery without the use of antibiotic therapy. *Journal of Veterinary Dentistry*.41(4):312–323. doi: 10.1177/08987564231207208.

Usmani, S., Choquette, L., Bona, R. et al. (2018) Transient bacteremia induced by dental cleaning is not associated with infection of central venous catheters in patients with cancer. *Oral Surgery, Oral Medicine, Oral Pathology, Oral Radiology* **125**(4):286–294. doi: 10.1016/j.oooo.2017.12.022.

3.18 Fella, 12-yo MN DSH: left for euthanasia

a) It is important to remember that Fella is likely to be in a lot of pain from his condition, and he is very stressed. You could give Fella some time to relax in his carrier. Placing him in a dark, quiet room with synthetic feline facial pheromone may help. You could offer Fella some high-value food. If he eats, you could provide oral gabapentin (100–200 mg PO per cat) or trazodone (50–100 mg PO per cat) in food.

b) Pre-euthanasia sedation or anaesthesia is considered best practice in the vast majority of euthanasias (Cooney 2020). If you are presented with a moribund patient for euthanasia, effectively heavily sedated by sickness or disease, then it may not be necessary to administer sedation, and doing so could compromise vascular access if blood pressure is low. But, in general, sedation reduces the need for restraint, which can exacerbate fear, anxiety and distress in cats. In Fella's case, this is important for both his comfort and his stress levels, and for the safety of the team. You may need to use a combination of oral and then injectable sedations. Patience is key to avoid unnecessary distress. You can administer the medication via IM or SC injection. Many combinations are possible. The following is an example:

- Butorphanol 0.4 mg/kg + acepromazine 2 mg/kg SC
- Wait 5 minutes
- Then tiletamine/zolazepam 6 mg/kg SC or alfaxalone CD 2–3 mg/kg IM

If injection is not possible, you could draw up one of the following and squirt it in Fella's mouth via syringe:

- Tiletamine/zolazepam 6 mg/kg + butorphanol 0.4 mg/kg + acepromazine 0.6 mg/kg
- Buprenorphine 0.02 mg/kg + medetomidine 0.04 mg/kg + ketamine 8 mg/kg

(Note: squirting these into Fella's mouth can cause hypersalivation, so if he is eating, follow up with food.)

c) Once Fella is sedated, if desired, an IV cannula can be placed, through which pentobarbital can be administered. This would ensure that the pentobarbital does not extravasate and cause preventable pain in Fella's final moments. However, experienced clinicians may also be comfortable giving pentobarbital by direct IV injection in a well-sedated cat, in a simple and smooth injection. When owners are present for euthanasia, taking the pet away to insert a cannula can be upsetting, as it separates them before the final goodbye. Using pre-euthanasia sedation creates a calm, pain-free experience for the pet and makes cannula placement easier. This avoids the need to take the animal away, allowing for a more peaceful and compassionate experience for both the pet, the owner, and the veterinary team. If Fella is anaesthetised, pentobarbital may be administered IV or via an organ such as the liver, kidney or – if required – heart (Cooney et al. 2022). Slow injection of euthanasia solution when administering IV helps to prevent agonal breathing and muscle spasm.

d) Performing euthanasia on an animal that has been dropped off can be upsetting. It is easy to assume that the owners 'don't care' if we can't imagine not wanting to be present for our own animals at this time. However, this kind of judgement can lead to cynicism and detract from our own wellbeing. Euthanasia is rarely an easy decision. The owner cared enough to bring Fella for euthanasia, but may have felt guilty about making that final decision, or be too distressed to remain during the euthanasia procedure. Sounding short or 'curt' might in fact have reflected extreme distress. If you have concerns about euthanasing this patient, you should attempt to contact the owners. It is important that veterinary team members can discuss ethical concerns with each other.

e) In this case, you did not meet the owners, so a phone call may not feel natural, although if you feel comfortable making such a call, there would be nothing wrong with doing so. Alternatively, you may wish to text, email, or send them a card to let them know that Fella passed peacefully after receiving gentle sedation and pain relief. We often want to make contact with owners after euthanasia, but perhaps hold off because we don't know what to say. Veterinary team members can normalise the grief that people feel over the loss of their animals by talking about it. A phone call the following day or a week later can make all the difference – it demonstrates that you care and that you do not expect them to be 'okay'. It gives the owner a chance to talk things through – people will often welcome the chance to talk about their pet with someone who understands how important the animal was. A follow-up call can give them the opening they need to ask you about the euthanasia. Owners are unlikely to call you to ask you, but if you reach out, they can put intrusive, anxiety-driven thoughts to rest. If you do not know what to say, then say that – 'I don't really know what to say, I just wanted to call and let you know that you're in our thoughts and we're here for you'.

REFERENCES

Cooney, K. (2020) Historical perspective of euthanasia in veterinary medicine. *Veterinary Clinics of North America: Small Animal Practice* **50**(3):489–502. doi: 10.1016/j.cvsm.2019.12.001.

Cooney, K. A., Coates, J. A., Leach, L. M. et al. (2022) The use of intrarenal injection of sodium pentobarbital for euthanasia in cats. *American Journal of Veterinary Research* **83**(1):95–99. doi: 10.2460/ajvr.21.08.0123.

3.19 Tully, 12-mo FE Lab: post-op wound check

a) Steps to prevent self-trauma in veterinary patients include the following:
    - Provide pre-, peri-, and post-operative analgesia
    - Careful surgical technique (see Halstead's Principles, Case 1.11)
    - Monitor patients for pain and provide rescue analgesia
    - Provide take-home, multimodal analgesia
    - Administer/dispense sedation if appropriate
    - Administer/dispense antipruritic medication if appropriate
    - Administer/dispense anxiolytic medication if appropriate
    - Cover the wound with an appropriate dressing and ensure this is changed/replaced regularly
    - Use clean, breathable fitted clothing to protect sites on the body
    - Clean the wound regularly, as required
    - Ensure that the patient has appropriate mental stimulation while minimising physical activity

It should be noted that Elizabethan collars, particularly if poorly selected (too small or large diameter) may cause or exacerbate self-trauma. The temperament of the patient and their acceptance (or not) of the collar are also important considerations. The size and material of Elizabethan collars should be selected carefully with these factors in mind. There are a variety of Elizabethan collars commercially available, including those made from soft plastic or other materials, that may be more suitable for some animals.

b) No. An uncomplicated seroma should reduce in size over time. Lancing and draining the site, even if using a sterile needle and syringe, risks inoculating agents from the skin into the site, leading to infection. The risk of infection increases with multiple aspirations. Ultrasonography of the swelling can be performed to determine the nature and contents, and guide sampling if required, but straightforward seromas are best left alone.

c) Systemic antibiotics are not indicated unless there is evidence of infection. While there remains a lack of consensus regarding diagnostic criteria for surgical-site infection in veterinary settings, an indicator of infection is purulent discharge from the wound (or positive culture). Wound infections are associated with cardinal signs of inflammation, including pain or tenderness at the site, localised swelling, redness or heat, pyrexia, or the presence of an abscess (Espinel-Rupérez et al. 2019). Seromas may be associated with swelling and erythema, but as Tully does not have any other signs of infection, and is otherwise bright and well, systemic antibiotics are not indicated. Furthermore, there are inherent risks to the use of antibiotics that outweigh the potential benefits. Antibiotic administration may lead to dysbiosis and subsequent gastrointestinal signs or antimicrobial resistance. If an abscess is suspected, in the absence of any surrounding signs of tissue infection, drainage and lavage of the cavity are indicated. Given that Tully has been able to lick the wound, it would be prudent to clean the wound using a topical aqueous antiseptic such as povidone-iodine solution or chlorhexidine.

d) Elizabethan collars can impact the behaviour of animals wearing them and may be perceived by owners as negatively impacting animal welfare (Shenoda et al. 2020). Table A3.19 provides a mnemonic 'ECOLLAR' that can be helpful when advising owners about managing animals with Elizabethan collars.

Table A3.19 The Elizabethan collar mnemonic for advising owners about managing animals with Elizabethan collars

MNEMONIC ELEMENT	COMMENTS
E	**Elizabethan collars** are applied to prevent self-trauma and protect surgical wounds as animals recover. One study found an association between lack of, or premature removal of, Elizabethan collars and surgical-site infections (Espinel-Rupérez et al. 2019). Furthermore, surgical-site infections prolonged recovery, and resulted in an increase of around 75% of veterinary costs (Espinel-Rupérez et al. 2019). Understanding why Elizabethan collars are used may increase owner adherence
C	**Comfort** is important. Collars should be fitted appropriately to ensure they remain in place. Owners should be shown how to place and remove the Elizabethan collar and confirm appropriate fit in case they need to remove the collar to facilitate activities such as eating and drinking
O	**Observe** animals whose collars have been removed continuously until the collar is replaced. Failure to observe animals whose collar has been removed, even for a short period, can allow significant self-trauma and associated complications, including wound dehiscence or infection, which may necessitate further veterinary intervention including surgery, thereby prolonging recovery and incurring further costs
L	**Life** at home may be challenging. Some animals may not be able to use dog or cat doors or navigate stairs while wearing the collar. Assistance or supervision from the owner or a carer may be required to avoid misadventure
L	**Look out!** Animals wearing Elizabethan collars may collide with objects or owners, with potential for injury or property damage. Animal access to some areas may need to be restricted while the collar is worn to avoid property damage or injury
A	**Assistance** with drinking, eating, or other activities may be required. Letting owners know allows them to plan time for these additional activities
R	**Ring** (telephone) or return to the veterinary hospital if there are concerns about the fit or the impact of the Elizabethan collar on the animal. Owners should feel comfortable that they have the support of the veterinary team. This might also reduce the risk of owners adapting or making their own Elizabethan collars or alternatives, which can be hazardous

REFERENCES

Espinel-Rupérez, J., Martín-Ríos, M. D., Salazar, V. et al. (2019) Incidence of surgical site infection in dogs undergoing soft tissue surgery: risk factors and economic impact. *Veterinary Record Open* **6**(1):e000233. doi: 10.1136/vetreco-2017-000233.

Shenoda, Y., Ward, M. P., McKeegan, D. & Fawcett, A. (2020) 'The cone of shame': welfare implications of Elizabethan collar use on dogs and cats as reported by their owners. *Animals* **10**(2):333. doi: 10.3390/ani10020333.

3.20 Womble, 6-yo MN English Bull Terrier: seizures

a) Oxygen should be delivered via mask over the nose or muzzle, or flow-by administration. With Womble restrained appropriately, an attempt should be made to place an IV catheter in a peripheral vein. If this is possible, blood can be collected to check blood glucose, electrolytes, and ionised calcium, and a CBC and biochemistry panel can be performed to detect metabolic causes of seizures and to guide fluid therapy. A benzodiazepine such as midazolam or diazepam can be given IV. If IV catheterisation is not possible, midazolam can be given intranasally (IN), or diazepam per rectum (Figure A3.20). When detected, hypoglycaemia and hypocalcaemia should be corrected as

seizures may continue otherwise.

Establish insofar as you can that Womble has a clear airway (remember that the jaws of animals who are seizuring tend to clamp down involuntarily, and it may be difficult to release the grip of an unconscious animal). It is important to measure the rectal temperature, as patients who are seizuring are at risk of hyperthermia. Active cooling of the patient may be required if the temperature is over 39 °C. Examples include putting a fan in front of the patient's face, wetting the coat with cool water, and giving a fluid bolus. Cooling measures can be stopped once the patient's temperature reaches 39 °C in order to avoid shivering.

Once seizures have abated, oxygen

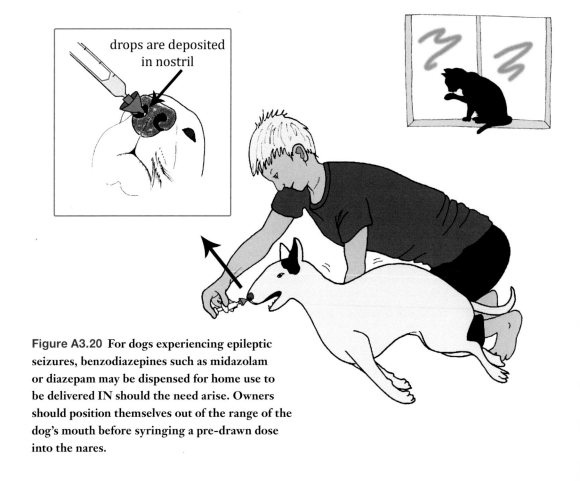

drops are deposited in nostril

Figure A3.20 For dogs experiencing epileptic seizures, benzodiazepines such as midazolam or diazepam may be dispensed for home use to be delivered IN should the need arise. Owners should position themselves out of the range of the dog's mouth before syringing a pre-drawn dose into the nares.

saturation can be measured via pulse oximetry. Suction of the mouth may be required if salivation is excessive, as there is a risk of aspiration in seizuring patients. Additional supportive care should be guided by findings (e.g. judicious fluid therapy for electrolyte derangements, vitamin B_1 supplementation for thiamine deficiency if suspected). If toxin ingestion is suspected, gastric lavage or an enema may be required.

b) There are many agents that are known to cause seizures in dogs. The American Society for the Prevention of Cruelty to Animals (ASPCA) lists six main categories (Table A3.20a). Do not be concerned if you have not identified all of these; the main point is to be aware of the wide range of possibilities and to make sure you take a good history once the patient is adequately stabilised to check for intended (e.g. new medication) or unintended access to drugs/agents. The potential for an agent to cause seizures may depend on the dose, the route of administration, and breed, e.g. ivermectin sensitivity in collies associated with a deletion mutation of the mdr1 gene (Mealey et al. 2001).

c) Status epilepticus is an emergency that can lead to brain damage, and is associated with a mortality rate of 25–39% (Charalambous et al. 2024). It is defined as seizure activity lasting 5 minutes or more (Charalambous et al. 2024). Without treatment, seizures can become self-sustaining and refractory

Table A3.20a **Agents known to cause seizures in dogs (adapted from Khan 2012 and ASPCA 2023)**					
MEDICATIONS	**PLANTS**	**FOOD/DRINK**	**RODENTICIDES, MOLLUSCICIDES, AND INSECTICIDES**	**OTHER DRUGS (INCLUDING ILLICIT DRUGS)**	**MISCELLANEOUS**
• 5-hydroxytryptophan (5-HTP) • Amitraz • Amphetamines • Avermectins • Baclofen • Benzodiazepines • Diphenhydramine • Fluorouracil (5-FU) cream • Fluoroquinolones • Ibuprofen • Isoniazid • Ivermectin • Lamotrigine • Metronidazole • Moxidectin • Phenylbutazone • Phenylpropanolamine • Penicillin G procaine • Selective serotonin reuptake inhibitors (SSRIs), e.g. fluoxetine, sertraline • Tricyclic antidepressants, e.g. amitriptyline, clomipramine • Vilazodone	• Brunfelsia ('yesterday-today-tomorrow') • Mushrooms • Sago palm	• Xylitol • Caffeine • Dark chocolate • Ethanol • Nicotine	• 4-aminopyridine • Bifenthrin • Carbamate pesticides • Metaldehyde • Organochlorine pesticides • Organophosphate pesticides • Strychnine • Zinc phosphide	• 4-aminopyridine • Amphetamines • Cannabis • Cocaine • Synthetic cannabinoids	• Bee sting • Ethylene glycol • Home-made play dough or salt dough • Lead • Mycotoxins • Propylene glycol

to anti-seizure medications. The American College of Veterinary Internal Medicine (ACVIM) recommends early, rapid, stage-based treatment, as outlined in Table A3.20b).

> Most general practices will not stock or use all of the medications given in Table A3.20b, so choices will be more limited and pragmatic. In status epilepticus, when seizures are not controlled with benzodiazepines or levetiracetam, any anaesthetic agent can be used initially, but it is important to remember to intubate these patients. Some clinicians prefer the use of alfaxalone CD to propofol in third-line treatments.

Table A3.20b Stage-based treatment of status epilepticus (adapted from Charalambous et al. 2024)

	STAGE 1: IMPENDING	STAGE 2: ESTABLISHED	STAGE 3: REFRACTORY	STAGE 4: SUPER-REFRACTORY
Time frame	5–10 minutes	10–30 minutes	>30 minutes	>24 hours
Treatment stage	First line	Second line	Third line	Fourth line
Treatment	Midazolam IN or IV *or* diazepam IV ± midazolam CRI ± levetiracetam IV ± phenobarbital IV	First-line treatments + levetiracetam IV ± phenobarbital IV ± fosphenytoin IV ± ketamine IV	First-line treatments + second-line treatments + ketamine CRI ± dexmedetomidine IV or CRI ± propofol IV or CRI ± phenobarbital IV or CRI ± inhalational anaesthetic	First-line treatments + second-line treatments + third-line treatments + other drugs as described in Charalambous et al. (2024) ± neurostimulation

d) Once the seizures are controlled, the next step is to look for an underlying cause, whether this is toxicity, metabolic disease, intracranial disease, or idiopathic epilepsy – a 'rule everything else out' diagnosis, as far as this is practicable in individual contexts. If no toxic or metabolic disease is found or suspected, empirical treatment with a longer-acting anticonvulsant such as levetiracetam or phenobarbital is appropriate. Anticonvulsants reduce the incidence of seizures in most dogs with epilepsy, but some dogs will become refractory to treatment.

e) It is important to perform a neurological examination when Womble has recovered (i.e. is not sedated or in a post-ictal state), which could be in a few hours or even a few days. It is difficult to give Womble a prognosis without further diagnostic information, but the following general principles may assist:

- Dogs with a normal neurological exam, no detectable metabolic abnormalities, and recurrent seizures who are younger than 6 years are more likely to have idiopathic or primary epilepsy
- Dogs with a normal neurological exam, no detectable metabolic abnormalities, and recurrent seizures who are 6 years or older are more likely to have an acquired (as opposed to inherited) intracranial disease. Imaging should be recommended but, regardless, Womble should be monitored closely. If neurologic signs develop between seizures, this is more

likely to indicate a brain tumour

- Dogs with a normal neurological exam, no detectable metabolic abnormalities, and recurrent seizures who are 6 years or older at the onset of seizures have at least a 50% probability of an underlying structural abnormality, including brain tumour
- Dogs with ongoing metabolic disease, toxicity, or progressive brain disease (e.g. brain tumour, encephalitis) are more likely to have abnormalities on neurological examination
- Dogs with worsening neurological signs are more likely to have progressive intracranial disease (e.g. brain tumour, encephalitis, neurodegeneration)
- Increase in the frequency of seizures alone may indicate that epilepsy is refractory to treatment, rather than indicating progressive disease

f) A suggested first line of treatment is midazolam (0.2–0.5 mg/kg IN), which can work within minutes (0.5–1.6 minutes) (Charalambous et al. 2021). If this is not available, an alternative is diazepam (0.5–2.0 mg/kg) administered per rectum. This may take slightly longer to take effect than midazolam, and absorption may be impaired by faeces. It is suggested that owners may find this route more difficult, and less acceptable, than the IN route. A third option is buccal or sublingual midazolam or diazepam; however, this route is not preferred due to a lack of evidence of clinical efficacy and safety, and the risk of the owner being bitten (Charalambous et al. 2021). Where it is legal to dispense these drugs for at-home use, caution should be exercised, as they can be misused. Dispensing benzodiazepines for at-home use should be reserved for an animal with a known history of repeated cluster seizure episodes (>2 self-limiting seizures over a 24-hour period [Charalambous et al. 2024]) and at least a tentative diagnosis (e.g. idiopathic epilepsy or intracranial disease). Any animal with continuous seizure activity should be taken to a veterinary hospital. Oral levetiracetam (60 mg PO initially) can be given to dogs that have a history of cluster seizures and to those that recover between episodes of status epilepticus such that oral medication can be given. It is likely to be active within 30 minutes.

REFERENCES

ASPCA (2023) Most common causes of seizures in dogs. Available at: www.aspcapro.org/resource/most-common-causes-seizures-dogs.

Charalambous, M. Volk, H. A., Van Ham, L. & Bhatti, S. F. M. (2021) First-line management of canine status epilepticus at home and in hospital-opportunities and limitations of the various administration routes of benzodiazepines. *BMC Veterinary Research* **17**(1):103. doi: 10.1186/s12917-021-02805-0.

Charalambous, M., Muñana, K., Patterson, E. E. et al. (2024) ACVIM Consensus statement on the management of status epilepticus and cluster seizures in dogs and cats. *Journal of Veterinary Internal Medicine* **38**(1):19–40. doi: 10.1111/jvim.16928.

Khan, S. A. (2012) Differential diagnosis of common acute toxicologic versus nontoxicologic illness. *Veterinary Clinics of North America Small Animal Practice* **42**(2):389–402, ix. doi: 10.1016/j.cvsm.2012.01.001.

Mealey, K. L., Bentjen, S. A., Gay, J. M. & Cantor, G. H. (2001) Ivermectin sensitivity in collies is associated with a deletion mutation of the mdr1 gene. *Pharmacogenetics and Genomics* **11**(8):727–733. doi: 10.1097/00008571-200111000-00012.

3.21 Rex, 8-yo ME Rottweiler: dental (extractions)

Veterinary team members are exposed to a variety of hazards and may suffer minor to serious injuries in their work (Johnson & Fritschi 2024). Critical workplace health and safety controls are important in minimising incidents and injuries.

Risks and mitigation strategies for a procedure like Rex's are given in Table A3.21.

Table A3.21 **Potential hazards, associated risks, and mitigation strategies for dental procedures in general, with specific notes on large-dog issues**

HAZARD	RISKS	MITIGATION STRATEGY
Dog	Bites/scratches	<ul><li>Minimise patient fear/anxiety and distress through gentle handling</li><li>Consider pre-visit pharmaceuticals to be administered by owner at home if required/safe to do so</li><li>Ask for assistance with handling</li><li>Muzzle if required</li><li>Use appropriate premedication/sedation</li><li>Provide pre-, peri-, and post-operative analgesia to minimise post-operative pain</li></ul>
Manual handling	Lifting a heavy patient onto a surgical table can lead to musculoskeletal injuries	<ul><li>Use a scissor lift, group lift, or hoist</li><li>Ask for assistance from multiple team members when repositioning the patient during the procedure</li><li>Plan lifting assistance in advance so people are ready and willing to help (this discourages 'just getting on with it' and attempting unsafe lifting)</li></ul>
Ergonomics (posture)	Poor/awkward posture, particularly over an extended period, can lead to musculoskeletal injuries and/or repetitive strain injuries	<ul><li>Take regular breaks to stand up and stretch</li><li>Use a comfortable chair or stool and, ideally, a height-adjustable dental table</li><li>Select appropriate instruments, and know the correct way to handle them</li><li>Ensure dental instruments are sharp</li><li>Stage procedures to minimise fatigue from lengthy operating time</li></ul>
Lighting	Poor lighting increases risks of eye strain, fatigue, and injury through lack of visualisation of where instruments are placed within the mouth	Ensure that you have bright, adjustable task lighting such as a wall or roof-mounted light, surgical loops, or a head torch, directed at the area of interest and redirected as needed
Zoonotic disease transmission	Bacteria and other organisms may become aerosolised during ultrasonic scaling or tooth sectioning	<ul><li>Wear appropriate personal protective equipment (PPE), which may include a face mask, face shield, or goggles; a long-sleeved gown; and gloves</li><li>Use chlorhexidine in irrigation fluids (proprietary products available as oral rinses or additives for dental machine water supply at appropriate dilutions)</li></ul>
Eye injuries	Eye injuries can occur due to projection of tooth fragments or tartar during ultrasonic scaling or tooth sectioning, leading to short- or long-term eye damage, including blindness	<ul><li>Wear a face shield and/or goggles</li><li>Use good operating technique</li></ul>

HAZARD	RISKS	MITIGATION STRATEGY
Hand injuries	• Hands or fingers may contact high-speed burrs or dental drills • May also occur with slipping of elevators or through contact with sharp instruments	• Maintain a high level of concentration when using powered equipment and direct instruments away from hands • Take breaks to reduce the impact of fatigue and strain • For a long procedure, and when working on large teeth in a big dog, it may be helpful to swap out with a colleague or stage the treatment into two or more procedures • Maintain instruments properly • Use appropriate sizes of instrument for the patient
Sharps	Sharps are defined as any implement that is capable of cutting the skin, including needles, stylettes, scalpel blades, and dental instruments	• Sharps should always be kept on an open part of the dental equipment tray where you can see them • The person who uses the sharps is responsible for disposal after use (failure to do this is a common cause of injury among support staff)
Anaesthetic gases	Exposure to anaesthetic gases has been linked to a variety of health issues; this is more likely during a dental procedure due to frequent patient repositioning	• Prior to anaesthetic induction, check anaesthetic circuitry (including leak testing) • Select the appropriate size endotracheal tube for the patient and ensure the cuff is inflated appropriately • Turn both anaesthetic gas and oxygen off when you disconnect the circuit temporarily to reposition the patient • Ensure that the anaesthetic vaporiser is regularly serviced
Clinical waste	Waste that has the potential to cause harm to humans or the environment, such as teeth, tissue, and blood-soaked gauze swabs	• Always handle with gloves • Dispose of clinical waste in the correct receptacle
Veterinary chemicals	Various cleaning and disinfection chemicals may be used to prepare instruments or clean them after use; these have the potential to cause skin reactions or other health issues	Read the safety data sheet of the chemical prior to use and follow all instructions, including the wearing of PPE if required
Electricity	There is a potential for electrocution, especially where electricity and water come into contact	• Visually inspect cords prior to use to ensure no internal wiring is exposed • Ensure all equipment is in good working order • Your building should have a surge protector or safety switch installed to protect you from a severe electric shock – ask your employer if you are unsure
Air compressor	Utilised to power high-speed dental equipment; small risk of explosion due to pressurised air; noise	• Ensure all users of the air compressor are trained on how to set up and use it correctly • If you need to raise your voice to be heard over the air compressor, wear hearing protection • When upgrading equipment, choose quieter compressors
Difficult clinical encounters	Clients may become upset or frustrated if expectations are not met	• Provide an estimate of fees and explain what this does and does not include • Explain that dentistry is difficult to estimate before comprehensive oral assessment has taken place • Document discussions regarding estimates on the patient records • Develop clear and consistent admission procedures • Check client contact details and ask if and to what extent you should proceed if they cannot be contacted during the procedure if priorities change • Update clients on costs during the procedure if possible • Develop a practice policy on managing abusive or hostile clients

Continued

Table A3.21 **(Continued)**

HAZARD	RISKS	MITIGATION STRATEGY
Workplace stress and fatigue	Dental procedures, especially those involving radiographs and complex or multiple extractions, may be extended	• Schedule enough time for the procedure to ensure that team members are not placed under stress • Consider staging procedures involving multiple extractions to minimise the risk of fatigue and ensure adequate time is available, e.g. perform comprehensive oral examination, radiographs, and cleaning during one appointment, and perform extractions on a different day; this will require two anaesthetics but may improve efficiency • Ensure that lunch and rest breaks are scheduled and taken, even if this means swapping with team members

REFERENCE

Johnson, L. & Fritschi, L. (2024) Frequency of workplace incidents and injuries in veterinarians, veterinary nurses and veterinary students and measures to control these. *Australian Veterinary Journal* **102**:431–439. doi: 10.1111/avj.13354.

TODAY'S CASE LIST

4.1 Gypsy, 2-yo FN Cross-breed: ate owner's tablet

4.2 Charlie, 3-yo MN Cross-breed: anxious, destroying things

4.3 Bella, 7-mo FE Cross-breed: spay

4.4 Cleo, 6-yo FN DSH: bleeding when eating

4.5 Gregor, 8-yo MN DLH: inpatient

4.6 Walter, 5-mo ME Miniature Dachshund: V ++ & D ++

4.7 Thor, 5-yo ME German Shepherd: off colour, no appetite

4.8 Maya, 17-yo FN DSH: vomiting & weight loss

4.9 Flora, 9-wo FE Cavoodle: passing blood

4.10 Walter, 5-yo ME Malinois Greyhound: swollen toe

4.11 Fluffy Friends Rescue Centre: site visit

4.12 Dusty, 6-yo ME Golden Retriever: annual vaccination

4.13 Kane, 14-yo MN Labrador: booster vaccination

4.14 Rusty, 2-yo ME Dachshund: vaccination

4.15 Shadow, 2-yo ME DSH: O thinks leg is broken

4.16 Peter, 6-mo ME Cross-breed: health check

4.17 On way in – see immediately: dog collapsed on walk

4.18 Cleo, 4-yo FN Cocker Spaniel: drinking & urinating lots

4.19 Seamus, 7-yo MN DSH; vomiting ++

4.20 Home time

Recipe: Mum's fresh lemon drizzle cake

4.1 Gypsy, 2-yo FN Cross-breed: ate owner's tablet

Ms Burstyn asks to speak to a vet urgently and the call is put through to your consulting room. Ms Burstyn is staying at a guest house in the remote countryside with her recently adopted dog Gypsy (Figure 4.1a). Ms Burstyn was about to take her medication for arthritis when Gypsy jumped up and ate it. You ask her to tell you the name of the product and the dose. Ms Burstyn replies that the active ingredient is meloxicam, and that Gypsy ingested a single 15-mg tablet (Figure 4.1b). Gypsy's most recently recorded weight (approximately 3 weeks ago) was 40 kg. She has been physically healthy since last seen and the owner does not think Gypsy has lost any weight.

a) What are the potential adverse effects of an overdose of an NSAID and how do these effects come about?
b) What factors should you consider before advising Ms Burstyn?
c) Would you advise differently if Gypsy ate the entire bottle of medication?

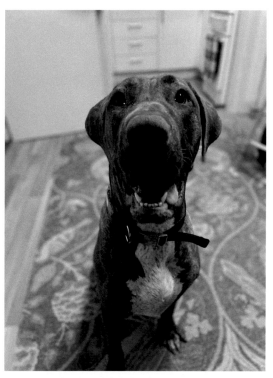

Figure 4.1a Gypsy, who weighs 40 kg, ate her owner's arthritis medication.

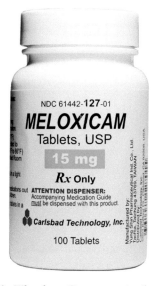

Figure 4.1b The dose Gypsy received was a single 15-mg tablet of human meloxicam.

4.2 Charlie, 3-yo MN Cross-breed: anxious, destroying things

Charlie's owner is concerned that Charlie is anxious when separated from the owner in the house and that he is destroying things at these times (Figure 4.2a,b). Outside the house, he is becoming less obedient and is also unsettled when travelling in the car. He is also barking much more. In the clinic, he is difficult to handle and showing aggression. This was noted in a comment at his last veterinary visit (an alert on the records reads: 'Care when getting

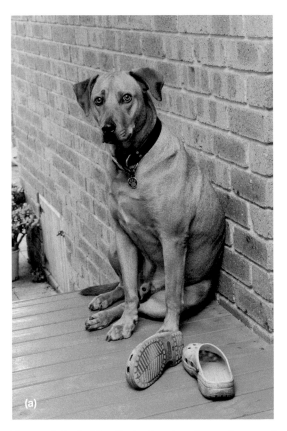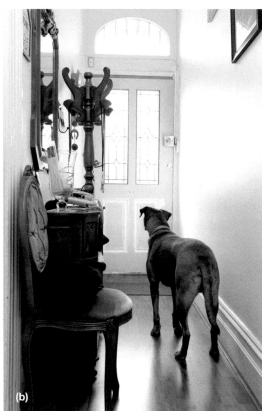

Figure 4.2a,b Charlie is showing signs of separation and generalised anxiety.

bloods!'). Charlie was diagnosed with Addison's disease (hypoadrenocorticism) 6 months ago.

a) What initial, general background questions will you ask of Charlie's owners? *Check your ideas against the answers before reading on.*

From these background questions, you find out that there are two adult owners and no other household pets. There were no concerns regarding Charlie's physical health until the diagnosis of Addison's. He responded well to reward based obedience training in class for 2 years and the owners are aware of the clicker as a training tool. There is, however, some evidence that aversive sprays have been used when Charlie was disobedient, and that a bark-activated collar spray has been used in attempts to deter barking. You also feel that Charlie's disobedience and demands for attention have been interpreted by the owners as an attempt to exert 'pack leadership'.

b) What specific questions would you now ask regarding his general demeanour and separation-related behaviour? *Check your ideas against the answers before reading on.*

The specific questions reveal that Charlie's anxiety-related problems are likely to be related to the onset of Addison's disease and subsequent treatment. It took some weeks for a diagnosis to be reached and for Charlie to be stabilised on medication, which involved multiple veterinary visits and invasive handling. His initial symptoms were most likely related to the as yet undiagnosed Addison's disease, coupled with owner confusion and concern regarding other apparently inexplicable behavioural changes, in particular the restlessness in the car and lack of response to the owner when at exercise. The fact that he responded well to reward-based training in the past made the sudden changes all the more frustrating. He was described as 'difficult to handle' for initial veterinary investigations. His behaviour has now deteriorated to the extent of requiring muzzling for routine blood tests to monitor treatment.

Charlie is now unable to relax and seems constantly on the alert to even small changes in his environment. This is particularly evident in the car. Surprisingly, it transpires that the 'separation anxiety', evidenced by chewing and destruction of household items, occurs only when the owners are at home and Charlie is confined by a child gate in the kitchen. When the owners were asked why they enforced this separation in the house, they say that when Charlie started being anxious, they believed that he needed 'his own territory to make him feel more secure'. Charlie is, however, content in the kitchen alone at night and when the owners leave the house. The owners have resorted to the aversive spray in attempts to get his attention and give him instruction on walks. The owners provide Charlie with treats when they leave the house.

c) How may Charlie's medical condition and treatment have affected his perceptions and behaviour?
d) What negative effect might Charlie's confinement in the kitchen be having?
e) How can Charlie's response to commands be improved and used to combat anxiety?
f) What are some key points to check regarding the owners' understanding of the clicker as a conditioned reinforcer?
g) How could the use of a long line on walks help Charlie's development?
h) How may Charlie's negative veterinary associations be reversed?

4.3 Bella, 7-mo FE Cross-breed: spay

Bella presents for ovariectomy. Upon intubation, you notice her mouth (Figure 4.3).

a) What is 'the rule of dental succession'?
b) What causes a primary tooth to be shed from the mouth under normal circumstances?
c) In general, what should you advise an owner if you see any retained primary teeth?
d) What are the clinical issues in Bella's case?
e) How would you treat Bella's mouth?
f) From what you see, what do you think of the prognosis, and why?

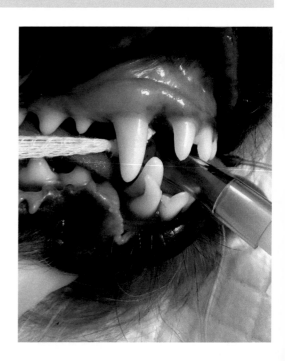

Figure 4.3 Bella's mouth has gone unnoticed until intubation for ovariectomy.

4.4 Cleo, 6-yo FN DSH: bleeding when eating

Cleo is brought in by her owner as they have noticed specks of blood in Cleo's food bowl for the past week. The owner has not been able to look inside Cleo's mouth, but advises you that she seems well, although she may be drooling a bit and chewing more on the right side of her mouth. On clinical examination, Cleo has lost 300 g (approximately 7% of body weight) in the 3 months since she was last seen for her vaccination, but presents in ideal body condition. You look in her mouth (Figure 4.4).

Cleo's submandibular lymph nodes do not appear enlarged or painful, and the remainder of her clinical examination is unremarkable.

a) Create a ranked problem list for Cleo, justifying the order you have chosen.

You anaesthetise Cleo to examine her mouth and, with permission from the owner, take a biopsy. Histopathology confirms a diagnosis of SCC. Despite this diagnosis, Cleo is doing well, and the owner wants to discuss options for treatment as they have read mixed reports of treatment options on the internet. To ensure that the client is fully informed and to aid shared decision-making, you decide to use a professional reasoning framework to prepare suitable options to discuss.

b) List the stakeholders impacted or involved in the creation of a treatment plan for Cleo.
c) For each of these stakeholders, explore the benefits (advantages) and costs

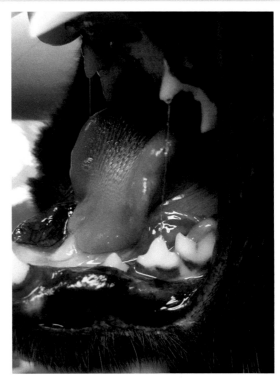

Figure 4.4 **Cleo has a lesion sublingually on the left side near the level of the lower molar.**

(disadvantages) of the following professional reasoning approaches, using current evidence-based medicine to support your answers:
- Do nothing
- Do something
- Do everything
- Euthanasia

4.5 Gregor, 8-yo MN DLH: inpatient

Gregor is an inpatient receiving IV fluids after falling from a third-floor apartment (Figure 4.5a,b). He is not eating or drinking owing to a fractured hard palate and is awaiting assessment for surgery. He weighs 4.0 kg.

Last night, Gregor's PCV was 37%. His IV catheter failed overnight; consequently, he received no fluids, and he has neither eaten nor drank. His PCV is now 49%. You place a new IV catheter successfully.

How much fluid does Gregor need over the next 24 hours?

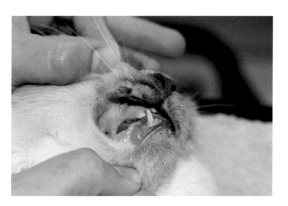

Figure 4.5a Injuries typical of a 'high-rise' cat after a fall: fractured 104 and a lip laceration cause by the lower canine on impact of his chin with the ground.

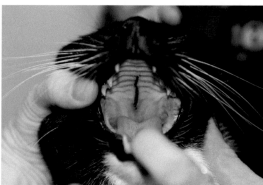

Figure 4.5b Gregor's hard palate fracture. His injury healed with conservative management, but more extensive fractures would probably need surgery.

'High-rise syndrome' is a pattern of injuries commonly seen in cats that have fallen from a height. Associated injuries include forelimb fractures and dislocations, pneumothorax, pulmonary contusions, rib fractures, fractured mandibular symphysis, temporomandibular joint fracture/luxation, hard palate fracture, and dental injuries. Cats that fall from a height should be checked for these injuries.

4.6 Walter, 5-mo ME Miniature Dachshund: V ++ & D ++

You consult at a local animal shelter on Thursdays. Walter was surrendered to the shelter today due to medical concerns and cost constraints. He was purchased online 4 days ago, and yesterday he started vomiting, became lethargic, and developed severe diarrhoea (Figure 4.6). His appetite also steadily decreased over the course of the day. The vaccine records from the breeder indicate that he was given one distemper–hepatitis–parvovirus–parainfluenza (DHPP) vaccination and one dose of pyrantel 2 weeks ago.

Physical findings:

- Demeanour: quiet, alert, reactive
- Temp: 39.5 °C
- CRT 3 s
- MMs pale pink
- HR = PR = 220 bpm, no murmurs

- Abdominal palpation: soft, possibly some pain on palpation

After the exam, Walter ate some puppy food that was offered by hand.

Shelter medicine is often considered to be small animal 'herd' medicine, because medical decisions not only affect the individual patient, but the entire shelter population as well. For instance, an infectious disease in an incoming patient could be detrimental to other animals in the shelter. In addition, each shelter has a finite capacity for care, dictated by the number of staff, funding, cage spaces, and number of adopters. In Walter's case, it is important to first rule out any potentially detrimental infectious diseases that fit Walter's signalment and history.

A parvovirus faecal antigen SNAP test is

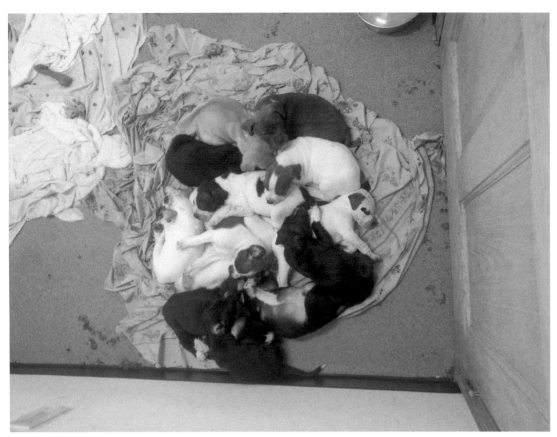

Figure 4.6 A litter of puppies in a shelter isolation facility with mild parvoviral enteritis (note evidence of diarrhoea in the environment). Strict biosecurity measures are essential to protect the wider shelter population from infectious diseases such as parvovirus.

a countertop enzyme-linked immunosorbent assay (ELISA) test that yields results quickly. The remainder of the stool sample can also be submitted for a faecal flotation test at the same time. Depending on the results of the parvovirus SNAP test, we can decide whether to run further diagnostics (e.g. blood work). Walter's results: parvovirus SNAP test: positive; faecal flotation: negative.

a) While Walter was being examined in the treatment room, a 4-week-old puppy was brought into the same room for her intake exam and vaccinations. This puppy is now considered exposed but not infected. Where should the puppy be housed after exposure?

b) What action should be taken if, instead, a 9-month-old dog is examined in the same treatment room as Walter?

c) What further diagnostics and treatment are indicated for Walter?

d) When is euthanasia considered for severely affected animals in a shelter?

e) When can Walter be made available for adoption?

4.7 Thor, 5-yo ME German Shepherd: off colour, no appetite

Thor, who weighs 42 kg, has been poorly for the previous 2 days. On presentation, he is quiet, alert, and responsive, with an HR of 126 and an RR of 30. Thoracic auscultation does not reveal any abnormalities; however, his MMs are pale and slightly tacky. His owner consents to more investigations, including haematology and biochemistry blood work, and abdominal imaging.

An abdominal ultrasound reveals a large splenic mass with some free fluid present (Figure 4.7a). You offer an exploratory laparotomy and splenectomy.

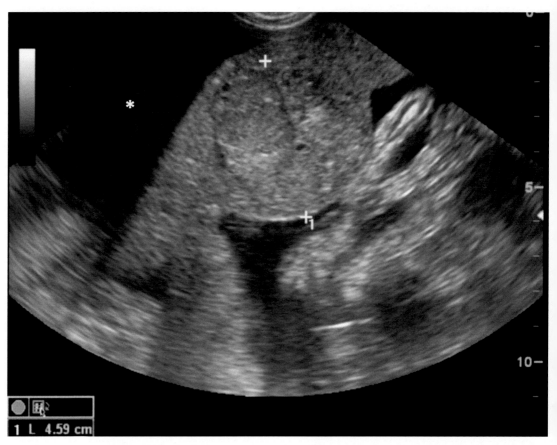

Figure 4.7a Ultrasound of Thor's abdomen shows free abdominal fluid and a splenic mass. The splenic mass is shown between the two + marks of the measuring calliper and free fluid is indicated by an asterisk.

a) While waiting for consent for surgery, Thor requires IV fluid therapy to help correct a presumed hypovolaemia. You opt for Hartmann's solution at a rate of 5 mL/kg/h. What rate do you set on your drip pump?

b) The drip pump is out of battery and refuses to work. How many drops per second do you set on your 20 drops/mL giving set?

c) You obtain consent for surgery and proceed to theatre. During the procedure the ECG shows the trace in Figure 4.7b. What is this trace?

d) Do you treat the abnormal ECG? If so, how?

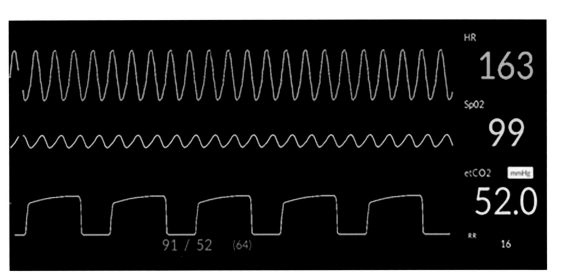

Figure 4.7b Image from the multi-parameter monitor during Thor's surgery.

4.8 Maya, 17-yo FN DSH: vomiting & weight loss

VISIT 1

The owner reports that lately Maya has been vomiting sporadically, every second to third day. She has also been a bit more vocal, mainly in the evenings. She is currently not on any medication and has a good appetite. There has also been some inter-cat conflict at home.

Maya is an indoor-only cat, vaccinated, wormed, and fed a renal diet. She lives with two younger cats who are sibling female neutered DSHs. Maya's weight had been stable at 5 kg for many years, but at her last vaccination a year ago it had dropped to 4.1 kg.

Maya had a blood test last year (Table 4.8a).

At the time of her bloods, an abdominal ultrasound revealed a suspected benign liver nodule and bacterial cholangitis. Bile culture revealed *Enterococcus* resistant to enrofloxacin, but susceptible to amoxycillin/clavulanate. Maya was not amenable to tabletting. She received injectable amoxycillin/clavulanate sporadically at home, and was not followed up.

Table 4.8a Maya's blood results from last year		
PARAMETER	**RESULT**	**NORMAL**
Haematocrit (HCT)	34%	0.25–0.48 L/L
Creatinine	130	80–200 µmol/L
Symmetric dimethylarginine (SDMA)	23	0–14 µg/dL
ALP	107	5–50 IU/L
AST	725	2–62 IU/L
ALT	1375	19–100 IU/L
GGT	4	0–5 IU/L
Cholesterol	10.3	2.2–5.5 mmol/L
Total thyroxine (TT4)	32	6–52 nmol/L

Maya's examination today is as follows:

- Weight: 3.91 kg
- BCS: 4/9
- Muscle condition score (MCS): 4/9, with pronounced muscle wasting in the hind legs (*https://wsava.org/wp-content/uploads/2020/01/Muscle-Condition-Score-Chart-for-Cats.pdf*)
- HR 188 bpm, no murmur, chest clear
- Abdominal palpation: lots of log-like faeces in distal colon, no bladder discomfort

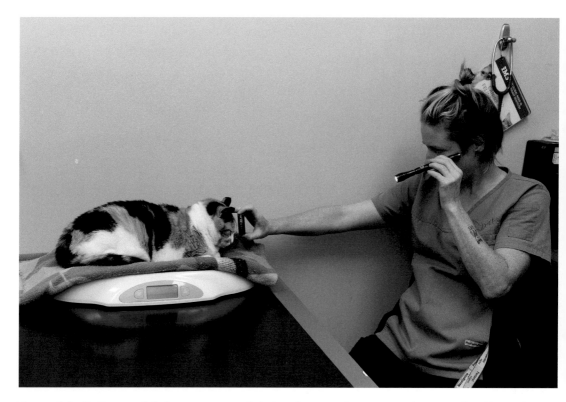

Figure 4.8a Indirect ophthalmoscopy revealed pinpoint spots in Maya's right eye and mild vessel tortuosity in the left eye.

- Pain on hip extension and elbow flexion
- Grade 1 tartar and mild gingivitis, no obvious dental pain
- Indirect ophthalmoscopy after tropicamide: a few pinpoint spots in her right eye and mild vessel tortuosity in the left eye (Figure 4.8a)

You ask about Maya's home environment. There is one heated bed in the laundry for the three cats to sleep in, and one large, high-sided litter tray outside a cat door. The owner believes that the cats like sleeping together. There are three food bowls in the kitchen, all placed together. On questioning, it is difficult for the owner to ascertain if Maya is passing faeces daily. The younger cats are also eating Maya's prescription kidney food.

a) How do you perform indirect ophthalmoscopy step by step?

b) Why is indirect ophthalmoscopy especially good for older, tricky-to-handle cats?

c) Maya's ophthalmoscopy showed blood vessel tortuosity. What is the next step?

d) Maya lives in a multi-cat household. What could you suggest to the owner to encourage Maya to eat more, and perhaps allow ease of urinating/defaecating?

e) You are not fully booked today and extend the appointment to allow serial BP measurements to be made. Maya seems relaxed during the process (Figure 4.8b). The average reading is 180 mmHg. After this, you attempt a jugular blood sample, but Maya seems uncomfortable on positioning for blood sampling, so you decide to delay this until the next visit. What treatment(s) will you give Maya today?

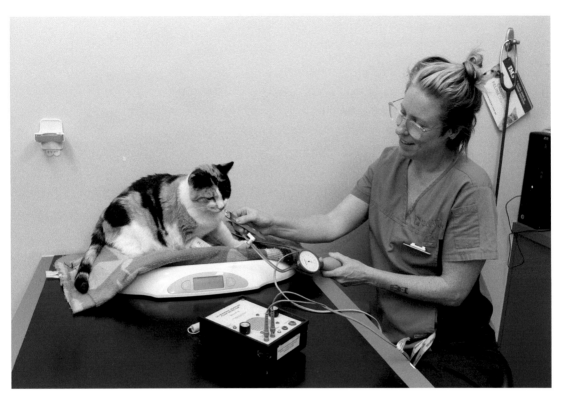

Figure 4.8b Maya getting treats while her BP is measured.

VISIT 2

Maya has her BP rechecked a week later. She is well managed and her readings now average 160 mmHg. Her abdomen palpates normally with no more log-like faeces. She has bloods taken following administration of gabapentin orally (2 hours before the visit) and EMLA™ cream applied 30 minutes prior to venepuncture (Leask 2021); a bent needle is used so as not to hyperextend her neck. The key results are in Table 4.8b.

a) What is your interpretation of these results?

b) What would be your next steps?

c) What other condition might you suspect in a cat with vomiting and a history of cholangitis?

Table 4.8b Maya's comparative blood test results

PARAMETER	TODAY'S RESULTS	PREVIOUS RESULTS	NORMAL
TT4	47	32	6–52 nmol/L
ALT	252	1375	19–100 IU/L
AST	182	725	2–62 IU/L
CK	700	200	64–400 IU/L

4.9 Flora, 9-wo FE Cavoodle: passing blood

Flora, a 1.75-kg Cavoodle puppy, was seen by a colleague this morning for a 24-hour history of frequent, watery diarrhoea, with the presence of fresh blood in the most recent stool. She was purchased from a pet shop 2 weeks ago, and vaccinated for parvovirus, distemper virus, and adenovirus soon after. No information was provided about worming. The owners reported that Flora was bright, eating well, and had not vomited. Her diet seems to be varied, as the inexperienced owners have spoiled Flora with a lot of treats. She was normothermic this morning and there was no indication of abdominal pain on examination. She was treated with an oral probiotic and bland diet, and prescribed a veterinary wormer.

It is now late afternoon and the owner has just returned to the clinic with a large worm that was passed in Flora's stool (Figure 4.9).

a) What kind of parasite is this?
b) How might the puppy have become infected?
c) How might older puppies and adult dogs become infected?

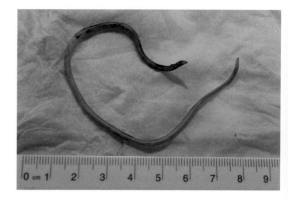

Figure 4.9 **Worm passed by Flora following administration of a worming tablet.**

d) Is it zoonotic?
e) How often should puppies be wormed?
f) Is this responsible for Flora's clinical signs?

4.10 Walter, 5-yo ME Malinois Greyhound: swollen toe

Three weeks ago, Walter presented with a 2-day history of left forelimb lameness following free exercise. He was treated conservatively with NSAIDs by a colleague at your clinic. There has been no improvement of his lameness. You palpate a swollen and displaced distal fifth digit (Figure 4.10).

a) What are the differential diagnoses for Walter?
b) How would you investigate Walter at this stage?
c) How would you treat the various conditions you are considering?
d) You decide Walter needs a permanent nail removal (ungual crest ostectomy [UCO]). Describe the procedure.

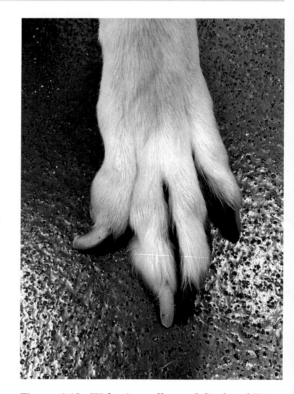

Figure 4.10 **Walter's swollen and displaced D5.**

4.11 Fluffy Friends Rescue Centre: site visit

Fluffy Friends is concerned that it has a lot of kittens showing sore eyes, sneezing, and lethargy. There have been two deaths. The rescue centre has 10 individual runs that they use for pregnant queens and kittens up to 6–8 weeks of age, and the rest of the adult cats and kittens are group-housed (Figure 4.11a). They currently vaccinate all kittens at 9 and 12 weeks of age, and vaccinate adult cats on entry (unless pregnant).

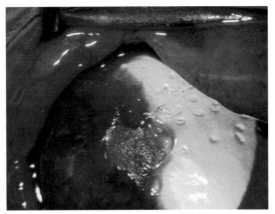

Figure 4.11b **A common presentation in shelter cats. The image shows a cat's cornea in close-up.**

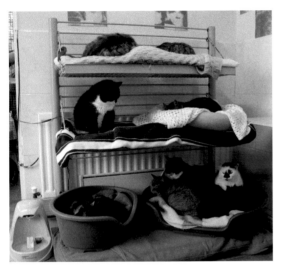

Figure 4.11a **At Fluffy Friends, cats are group-housed.**

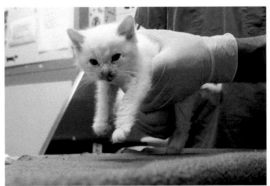

Figure 4.11c **This kitten has marked nasal congestion with bilateral nasal and ocular discharge. She is sneezing frequently, has crackles and rales on lung auscultation, and has a rectal temperature of 39.8 °C.**

a) Which vaccine-preventable pathogens are most commonly implicated in feline upper respiratory tract disease ('cat flu')?
b) What management changes would you implement to reduce new cases at Fluffy Friends?
c) When would you consider diagnostic testing to identify the pathogen(s)?

d) What pathogen is the condition shown in Figure 4.11b typical of? How would you treat this?
e) What treatment options would you consider for the kitten in Figure 4.11c?

4.12 Dusty, 6-yo ME Golden Retriever: annual vaccination

Wilson has brought his healthy retriever, Dusty, in for annual vaccination. During the consultation, he mentions how impressed he is that the clinic has solar panels and an electric

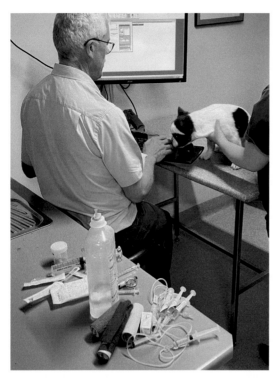

Figure 4.12a Medical consumables, particularly plastic, produce high CO$_2$-equivalent emissions. Conscious monitoring of the use of medical consumables, and reduction of this use, can reduce a practice's carbon footprint.

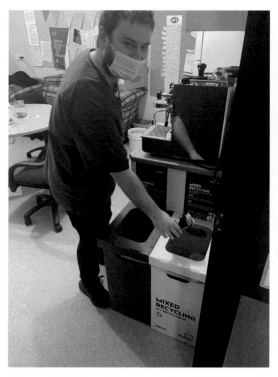

Figure 4.12b Practices can reduce their footprint by encouraging waste separation and recycling, e.g. by placing appropriate bins in consultation rooms, treatment areas, and the staff room.

vehicle charging station. However, upon noticing the plastic syringe and packaging, Wilson comments that a lot of waste must be generated by vet practices (Figure 4.12a,b), reflecting that the COVID-19 pandemic has raised his awareness of medical waste.

a) What factors contribute to the environmental footprint of a veterinary practice?
b) Why should veterinary practices take steps to reduce their environmental impact?
c) What can practices do to reduce their environmental impact?

4.13 Kane, 14-yo MN Labrador: booster vaccination

Kane (Figure 4.13) is a Labrador who struggles to get to his feet in the waiting room when called in. You help him by lifting his hindquarters using a towel sling under the abdomen. He makes his way to your consult room with some difficulty. Kane has advanced elbow dysplasia and atrophy of the muscles in his hindquarters. As soon as he is in the consultation room, he lies back down, which is an uncomfortable-looking process, with lots of shifting. He seems disinterested in his surroundings, but he does take treats with typical Labrador enthusiasm.

a) What questions do you wish to ask the owner having observed Kane's progress into the consulting room?
b) What concerns do you have for Kane and how will you go about expressing them to his owner, who has just booked him in for a simple vaccination?
c) What diagnostics and treatment, if any, do you want to offer?
d) What factors might limit diagnostic/treatment options?
e) Is it acceptable to bring up the topic of euthanasia? How will you go about doing so?

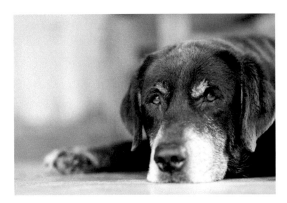

Figure 4.13 **Kane had to be helped into the consulting room.**

4.14 Rusty, 2-yo ME Dachshund: vaccination

Rusty presents for a vaccination when the owner reports that, over the past month, Rusty has had periods of being 'not quite right' – lethargic and 'moping', but then seems to recover.

Physical examination findings:

- BAR
- BCS: 3.5/5
- HR 144 bpm, with a regular rate and rhythm and no audible murmur
- RR: panting
- Lung fields: difficult to auscultate as Rusty barks frequently
- Lymph nodes: no abnormalities detected
- Abdominal palpation: slightly reactive when mid-abdomen is palpated, with no mass effect
- Gut sounds: normal
- Testicular palpation: both testes are present in scrotum. The right testicle is harder on palpation, feels heavier, and is grossly larger than the left (Figure 4.14a). Rusty does not react to palpation
- Temp: 38.7 °C
- Rectal examination: no abnormalities detected

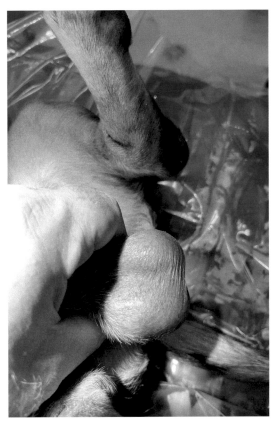

Figure 4.14a **Rusty's right testicle is larger than the left and hard on palpation.**

A routine, open castration is performed on the same day. The left testicle is normal. The right testicle appears dark red in colour and is torsed (Figure 14.4b).

a) What are the key differentials for an enlarged testicle in the dog?
b) What structures does the spermatic cord contain? What are the likely sequelae of its torsion?
c) Why is it important to perform a rectal examination in dogs with testicular masses?
d) What conditions increase the risk of testicular torsion?
e) What other clinical signs are associated with testicular torsion?
f) What is the recommended treatment for unilateral testicular torsion?

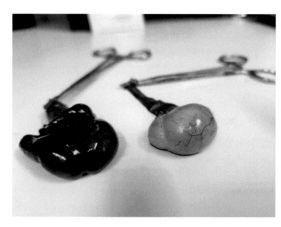

Figure 4.14b Rusty's testicles immediately after surgery.

4.15 Shadow, 2-yo ME DSH: O thinks leg is broken

Shadow presents non-weight-bearing on his right hindlimb after being missing for 2 days. On examination, Shadow is BAR, with tacky MMs, mild tachycardia, and scuffed nails. He vocalises whenever you try to manipulate his right hindlimb. The rest of his clinical examination is unremarkable.

a) What immediate action would you take to manage Shadow? Justify your reasoning.

Following initial treatment, Shadow is anaesthetised for radiographs (Figure 4.15).

b) Comment on the radiographic findings.
c) What is your diagnosis and interpretation of the lameness?
d) What treatment is used initially?
e) If the first treatment method fails, what alternatives can be offered?

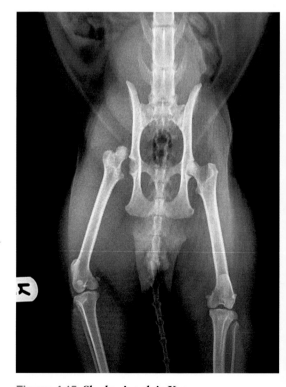

Figure 4.15 Shadow's pelvis X-ray.

4.16 Peter, 6-mo ME Cross-breed: health check

You are seeing Peter for a health check. In your overall preventive medicine discussion, you bring up the topic of gonadectomy (Figure 4.16). The owner, who also has a young female dog, responds that they have been doing some reading and are finding conflicting information about timing and even whether or not we should do this procedure at all.

a) What factors will impact your recommendation?
b) What is your recommendation for timing of gonadectomy if the dog is female?
c) What is your recommendation for timing of castration if the dog is male?

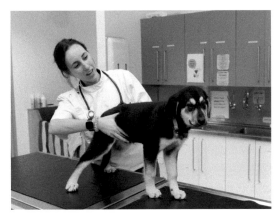

Figure 4.16 **During the puppy health check, you discuss the topic of gonadectomy.**

4.17 On way in – see immediately: dog collapsed on walk

You are presented with Deano, a 9-year-old Hungarian Vizsla who collapsed on a walk and has been rushed in by the owner. Deano is unresponsive to stimuli, although there is a weak femoral pulse. Following a brief examination, you intubate Deano to provide supplementary oxygen and connect some monitoring, including an ECG and capnography, which result in the trace shown in Figure 4.17.

a) What is the ECG trace displayed above?
b) What treatment would you commence immediately?
c) How long would you continue with this treatment?

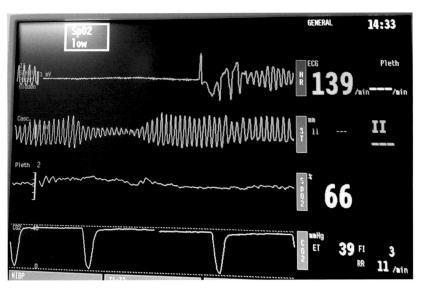

Figure 4.17 **Monitor display from Deano immediately after admission.**

4.18 Cleo, 4-yo FN Cocker Spaniel: drinking & urinating lots

Cleo has been drinking and urinating excessively for the last 3–4 weeks (Figure 4.18a). The owner also mentions that she has been trembling intermittently and is a bit quieter and more picky with her food in recent weeks. She had some diarrhoea and one vomit yesterday, but none prior to this. You notice Cleo's weight is 10.8 kg today. At her last vaccination almost a year ago, it was 11.6 kg.

You also took the time to read through Cleo's history prior to the consultation, and noticed that, 5 months ago she had markedly decreased sodium and chloride levels on a blood test. However, this blood test was performed when she presented for acute onset vomiting, which turned out to be due to a corncob obstructing her jejunum (Figure 4.18b,c). This was surgically removed via enterotomy, and Cleo made a slow but full recovery from her surgery. A repeat blood test after surgery, and again 1 month later, revealed sodium and chloride levels that had increased almost back into the normal reference range, so no further blood work has been performed since. The owner agrees with your recommendation to run bloods on Cleo again today. Her results are shown in Tables 4.18a,b (see page 208 for Table 4.18b).

a) What disease does Cleo's blood work make you suspicious of, and why?
b) What test do you need to perform to definitively diagnose this disease?
c) What is the prognosis for this disease and how will you explain Cleo's disease to her owners?
d) What treatment is required for Cleo?
e) Why do you think this condition is so easily missed?
f) What aspects of Cleo's presenting signs are not typical of the condition and what other diseases could she have been suspected of having?

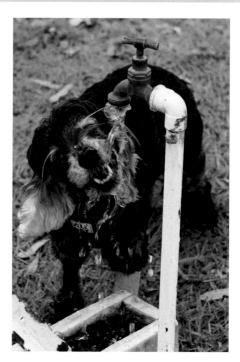

Figure 4.18a Cleo has been drinking a lot for 3–4 weeks.

Table 4.18a Cleo's haematology results. Values outside the reference ranges are in red

PARAMETER	RESULT	REFERENCE RANGE
RBC	7.57	5.5–8.5 × 10^{12}/L
Hb	170	120–180 g/L
PCV	0.44	0.37–0.55 L/L
MCV	58	60–77 fL
MCH	23	19–25 pg
MCHC	386	320–360 g/L
Leukocytes	12.59	6.0–17.0 × 10^9/L
Neutrophils	6.39	3.6–13.10 × 10^9/L
Lymphocytes	5.79	0.72–2.21 × 10^9/L
Monocytes	0.28	0.00–1.7 × 10^9/L
Eosinophils	0.12	0.00–1.7 × 10^9/L
Basophils	0.01	0.00–0.36 × 10^9/L
Total plasma protein (TPP) (refract)	61	58–84 g/L
Platelets	212	200–500 × 10^9/L
Plasma appearance	Normal	

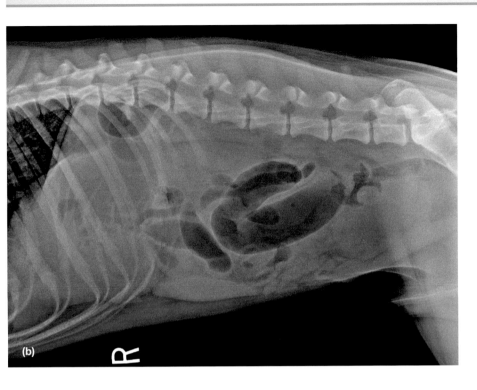

(b)

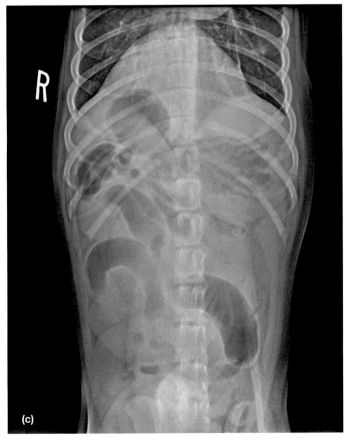

(c)

Figure 4.18b,c Cleo's acute vomiting episodes were attributed to a corncob foreign body, not easily visible here. However, note the obstructive gas pattern. For dogs, intestinal diameter of over 1.6× the height of the midsection of the L5 vertebra is suggestive of intestinal dilation and may indicate obstruction, while in cats, an intestinal diameter of >2× the height of L2 is suggestive of intestinal dilation and may indicate obstruction. The corncob was surgically removed via enterotomy.

Table 4.18b **Cleo's biochemistry results. Values outside the reference ranges are in red**

PARAMETER	RESULT	REFERENCE RANGE
CK	64	<400 U/L
AST	16	<80 U/L
ALT	16	<80 U/L
ALP	12	<120 U/L
Total bilirubin	3.0	<10 µmol/L
Cholesterol	2.56	3.49–7.18 mmol/L
Creatinine	78	47–128 µmol/L
Urea	6.3	4.3–7.1 mmol/L
Glucose	5.8	3.9–6.9 mmol/L
Phosphate	1.63	0.84–2.00 mmol/L
Calcium (uncorrected)	2.56	1.9–2.8 mmol/L
Serum protein	63	54–78 g/L
Albumin	37	23–40 g/L
Globulin	27	27–41 g/L
Albumin:globulin ratio	1.37	0.59–1.11
Sodium	111	144–160 mmol/L
Potassium	4.7	3.6–5.8 mmol/L
Chloride	90	110–125 mmol/L
C-reactive protein	<1.0	0.00–10.00 µg/mL
Serum/plasma appearance	Normal	

4.19 Seamus, 7-yo MN DSH: vomiting ++

Seamus (Figure 4.19a) presents with an acute history of projectile vomiting. The owner came home from a 12-hour overnight work shift to find several piles of vomit. Seamus was hiding under the bed, which was highly unusual, compared with his normally gregarious, greedy self. When picked up, Seamus projectile vomited and continued to do so once placed in his carry cage on the way to the clinic. On physical examination, marked dehydration and a painful mid-abdominal mass are noted. Seamus weighs 5.8 kg and is otherwise in good body condition (BCS 3/5).

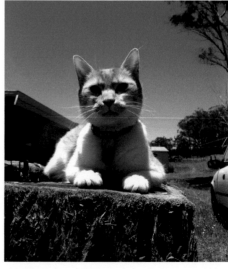

Figure 4.19a **Seamus in a happier state than on presentation today.**

a) What are your differentials for a painful mid-abdominal mass in a 7-year-old cat?
b) You decide to put the ultrasonography probe onto the mass to investigate further. Describe what you see (Figure 4.19b), and the most likely diagnosis indicated by this finding.
c) How would you treat Seamus?
d) How would you investigate the underlying cause of this condition?

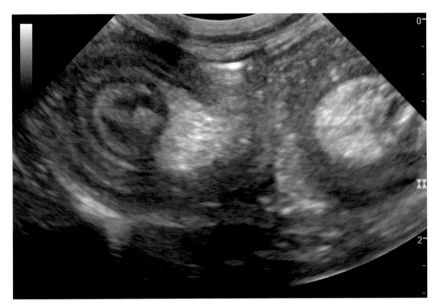

Figure 4.19b The image when the probe is applied to Seamus's abdomen.

4.20 Home time

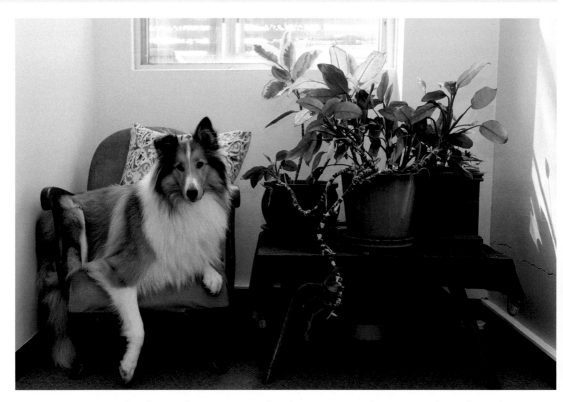

Figure 4.20 Canine family members are attuned to home time. Perhaps we can learn from them.

It can be difficult for veterinarians to 'switch off' after work. We care about our patients and their humans, and the job is full of challenges: clinical, ethical, and emotional. It is part of what makes being a veterinarian so absorbing, but such deep investment can prevent us from being fully present in our personal lives, with potentially negative impacts on wellbeing and personal relationships. Make a list, or a drawing, of things you can do that will help you change your focus from work to home at the end of the working day.

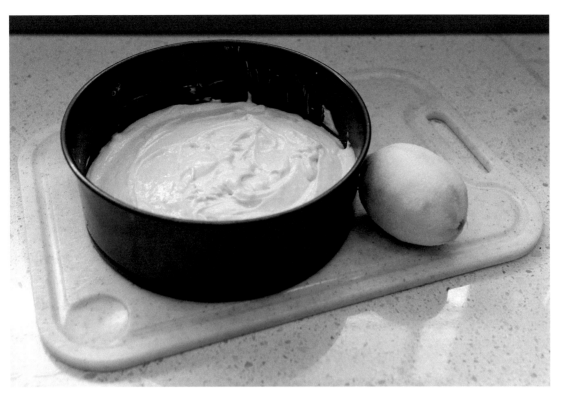

Figure 4.21a **The ingredients after mixing.**

MUM'S FRESH LEMON DRIZZLE CAKE

This easy cake is incredibly moreish. If you add in extra lemon, and even some lime, it gives it a special zingy deliciousness.

Ingredients

Cake

Approximately 112 g soft margarine
1 level teaspoon baking powder
170 g self-raising flour
170 g caster sugar
2 free-range organic eggs or substitute
4 tablespoons milk or substitute
Grated rind of a lemon (but you can add more of this, and also lime rind)

Icing

Juice of one lemon (and lime if desired)
112 g caster sugar

Equipment

Oven
Large mixing bowl
Electric or hand mixer
20-cm cake tin (springform is ideal as this makes the cake easier to remove)

Method

1. Preheat oven to gas 4/350 °F/180 °C.
2. Put all cake ingredients into a bowl and mix by hand or electric mixer (2 minutes) (Figure 4.21a).
3. Grease or line a 20-cm cake tin, then pour in cake mix.
4. Bake the cake for 50–60 minutes.
5. While the cake is cooking, mix lemon juice (and optional lime juice) and sugar to create a paste.
6. Remove the cake from the oven and drizzle the icing on the cake while the cake is hot (Figure 4.21b).
7. Leave cake to cool on a wire cooling rack.
8. Enjoy with some English Breakfast or Australian Afternoon Tea.
9. When the cake is finished: repeat.

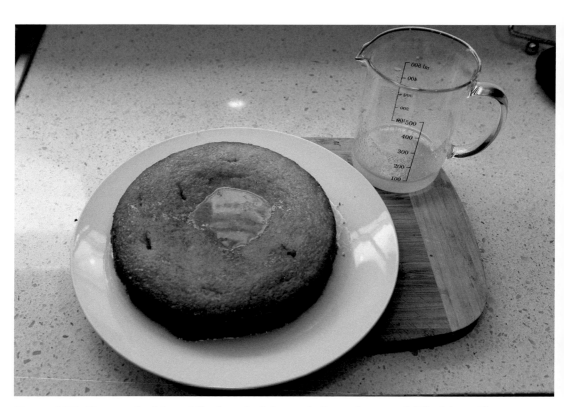

Figure 4.21b Pour on the icing while the cake is hot and allow cake to cool. The icing will create a delicious frosting on top and down the sides.

Name	species breed	sex	Age	Weight	Procedure	Switch +O2
Pepper Fern	Lizard B.J.	?	1yr	312g	+axing Xrays — its a boy :)	
Zombie Green	Cat DSH	FS	11yr	4.2kg	Grade IV dental inc teeth	☑ Pregn Bloods ☑ Fluids
Florence O'Reilly	K9 Mini Daschund	F	6m	3.6kg	Spey	✓ ☑ Fluids
Ginger Hall	K9 min Poodle	M	6m	6.7kg	Castration + Microchip	✓
Teddy Stephens	K9 Pomranian	M	6m	3.2	Castration	✓
Fuk Fuk Lee	Cat DSH	M	4m	2.6	Castrate + F3	✓
Hooch Crosbie	K9 Pitbull x	M	6yr	38kg	Eyelid Mass removal - estimate given + grade 2 dental	Fluids ✓
Flutfy Buns Smith	Rabbit Lop x	M	3m	1.2kg	Rabbit Castrate	☑ critacare

4.1 Gypsy, 2-yo FN Cross-breed: ate owner's tablet

a) Adverse effects of NSAIDs, at both on-label and off-label doses, can range from mild gastritis and vomiting to severe GIT ulceration and bleeding, kidney injury, and both dose-dependent and idiopathic hepatotoxicity, as well as central nervous system signs (Walton et al. 2017, Chalifoux et al. 2023). These adverse effects are believed to be due to the inhibition of COX-1, a 'housekeeping enzyme' that protects the gastrointestinal mucosa, maintains renal blood flow, and helps maintain homoeostasis. NSAIDs such as meloxicam act by preferentially inhibiting COX-2, which facilitates the production of inflammatory prostaglandins. But COX-2 selectivity diminishes at higher doses of these NSAIDs (Walton et al. 2017).

b) The following are factors to consider:

i) The maximum possible dose of exposure. For Gypsy, this is 15 mg in a 40-kg dog: 15/40 = 0.375 mg/kg.

ii) Is the active ingredient registered for use in dogs? If so, is it within the normal dose range? Meloxicam is also registered for use in dogs, albeit at different dose rates than in humans. The label dose for meloxicam is 0.2 mg/kg IV or SC, followed by 0.1 mg/kg PO q24h. Following oral administration or ingestion, the drug is well absorbed and almost 100% bioavailable (Walton et al. 2017). Gypsy has received a dose just under double that of the maximum label dose.

iii) If the drug was outside the normal dose range, are there safety studies? In such cases, it may be quicker to contact the product manufacturer technical services veterinarian for data from safety studies in which products may have been administered at higher doses. In this case, you learn that dogs administered the drug at five times the labelled maintenance dose (0.5 mg/kg/PO q24h) for 6 weeks had occurrences of diarrhoea and vomiting, with no occult faecal blood detected (Boehringer Ingelheim Vetmedica Inc. 2003). In light of this, it seems unlikely that a healthy dog receiving a single dose not quite four times the maintenance dose would develop clinical signs. Of course, the risk of an idiosyncratic reaction cannot be ruled out.

iv) The health condition of Gypsy. In addition to dose, factors that may predispose dogs to adverse effects from NSAIDs include concurrent disease (particularly pre-existing renal disease), dehydration, hypotension, young or advanced age, concurrent medication or drug interactions, and anaesthesia (Walton et al. 2017). Gypsy is in excellent health and not taking medications. It is also useful to know if Gypsy has eaten a meal recently, as NSAIDs are typically administered on a full stomach.

> Any advice given by telephone, including the information provided by Ms Burstyn, your estimation of the exposure, recommendations about whether to seek veterinary care immediately or monitor, and what you advise Ms Burstyn to monitor (e.g. reduced appetite, increased thirst, dull demeanour, vomiting, diarrhoea or the presence of blood in the stool) should be recorded in Gypsy's record.

c) Yes. Depending on the dose and the condition of the patient, management of NSAID intoxication may include gastrointestinal decontamination, administration of gastroprotectants (e.g. H_2 antagonists such as famotidine, proton-pump inhibitors such as omeprazole, and ulcer binding agents such as sucralfate), prostaglandin analogues (such as misoprostol), judicious fluid therapy, and, in more severe cases, IV lipid emulsion or referral for therapeutic plasma exchange (TPE). If she has ingested the full bottle of meloxicam, Gypsy should be taken to the nearest veterinarian immediately for prompt decontamination and assessment.

REFERENCES

Boehringer Ingelheim Vetmedica Inc. (2003) Freedom of information summary, new animal drug application NADA 141-219 METACAM (meloxicam) 5 mg/mL solution for injection. Boehringer Ingelheim Vetmedica Inc. Available at: https://animaldrugsatfda.fda.gov/adafda/app/search/public/document/downloadFoi/751.

Chalifoux, N. V., Butty, E. M., Mauro, K. D. et al (2023) Outcomes of 434 dogs with non-steroidal anti-inflammatory drug toxicosis treated with fluid therapy, lipid emulsion, or therapeutic plasma exchange. *Journal of Veterinary Internal Medicine* **37**(1):161–172. doi: 10.1111/jvim.16603.

Walton, S., Ryan, K. A., Davis, J. L. & Acierno, M. (2017) Treatment of meloxicam overdose in a dog via therapeutic plasma exchange. *Journal of Veterinary Emergency and Critical Care* **27**(4):444–450. doi: 10.1111/vec.12607.

4.2 Charlie, 3-yo MN Cross-breed: anxious, destroying things

a) Initial, general background questions should include the following:
   - At what age and from where was Charlie acquired?
   - What is his personality like?
   - Family set-up and habits. Are there other pets?
   - General health/daily routine/exercise/diet/feeding times?
   - What is Charlie's training history?
   - What techniques have been used to modify Charlie's behaviour in the past?

b) Specific questions to ask regarding Charlie's general demeanour and separation-related behaviour include the following:
   - When did the various components of his problematic behaviour begin?
   - Has his response to everyday events changed?
   - When is he destructive?
   - What measures are being used to limit destruction and his other unwanted behaviours?

c) Although Charlie's problems may have arisen without the complication of Addison's disease, his medical condition may have contributed to his behaviour in the following ways:
   - A reduction in cortisone results in a disrupted stress (fight–flight) response, meaning that Charlie would have been less able to cope with normal, healthy 'ups and downs' of life
   - Cortisone has been shown to enhance the memory of unpleasant events, which is a survival mechanism to allow avoidance of danger. In Charlie's case, administration of exogenous cortisone, although essential for treatment, may have, in turn, increased his anxiety in the face of normal everyday events
   - Veterinary handling is, by its very nature, often invasive and threatening to dogs. For Charlie, the worse he has felt, the more handling was needed
   - The human attention given to dogs when they are ill, as well as anxious, risks giving the appearance that owners are also anxious. It may be that some inconsistency has arisen in communication with Charlie and in his management when he has been unwell – at the very times when, in fact, he needed the most clear and consistent guidance

It should be stressed that, in view of Charlie's illness and the effects it potentially has had upon his perception of the world, a guarded prognosis regarding behavioural improvement should be given.

d) There is no basis for considering the kitchen as a territory that Charlie needs to have to make him feel more secure. Instead of placing him there, the owners should spend more time with Charlie, to routinely practise all the behaviours that they need him to demonstrate elsewhere. The more separated Charlie is from his owners, the fewer opportunities there are to rehearse positive behaviours at a time when Charlie is in a relaxed frame of mind and able to learn to the best of his ability. The confinement has also created needless times of stress and upset, such as when the owners go up and down the stairs. This does not mean that the owners' routine at night and when they leave the house should change in any way, as Charlie only seems to be upset by separation when the owners are at home. Their absence from the house and at night should be associated with rewards in the same way as always.

e) The owners already use reward-based training methods, but their frustration and concern has inevitably impacted negatively on Charlie. The reward-based work they have already done should be commended. They also need to be warned how human emotion and untoward response may worsen Charlie's anxiety. Their attention, as well as food, must be used as reinforcers, giving these for appropriate, calm behaviour and withholding attention and food rewards if Charlie is stressed or anxious. Simple obedience commands, instilled using positive reward-based methods, change emotion as well as behaviour for the better, and therefore can be looked upon as 'antidotes to anxiety'. Eliminating the frustration Charlie may feel at home in being kept separated from his owners will give far more opportunity for rehearsal of all the simple obedience tasks (to come, sit, 'watch me', 'lie down', and 'stay') needed to assist him when he is anxious. The more these are rehearsed before Charlie is emotionally upset, the better.

Whose idea is it anyway?

To remind owners to rehearse obedience responses in advance, it is useful for them to consider whose idea it is for Charlie to behave like this (i.e. is his behaviour the owners' idea or his own?). Routinely changing Charlie's mind with simple requests throughout the day, whether or not the owners need to, will ensure that the necessary rehearsal is carried out. This will also imply that they do not give Charlie attention on demand, which risks 'drip-feeding' anxiety, particularly during greetings. Here, they should remain calm and aloof to ensure that arousal and excitement are not accidentally rewarded. In so doing, rather than fulfilling any concept of 'pack leadership', the owners will become more consistent in their behaviour and response, which will help stabilise Charlie's expectations in a more positive frame of mind.

f) It is not uncommon to find that the clicker has been used to create a sound that simply means to a dog, 'Food available if you run this way'. The sound causes a dog to decide to run in the appropriate direction, but often only if nothing more salient is in the environment. Owners frequently need reminding that the clicker is not a controlling device but produces a distinct sound that, once firmly associated with the arrival of a titbit, becomes something that Charlie will want and work to hear.

> If used correctly, the clicker's **click** marks the behaviour a dog performs to make the click happen.

As a positive-reward sound, the clicker can be used to override other extraneous sounds to which Charlie may react and to inform Charlie that he is approved of, whether or not he has been given an instruction. It may be more effective to simply 'click and treat' absence of excitement or looking worried than deliberately used obedience commands, e.g. whenever Charlie is lying down in the house or walking calmly with a loose lead of his own volition. If he is asked to 'sit–stay' at the bottom of the stairs at home or at a distance in the park, his owners should click to predict the food when they are at the furthest point from him and return to him to give the food rather than asking him to come to them. He must learn that only by staying put will he gain their company.

g) A long line on walks will allow both the owners and Charlie to relax. It will reduce the owners' dependence upon a lead for control and also reduce Charlie's perception that they will always follow him wherever he goes. Meaningful cues already in place on walks, e.g. 'I'm going' or hiding behind a tree to encourage him to seek and follow them, and 'Uh-uh' to warn him he is about to make a mistake, can be rehearsed with more confidence in the knowledge that they cannot lose him. The negative punishment effect of the owners turning away from him in a 'couldn't-care-less' fashion is extremely important. Friends and their dogs can be used to provide extra behavioural leverage as they all walk away from him. To maintain effectiveness of any words or signals, they must be delivered before Charlie is distracted. This means that walks may have to be kept very short and unexciting for the time being, with the emphasis being on mental rather than physical exercise.

h) If there is any worry that Charlie may feel the need to bite at the vets, he should be properly muzzle-trained, rather than forcing a muzzle on him when he is already fearful and potentially aggressive. He and his owners should come to think of a basket-type muzzle as a food dispenser rather than a bite preventer, and owners should routinely practise placing one on his head at home in preparation for veterinary visits. Exceptionally tasty food should be used as reward for compliance in the surgery and the owners' own body gestures kept predictive of reward, i.e. poised and alert to a reward being offered while the muzzle is offered. Taking the clicker with them will help to make Charlie feel more hopeful. The most important commands for veterinary intervention are simply to sit and to 'watch me', using the clicker and a continual supply of treats to maintain his focus. If possible, injections or blood tests should be carried out where Charlie least expects them, e.g. in low-stress places such as the car park or on grass. This will require support from veterinary staff, but most vets and nurses will understand this approach.

4.3 Bella, 7-mo FE Cross-breed: spay

a) The 'rule of dental succession' states that there should never be two teeth of the same type in the same place in the mouth at the same time. In other words, it is not part of normal tooth shedding to see both primary ('milk') and secondary ('adult') teeth together in the mouth at any time.

b) A primary tooth is shed as the incoming

permanent tooth triggers root resorption of the primary tooth by osteoclasts. This is why primary teeth, when lost from the mouth, can look shell-like and incomplete. This 'partial' tooth appearance does not mean that a part of the primary tooth remains stuck within the alveolus. The permanent tooth is actually 'pulled into' the correct location along a pathway as the primary tooth root resorbs to make way for it.

c) The retained teeth should be removed as soon as possible (Bellows et al. 2019). Leaving them in situ may mean that the permanent tooth comes in at an abnormal orientation, causing a malocclusion that could be expensive to fix (Figure A4.3). While it is common to delay removal of persistent deciduous teeth until neutering, this is not recommended.

d) Applying the four-step malocclusion check (see also Case 2.6), we note the following:
1. The upper incisors appear to be going to sit just rostral to the lower incisors. Note

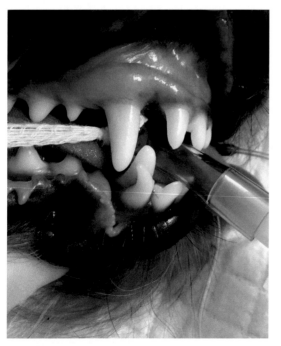

Figure A4.3 Bella's malocclusion.

that the endotracheal tube would need to be removed to check this. This *appears* correct (but see 3 below).

2. The right lower permanent canine (404) appears to be going to sit between the third upper right incisor (103) and the upper right canine (104). This is the correct relationship, but the canine appears medially displaced due to a retained primary right lower canine (804). **This is incorrect. The left lower canine should now be checked**.

3. The premolars sit directly on top of each other, without interdigitating in pinking shear fashion. **This is incorrect** and suggests slight discrepancy in jaw length between mandible and maxilla caused by the medially displaced canine (404) touching the hard palate and arresting forward growth of the mandible (= brachygnathism, 'short mandible').

4. It is not possible to see if the upper cheek teeth sit lateral (= buccal) to the lower cheek teeth, which would be the correct formation.

e) Bella should immediately have the retained lower right primary canine (804) removed. Note that it is likely that the equivalent left tooth (704) will be similarly retained and need removal. A clinical judgement will then need to be made regarding the degree of medial displacement of the permanent lower canines (304 and 404). Clearly, some interruption of horizontal jaw growth has already occurred. Depending on the degree of displacement of the permanent canines, there are various treatment options to try to minimise further problems (see Case 2.6 for details).

f) Had there been no discrepancy in jaw length (indicated by normal premolar interdigitation), the prognosis after simple removal of the retained deciduous canine(s) might have been good. However, the fact that the mandible has been arrested in forward growth suggests that the medial displacement(s) may warrant surgical intervention. This could be a simple technique (e.g. orthodontic ball of the correct size) or a more invasive procedure such as gingivectomy or gingivoplasty to try to prevent the development of a worsening malocclusion (Ringen et al. 2024) or crowding, which can exacerbate periodontal disease (Bellows et al. 2019).

REFERENCES

Bellows, J., Berg, M. L., Dennis, S. et al. (2019) AAHA Dental Care Guidelines for Dogs and Cats. *Journal of the American Animal Hospital Association* **55**(2):49–69. doi: 10.5326/jaaha-ms-6933.

Ringen, D., Hoyer, N. & Vall, P. (2024) Outcome of permanent canine teeth following extraction of linguoverted deciduous mandibular canine teeth in 28 dogs. *Journal of Veterinary Dentistry* **41**(3):217–224. doi: 10.1177/08987564231206036.

4.4 Cleo, 6-yo FN DSH: bleeding when eating

a) 1. Oral discomfort/pain
   2. Oral mass/lesion
   3. Bleeding when eating
   4. Drooling/ptyalism
   5. Weight loss

From a welfare perspective, the most pressing concern is pain. From a causal perspective, the most pressing concern is the oral mass/lesion, which is most likely the cause of the oral pain, bleeding, and ptyalism. Weight loss may be due to decreased food intake (secondary to pain), or decreased absorption of nutrients due to cachexia of systemic disease.

b) Stakeholders are entities with an interest or concern in a specific situation. In this case, the stakeholders include the following:
   - The animal (Cleo)
   - The owner
   - The vet (and team) treating the animal
   - The business (practice where the animal is being treated)
   - The profession (as a whole, and, in this case, referral veterinary teams that may help with treatment)

We can also consider additional stakeholders who would play a lesser role in this situation, such as the public and regulators (e.g. the Royal College of Veterinary Surgeons [RCVS] in the UK, regulatory authorities, animal welfare inspectors, or police).

c) In this professional reasoning framework, treatment options fall under one of four categories (more categories or combinations could be added). The impact on different stakeholders can be explored using the framework, which can aid in providing a balanced approach to shared decision-making, supported by evidence from the literature, as well as supporting the opportunity for reflection in challenging situations. It should be noted that the veterinary business as a stakeholder requires a balance of generating income to operate sustainably while inspiring confidence among the public and their clients in the services provided.

> Use of a professional reasoning framework is highly contextualised. You may identify different advantages and disadvantages depending on your own professional values and situation. Those given here are not definitive. Despite this, a framework exercise can be useful in exploring options and revealing unexpected advantages and disadvantages.

Do nothing

This approach would result in Cleo receiving no medication or surgery, and no further diagnostic testing (Table A4.4a).

Table A4.4a 'Do nothing' stakeholder analysis

STAKEHOLDER	ADVANTAGES	DISADVANTAGES
Cleo	• No painful procedures or stress of being brought to the clinic • No potential side effects from medication	• Cleo is in pain; doing nothing is unacceptable on welfare grounds • Conflict with veterinary professional/ethical obligations
Owner	• Owner thinks Cleo seems well; they may feel comfortable not intervening • Prevents further costs to owner • Prevents potential damage to human–animal bond from repeated vet visits and giving medications	• Owner will see disease progress and pain become more evident • May feel guilty watching Cleo struggle • May later regret not intervening sooner
Vet (+ team)	• No additional work to be managed	• Unrewarding as no opportunity to use skills • Conflict with professional values knowing disease will progress and intervention may aid QOL
Practice	• Less workload straining staff resources and time with a 'difficult' case	• No additional income • May damage practice reputation as a registered animal is 'left suffering'
Profession	• Profession 'knows when to stop' with treatment	• Could damage overall reputation as an animal is left suffering whereas a human would be treated

Do something

This approach has the broadest scope of options along a spectrum of care, such as palliative analgesia/anti-inflammatories, placement of a feeding tube, surgical resection, radiotherapy, or toceranib phosphate (Table A4.4b).

Table A4.4b 'Do something' stakeholder analysis

STAKEHOLDER	ADVANTAGES	DISADVANTAGES
Cleo	• Palliative care with analgesia would help maintain Cleo's QOL • An oesophageal feeding tube ensures nutrition and avoids pain on eating • Radiotherapy with or without surgery has been reported to improve median survival times (12–24 weeks) • Toceranib phosphate alongside NSAIDs has been shown to extend median survival times (20–28 weeks, compared with 6 weeks without treatment); it is non-invasive and involves shorter trips to the vets	• Palliative care may not extend Cleo's quantity of life • An oesophageal feeding tube is invasive and involves risks associated with general anaesthetic • The challenges, common occurrence of complications, and limited improvement in survival times reported with surgery alone mean it is unlikely to benefit Cleo • Radiotherapy involves multiple trips/stays at the vets and associated side effects, which would need to be managed • Toceranib phosphate commonly causes mild myelosuppression and gastrointestinal side effects, and may be associated with severe side effects such as hepatotoxicity; Cleo may require regular blood tests

STAKEHOLDER	ADVANTAGES	DISADVANTAGES
Owner	• A feeding tube provides a non-oral route for medication, which helps maintain the owner's bond with Cleo as the mouth becomes progressively more painful • Radiotherapy may prolong Cleo's quantity of life and time spent with her owner • Toceranib phosphate alongside NSAIDs may prolong Cleo's life with her owner, take up less of the owner's time going to the vets, and be cost-effective	• A feeding tube involves additional time for the owner, as well as adherence to its correct use and the cost of placement • Oral SCC surgery (e.g. hemimandibulectomy) can result in disfigurement and dysphagia, which may be difficult for the owner to manage • Radiotherapy is expensive and time-consuming for the client, who will often need to travel to a referral centre • Toceranib phosphate commonly causes mild side effects, plus the cost of regular blood tests for monitoring
Vet (+ team)	• Treatment involves the veterinary team that is caring for Cleo building rapport with the owner and improving job satisfaction, which, in turn, benefits the practice • Treatment provides an enriching case if it can be performed in-house • Treatment would allow the vet to feel that they are taking positive action in treating Cleo's condition • Fosters the vet–client relationship	• Surgery/radiotherapy may require referral, reducing the opportunity for in-house patient care and team development • Some may feel that certain interventions are going too far and extending life solely for the benefit of Cleo's owner
Practice	• Treatment improves job satisfaction, thereby improving staff wellbeing • All treatment options create revenue if done in-house	• Revenue is lost at the point the case is referred • Staff development is reduced at the point the case is referred
Profession	• Referral needed for radiotherapy (and possibly surgery) allows rapport between veterinary teams • Advanced level of care reflects well on the profession	• Advanced cancer care for animals may be seen as inappropriate, depending on viewpoint

Do everything

This approach would include further diagnostic testing to determine the extent of disease, ideally imaging to assess any potential metastases (10–31% of cases metastasise); radical surgical removal of the mass; and adjunctive treatments such as radiotherapy. The impact on the vet and the practice will vary depending on the capability and resources available (Table A4.4c).

Table A4.4c 'Do everything' stakeholder analysis		
STAKEHOLDER	ADVANTAGES	DISADVANTAGES
Cleo	• A fully tailored treatment plan should extend Cleo's lifespan as much as possible (with around 10% of cases surviving 1 year or longer)	• Requires a variety of veterinary visits with varying degrees of stress/pain and risk of complications or side effects
Owner	• A fully tailored treatment plan should extend Cleo's lifespan, giving her longer with her owner	• This approach will be the most expensive and time-consuming • Some owners may feel guilt at putting their pet through treatment if the animal experiences pain/side effects

Continued

Table A4.4c **(Continued)**

STAKEHOLDER	ADVANTAGES	DISADVANTAGES
Vet (+ team)	• Will provide an enriching case for the vet (and team) for any aspects done in-house • Fosters the vet–client relationship	• May create team conflict if professional/personal values do not align with intensive treatment that the animal patient cannot consent to
Practice	• Creates revenue for the business for everything done in-house • Team job satisfaction can be improved • Practice builds rapport with the client by facilitating treatment/referral	• Revenue is lost at the point the case is referred to another practice • Staff development is reduced at the point the case is referred
Profession	• Fosters interprofessional relationships if/when referral is needed, which may include a degree of learning for the vet/team • Good for overall reputation as aiding an animal in need	• Referral decreases the degree of hands-on learning for the vet/team • Potential to be perceived as 'going too far' by carrying out expensive treatment with potentially little gain in life expectancy

Euthanasia

Given the average life expectancy for cats with oral SCCs is 6–12 weeks with only palliative care, euthanasia is an important option to consider for Cleo (Table A4.4d).

Table A4.4d **'Euthanasia' stakeholder analysis**

STAKEHOLDER	ADVANTAGES	DISADVANTAGES
Cleo	• Ends Cleo's life before she suffers further • Will not be put through additional painful procedures or have repeated stressful visits to the vet practice	• Despite her current pain, Cleo may have good QOL overall, or regain this, so this route may not yet be suitable • In ending Cleo's life, she avoids future negative welfare, but she cannot enjoy future positive welfare
Owner	• Prioritises Cleo's welfare over their own attachment • Gives the owner the chance to say goodbye on 'good terms', which can aid in their bereavement	• The owner will have less time with their pet • May feel guilty about making the decision when treatment is theoretically possible
Vet (+ team)	• Can align with professional values on animal welfare given knowledge of the disease and poor prognosis • If handled well, can foster the vet–client relationship	• May give rise to mixed opinions depending on everyone's professional values • If the vet's values do not align with the owner's, discord could damage the vet–client relationship
Practice	• If handled well and vet–client relationship is bolstered, can lead to future business (with this client or others through word of mouth)	• Less income generated compared with most treatment options
Profession	• Good for overall reputation as animal pain/suffering is ended where there is a poor prognosis	• May suggest veterinary medicine is less advanced or caring than human medicine in serious disease

REFERENCES

Armitage-Chan, E. (2022) Principles of Professional Reasoning and Decision-Making. In: Maddison, J. E., Volk, H. A. & Church, D. B. (eds) *Clinical Reasoning in Veterinary Practice*, 2nd edition. Oxford: Wiley-Blackwell.

Moore, A. S. (2009) Treatment choices for oral cancer in cats: What is possible? What is reasonable? *Journal of Feline Medicine and Surgery* **11**(1):23–31. doi: 10.1016/j.jfms.2008.11.010.

Pellin, M. & Turek, M. (2016) A review of feline oral squamous cell carcinoma. *Today's Veterinary Practice* **6**:24–31.

4.5 Gregor, 8-yo MN DLH: inpatient

Gregor's PCV has increased by 12%.

For each increase in PCV of 1%, there is a fluid requirement of approximately 10 mL/kg, meaning Gregor needs $4 \times 10 \times 12 = 480$ mL on top of maintenance.

Maintenance for Gregor over 24 hours is 50 mL/kg = $50 \times 4 = 200$ mL.

Gregor therefore needs $480 + 200 = 680$ mL over 24 hours, which equates to approximately 28 mL/h.

4.6 Walter, 5-mo ME Miniature Dachshund: V ++ & D ++

a) A puppy under 5 months of age is considered 'high risk exposed' even if vaccinated. This is due to the presumed impact of maternal antibodies on the efficacy of the vaccine. For this reason, this exposed puppy should be quarantined for 14 days (the maximum incubation period for parvovirus). The quarantine can be implemented either in the shelter or off-site with a trained foster carer. The latter option is often preferable for puppies to promote healthy behavioural development in a home environment.

b) Exposed dogs older than 5 months or without adequately documented vaccine histories can be considered 'moderate risk exposed'. These dogs can either be quarantined or an antibody titre test used for risk assessment before clearing for adoption.

c) Walter should be placed in an isolation room for treatment and remain there until clinical signs have resolved. Shelter treatment rooms and isolation facilities should have strict biosecurity policies to prevent disease spreading to the general population, and protocols should be implemented to prevent the exposure of new animals entering the shelter to those already there. Depending on the finances of the shelter, either a basic blood-work panel (e.g. PCV/TP, blood glucose, blood smear) or full in-house blood work (e.g. CBC, biochemistry, electrolytes) can be used to guide treatment. Treatment of a stable patient should include three components:

1. IV isotonic crystalloid and occasionally colloid fluid therapy (SC fluid therapy may be suitable for stable cases).
2. Medications including anti-nausea therapy (maropitant, ondansetron, or metoclopramide CRI), opioid pain relief, and judicious use of broad-spectrum antibiotics appropriate to the degree of neutropenia. It is also prudent to include a course of anthelmintics such as fenbendazole and ponazuril or toltrazuril, as a concurrent worm burden may exacerbate clinical illness.
3. Nutritional support, either by encouragement, syringe feeding, or feeding tube of a high-caloric diet. Regular (at least daily) veterinary recheck examinations should guide the treatment plan (Mazzaferro 2020).

d) While the mortality rates of untreated parvovirus cases approach 90%, most puppies recover from parvovirus if treated (Horecka et al. 2020). An important consideration in the shelter environment is whether the shelter has the capacity to provide or fund treatment for affected patients appropriately, without contaminating the entire facility and putting healthy animals at risk. The second consideration is how Walter responds to treatment and whether there are other concurrent illnesses or complications (such as intussusception) that may worsen his prognosis and limit the opportunity for adoption or transfer to another rescue organisation. These would inform any decisions about euthanasia.

e) After resolution of clinical signs, the shelter may authorise a repeat parvovirus SNAP test before rehoming Walter. However, depending on the risk tolerance of the shelter, it is also reasonable to forgo testing due to its low sensitivity. It is important to note that infectious levels of parvovirus can continue to shed for 12 days after resolution of clinical signs. For this reason, it is recommended that Walter is adopted with a disclosure outlining that he should interact only with fully vaccinated adult dogs during this period, after which he is considered to be fully recovered. Before moving out of isolation, Walter should also be bathed and dried thoroughly and vaccinated according to schedule; he can then be made available for adoption as soon as possible.

REFERENCES

Horecka, K., Porter, S., Amirian, E. S. & Jefferson, E. (2020) A decade of treatment of canine parvovirus in an animal shelter: a retrospective study. *Animals* **10**(6):939. doi: 10.3390/ani10060939.

Mazzaferro, E. M. (2020) Update on canine parvoviral enteritis. *Veterinary Clinics of North America Small Animal Practice* **50**(6):1307–1325. doi: 10.1016/j.cvsm.2020.07.008.

4.7 Thor, 5-yo ME German Shepherd: off colour, no appetite

a) The drip pump rate is 42 kg × 5 mL/kg/h = 210 mL/h.

b) There are many different ways of performing this calculation. Here is one:

$$210 \text{ mL/h} \div 60 \text{ minutes} = 3.5 \text{ mL/min}$$

The giving set is 20 drops/mL; therefore:

$$3.5 \text{ mL/min} \times 20 \text{ drops/mL} = 70 \text{ drops/min}$$

This suggests that the rate will be roughly 1 drop per second:

$$70 \text{ drops/min} \div 60 \text{ seconds}$$
$$= 1.16 \text{ drops/s or 12 drops over 10 seconds}$$

c) This ECG trace shows ventricular tachycardia. It is not sinus rhythm as there is no P wave for the QRS complex. The complex is wide and bizarre, suggesting it originates from below the annulus fibrosus, i.e. the ventricle. The rate is above 160 bpm, which is classified as ventricular tachycardia in most veterinary texts. Intra- and perioperative ventricular arrythmias are more frequent in dogs whose splenic masses have ruptured. In addition, in one study, dogs undergoing splenectomy with intra- and perioperative ventricular arrythmias had higher rates of in-hospital mortality than those without arrhythmias (Michael et al. 2023).

d) As the BP is currently acceptable, it is alright to observe this rhythm for 20–30 seconds in case it is self-limiting due to manipulation of the spleen; however, some people opt to treat straight away. The currently recommended treatment is 2 mg/kg (preservative and adrenaline free) lidocaine given as an IV bolus.

REFERENCE

Michael, A. E., Grimes, J. A., Rajeev, M. et al. (2023) Perioperative ventricular arrhythmias are increased with hemoperitoneum and are associated with increased mortality in dogs undergoing splenectomy for splenic masses. *Journal of the American Veterinary Medical Association* **261**(12):1–6. doi: 10.2460/javma.23.05.0289.

4.8 Maya, 17-yo FN DSH: vomiting & weight loss

VISIT 1

a) Indirect ophthalmoscopy is quick and easy and can give you valuable information related to BP (Figure A4.8). We need to look at retinas routinely – look at retinas in all the cats you examine, know what a normal retina looks like! The step-by-step process is as follows:

1. Dilate the pupil with one drop of tropicamide 1%.
2. Take a condensing lens, e.g. 20 D, and a focal light source such as a pen torch.
3. Hold the lens 2–8 cm from the cat's eye and use the fingers of the same hand to rest lightly on the cat's head (middle fingers to little finger) (see page 198).
4. Hold the focal light source behind your ear, 50–80 cm away from the cat's head.
5. What you see is a magnified and inverted image, which gives you a wide view and a good image of the retina to check for vessel abnormalities or retinal blow-outs ('sheet blowing in the wind').

b) Indirect ophthalmoscopy is a good hands-off approach to get a feel for whether BP is elevated in older, tricky cats in whom you cannot measure BP by Doppler. It can be done without causing too much stress.

c) BP measurement comes next. Hypertension is common in older cats and is often overlooked, resulting in target organ damage leading to red eyes, blindness due to retinal detachment, left ventricular hypertrophy, neurological signs such as seizures, or kidney disease. Where systolic blood pressure is under 150 mmHg, the risk of target organ damage is considered low, but systolic pressures consistently above 180 mmHg are associated with risk of target organ damage. To ensure accurate reading, it is important that cats are calm and comfortable when indirect BP

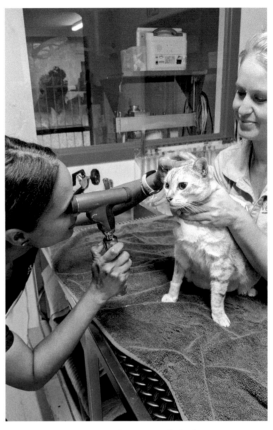

Figure A4.8 Use of the pan ophthalmoscope is another way of gaining a wide overview of the retina for screening purposes.

measurements are taken. The International Society of Feline Medicine has published online practical recommendations for indirect measurement of feline blood pressure (*https://icatcare.org/app/uploads/2020/05/ISFM-BP-recommendations.pdf*).

d) It is important to separate cats at feeding time, especially if one is losing weight. Cats are not social feeders! Microchip feeders and visual separation were recommended in this case. Older, arthritic cats may struggle to climb into a litter tray, and as a result may 'hold on' to their urine or faeces, leading to constipation or urinary issues. Having one litter tray per cat plus one extra is recommended for indoor cats, as well as ensuring that there are trays with lower sides for the older cat to use (seeding trays or cut-out storage containers can be a good alternative to commercially available litter trays) (Rodan et al. 2024).

e) Maya is hypertensive and should be treated to minimise the risk of (additional) target organ damage. The calcium channel blocker amlodipine besylate is recommended as the first line of treatment (Taylor et al. 2017). The drug is a peripheral arterial dilator that works directly on the smooth muscle of blood vessels, causing a reduction in stroke volume and BP, with minimal impact on the heart. It can reduce systemic BP by 30–70 mmHg. The recommended starting dose is 0.625 mg per cat (this approximates to 0.125 mg/kg) once per day, though cats with systolic BP over 200 may benefit from 1.25 mg PO q24h (approximately 0.25 mg/kg) (Taylor et al. 2017). Maya should be rechecked 1–3 weeks following commencement of therapy, or sooner if she deteriorates.

For presumed orthopaedic pain, Maya can start some analgesia. Low-dose gabapentin is suitable because her kidney status is uncertain (a lower dose is used because gabapentin is renally excreted), as is an injection of monoclonal antibody targeting nerve growth factor (frunevetmab). Changes to Maya's environment are also recommended, including a bed for each cat in the house, ramps or steps to help her reach elevated resting places, an elevated food bowl, and a laxative for constipation.

VISIT 2

a) Maya's thyroid result is 47, which is within normal limits, albeit at the higher end of the reference range. Previously the result was 32. Why is this important? With concurrent conditions, the thyroid will be artificially suppressed, so hyperthyroidism cannot be ruled out. Hyperthyroid cats lose weight (by measurement of weight, but also muscle loss, which may lead to an elevated CK level), have a higher incidence of hypertension, and appear quite strong/energetic for their age.

The next area of interest is Maya's liver. We know previously she has had bacterial cholangitis and elevated liver enzymes, so it is no surprise that there are elevated liver enzymes and occasional vomiting – perhaps the disease is recurrent, or had never fully resolved, though levels are not as high as previously.

ALT in cats has a short half-life of 2–6 hours and can indicate conditions such as cholangitis, liver neoplasia, malabsorption, biliary cysts, cholecystitis, and extrahepatic biliary duct obstruction. AST is deeper in the cells, so is a more sensitive indicator of liver disease; it is also present in muscle injury. Its half-life is 1.5 hours.

Her CK is fairly high at 700 (normal <400). It was 200 when she was sick with cholangitis previously, so muscle breakdown is happening. This could be due to weight loss or concurrent hyperthyroidism.

b) To investigate the possibility of hyperthyroidism, you can request a free T4 by equilibrium dialysis. Alternatively, you can recheck Maya's total T4 in a month or so and see if it is increasing, which would raise suspicion of hyperthyroidism. There is no real rush here as her BP is stable and hyperthyroidism is hormonal – so no fast changes are expected. Regarding Maya's hepatopathy, sonographic examination would be useful. We don't know if she is suffering from unresolved bacterial cholangitis, or whether this is recurring. Symptomatic treatment involves anti-emetics such as maropitant (1 mg/kg PO SID – compounded into a liquid to facilitate dosing), and liver support in the form of S-adenosyl-methionine (SAMe) and ursodiol.

c) Triaditis is the term for inflammation of the liver, intestine, and pancreas. Often, due to the physical proximity of the duodenum, gallbladder, and pancreas in cats (linked by the common bile duct), inflammation in one of these areas can cause disease in another. It would be prudent to monitor the pancreas and also keep an eye out for symptoms of inflammatory bowel disease such as vomiting and diarrhoea. Addition of a DGGR lipase or feline-specific pancreatic lipase (fPL) to the next blood test would be prudent, as would monitoring cobalamin levels and supplementing as required. Any cat with PU/PD has the risk of also being low in water-soluble vitamins such as B12. Combining a blood test with a repeat ultrasonography at her next recheck, Maya had a normal fPL and a stable TT4, but her B12 levels were low, so she was supplemented with injectable B12 weekly for 6 weeks.

REFERENCES

Leask, E. (2021) Efficacy of EMLA™ cream for reducing pain associated with venepuncture in felines. *Veterinary Evidence* **6**(3). doi: 10.18849/ve.v6i3.456.

Rodan, I., Ramos, D., Carney, H. et al. (2024) AAFP intercat tension guidelines: recognition, prevention and management. *Journal of Feline Medicine and Surgery* **26**:1098612X241263465. doi: 10.1177/1098612X241263465.

Taylor, S. S., Sparkes, A. H., Briscoe, K. et al (2017) ISFM consensus guidelines on the diagnosis and management of hypertension in cats. *Journal of Feline Medicine and Surgery* **19**(3):288–303. doi: 10.1177/1098612X17693500.

4.9 Flora, 9-wo FE Cavoodle: passing blood

a) This is an adult female roundworm, *Toxocara canis*.

b) Routes of infection are illustrated in Figure A4.9. Puppies are particularly vulnerable to infection *in utero*, and it should be assumed that all puppies <12 weeks of age with no history of worming are infected with *T. canis* (Yabsley & Sapp 2023). Infection of puppies is largely transplacental, but can occur following parturition when smaller numbers of reactivated larvae are shed in the dam's milk. Puppies may also become infected via ingestion of eggs or paratenic hosts containing infectious larvae (Bowman 2021).

In puppies <3 months old, infection follows a standard tracheal migration common to most ascarids. That is, third-stage larvae (L3) emerge from eggs in the gut, migrate in the blood via the liver to the lungs, where they are coughed up and swallowed. In the stomach, they moult to L4, before migrating to the small intestine where they moult to L5, and develop to sexual maturity. Unembryonated eggs are passed in dog faeces from 2–5 weeks post-infection and eggs take 2–4 weeks to become infectious (contain L3). Embryonated eggs can survive in the environment for up to 14 months, and are typically resistant to freezing.

c) In puppies >3 months old, migrating larvae increasingly undergo somatic migration, and the number developing to sexual maturity in the gut decreases. During somatic migration, larvae are returned to the heart by the pulmonary veins and are carried by the circulation until they are deposited in tissue (e.g. the kidney or muscle) where they encyst and undergo hypobiosis (arrested development). Some age-related resistance occurs, so that puppies may spontaneously lose worms from 6 weeks of age.

Adult dogs may acquire infection via ingestion of embryonated eggs (containing infectious L3) or paratenic hosts (containing

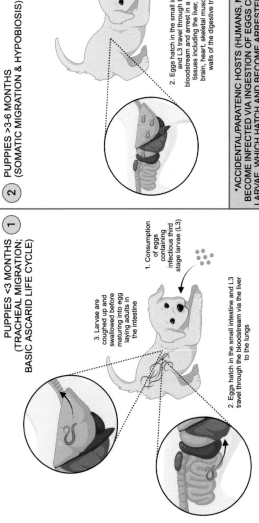

PUPPIES >3-6 MONTHS (2)
(SOMATIC MIGRATION & HYPOBIOSIS)

1. Consumption of eggs or paratenic hosts* containing infectious third stage larvae (L3)

2. Eggs hatch in the small intestine and L3 travel through the bloodstream and arrest in a range of tissues including the liver, lungs, brain, heart, skeletal muscle and walls of the digestive tract

*ACCIDENTAL/PARATENIC HOSTS (HUMANS, MICE, RABBITS ETC),
BECOME INFECTED VIA INGESTION OF EGGS CONTAINING INFECTIVE
LARVAE, WHICH HATCH AND BECOME ARRESTED IN TISSUES, SERVING
AS A SOURCE OF INFECTION FOR PREDATOR SPECIES

SUCKLING PUP (4)
(TRANSMAMMARY INFECTION; RARE)

1. After parturition, a small number of mobilised larvae may be shed in the milk, infecting suckling pups

2. Larvae ingested in milk travel to the intestines of pups via the trachea and mature into egg-laying adults

PUPPIES <3 MONTHS (1)
(TRACHEAL MIGRATION; BASIC ASCARID LIFE CYCLE)

1. Consumption of eggs containing infectious third stage larvae (L3)

3. Larvae are coughed up and swallowed before maturing into egg laying adults in the intestine

2. Eggs hatch in the small intestine and L3 travel through the bloodstream via the liver to the lungs

PREGNANT BITCH (3)
(TRANSPLACENTAL INFECTION; COMMON)

3. Some mobilised larvae will complete the basic ascarid life cycle in the bitch and result in a transient population of sexually-mature adult worms in the gut and an associated increase in faecal egg output

1. Pools of arrested larvae mobilise ~3 weeks prior to parturition and migrate to the lungs of the foetus

OR

Bitches may become infected during late pregnancy and somatic migration (2; above right) of L3 leads to infection of the developing foetus

2. Shortly after birth, migrating larvae travel to the intestine of pups via the trachea, where they mature into egg laying adults

AN INFECTED BITCH USUALLY HARBOURS SUFFICIENT NUMBERS OF
ARRESTED LARVAE TO INFECT ALL SUBSEQUENT LITTERS

Figure A4.9 Egg shedding due to patent *T. canis* infections are commonly seen in puppies <6 months old. Adult worms are typically 10–15 cm long. This figure describes the four main routes of infection. Note that *T. canis* is zoonotic, and care should be taken when disposing of faeces from potentially infected animals.

arrested larvae). Infection during adulthood usually results in somatic migration and hypobiosis of larvae in tissues, although, in rare circumstances (including shortly after parturition), adult dogs may experience tracheal migration resulting in a transient pool of sexually mature adults in the gut and an associated rise in faecal egg output. A single infection is sufficient to generate a pool of arrested larvae able to infect all subsequent litters; in addition, nursing bitches may swallow eggs when cleaning their puppies and their faeces in the environment, adding to their pool of arrested larvae.

d) Yes. Embryonated *T. canis* eggs and undercooked paratenic hosts can be ingested by humans, in some cases leading to visceral larva migrans or ocular larva migrans. Strict hand hygiene and appropriate environmental hygiene should be observed.

e) Treatment should be commenced with a licensed product from 2 weeks of age, and repeated every 2 weeks until the puppy is 3 months old, then placed on a monthly preventive that is active against *T. canis*, until the age of 6 months. Dogs may be wormed regularly, at intervals appropriate to the product used, though increasingly a 'test and treat' approach is recommended. Bitches should be treated late in pregnancy with a registered anthelmintic with activity against *T. canis*.

f) *T. canis* may cause diarrhoea, but not usually bloody diarrhoea. It is important to rule out parvovirus in a puppy with bloody diarrhoea. Puppies with heavy *T. canis* may present with abdominal tenderness, poor body condition, lethargy, vomiting (in some cases, bringing up adult worms) or cough, and may have a pot-bellied appearance. Adult worms can cause intestinal obstruction or intussusception. However, it is possible that the primary reason for Flora's gastrointestinal signs is dietary change. Regardless, small puppies can deteriorate rapidly, and her progress should be followed up with the owners. If she fails to improve within 24 hours or worsens at any point, she should be re-evaluated.

REFERENCES

Bowman, D. D. (2021) Helminths. In: Bowman, D. D. (ed.) *Georgis' Parasitology for Veterinarians*. St Louis, MO: Elsevier, pp. 135–260.

Yabsley, M. J. & Sapp, S. G. H. (2023) Ascarids. In: Sykes, J. (ed.) *Greene's Infectious Diseases of the Dog and Cat*. St Louis, MO: Elsevier, pp. 1418–1435.

4.10 Walter, 5-yo ME Malinois Greyhound: swollen toe

a) Common differentials for a swollen distal digit are shown in Table A4.10a.

Table A4.10a Common differentials for a swollen digit

FRACTURES	DISLOCATIONS	OTHER
• Fracture of second phalanx (P2) • Fracture of the third phalanx (P3) • Fracture of the ungual process	• Luxation or subluxation of the distal interphalangeal (DIP) joint • Open subluxation of the DIP joint	• Infection of the DIP joint • Osteomyelitis of P3 • Benign or malignant neoplasia

Benign neoplastic disease can include subungual keratoacanthoma, histiocytoma, melanocytoma, inverted squamous papilloma, sebaceous gland tumour, infiltrative lipoma, and osteochondroma, while examples of malignant neoplasia can include SCC, melanoma, soft tissue sarcoma, and mast cell tumour (Grassinger et al. 2021).

b) After a duration of 3 weeks, thorough investigation requires general anaesthesia (Table A4.10b).

Table A4.10b **Investigations and findings for various conditions causing swollen digit**	
CONDITION	**INVESTIGATION AND FINDINGS**
DIP joint luxation or subluxation	• Instability on careful manipulation of the joint • Stressed radiographs will demonstrate the (sub)luxation (Figure A4.10a)
Ungual crest fracture	• Loose nail on palpation
Osteomyelitis or joint infection	• Swelling, broken nail and discharge from the nail bed is seen • Using a 23-G needle, and approaching the DIP joint laterally, a synocentesis (joint aspiration) will show leukocytosis and predominantly polymorphic cells • Nail bed swab is sent for C&S to guide antimicrobial use
Open subluxation of the DIP joint	• A small wound on the lateral aspect of the DIP joint that opens each time the dog runs (Figure A4.10b)
Fracture of P2 or P3	• Orthogonal radiographs will diagnose fractured P2, but are not sensitive for fractures of P3
Neoplasia	• Incisional or excisional biopsy, with additional staging (e.g. cytology of aspirates of regional lymph nodes, thoracic radiographs)

c) Most of the conditions will require permanent nail removal, which is achieved by performing a UCO. There are three types or degrees of instability of the DIP joint (Table A4.10c).

Table A4.10c **Treatment of DIP joint instabilities**		
TYPE	**FEATURES**	**TREATMENT**
1	Little or no palpable instability	Shorten nail; rest
2	Luxation palpable	UCO
3	Unstable joint	UCO and tightening of periarticular tissue with mattress suture (absorbable material); primary ligament repair is not necessary; periarticular fibrosis creates stability

Fracture of P3 or the ungual bone heals rapidly after UCO.

Osteomyelitis of P3, usually a sequel to ungual bone fracture, will heal after UCO, thereby removing the nidus of the infection. A course of a suitable antibiotic is required.

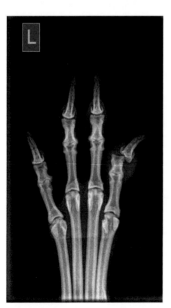

Figure A4.10a Luxation of the DIP joint.

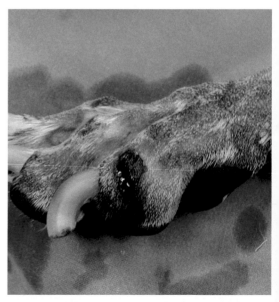

Figure A4.10b Lateral wound in the case of open subluxation of the DIP joint.

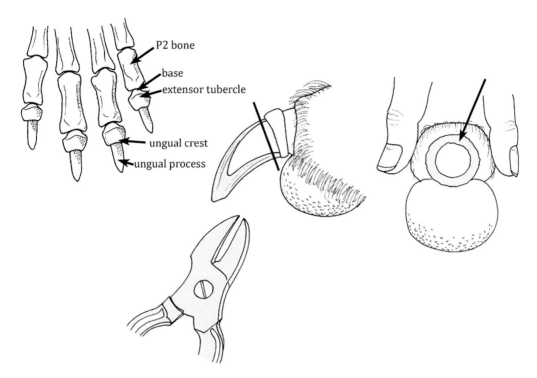

Figure A4.10c The middle diagram shows the direction of the cut after the skin has been incised around the nail and peeled away to expose the dorsal joint area. The arrow in the right diagram points to the nail remnants requiring excision with rongeurs. The central circle is the bone of the ungual process.

UCO works for all these conditions because it reduces the lever arm effect of the nail, relieving pain and allowing healing (Guilliard 2012).

Treatment of neoplasia should be guided by a tissue diagnosis (histopathology) and staging as appropriate.

d) To perform a UCO:
- The skin and pad are incised around the nail bed, exposing the dorsal aspect of the DIP joint
- With P3 tightly grasped between forefinger and thumb, the nail is removed with bone cutters, leaving remnants of the nail around the exposed ungual process (Figure A4.10c)
- All the nail is removed along with the ungual crest using rongeurs

- Enough bone is removed to allow tension-free skin closure
- Occasionally, the dorsal joint is damaged, but this is not of any consequence
- UCO allows normal contact between the pad and ground, and thus relieves pain

REFERENCES

Grassinger, J. M., Floren, A., Müller, T. et al. (2021) Digital lesions in dogs: a statistical breed analysis of 2912 cases. *Veterinary Science* **8**(7):136. doi: 10.3390/vetsci8070136.

Guilliard, M. (2012) *The Nature, Incidence and Response to Treatment of Injuries to the Distal Limbs in the Racing Greyhound. A thesis for Fellowship of the Royal College of Veterinary Surgeons.* Fellowship T/736. London: RCVS.

4.11 Fluffy Friends Rescue Centre: site visit

a) Feline calicivirus (FCV), FHV, *Chlamydia/Chlamydophila felis*, and *Bordetella bronchiseptica* are the vaccine-preventable pathogens in cat flu. (Note that the last two are not universally available as vaccines.)

b) There are many possible management changes. Important suggestions include the following:

- Pause intake of new kittens to avoid increasing population density
- Stop mixing cats from different households
- Reduce population density if possible (arrange off-site foster care of cats)
- Check hygiene, e.g. are areas being appropriately cleaned with detergent and then disinfected? Are staff using appropriate hand hygiene and PPE, and cleaning the cleanest areas first, followed by the dirtiest?
- Promptly isolate clinically infected cats
- Consider vaccinating earlier (licensing varies by region, but, if appropriate, can be started from 4 weeks of age – see WSAVA [Squires et al. 2024] and ASV [2022] guidelines for details)
- Consider vaccinating pregnant queens on entry (again, licensing varies – also may wish to consider spaying pregnant queens if acceptable locally)
- Reduce stress – ensure all cats have more than enough resources such as hiding places, beds, and feeding stations

c) Many cat flu pathogens are ubiquitous. This means it is often more important in a shelter situation to sort out environmental factors that lead to high levels of disease before worrying too much about individual pathogens. It is only worth diagnostic testing in a shelter if the results are going to change management. So, for example, if considering a change of vaccine to include a wider range of pathogens, sampling may inform the necessity for this. Many of the pathogens are viral; however, if *C. felis* is suspected, treatment involves 4–6 weeks of doxycycline for the infected cat AND all in-contact cats, so should only be done with a confirmed diagnosis. This would be another reason for testing.

d) This dendritic ulcer is typical of FHV. If ulcers are not obvious with fluorescein staining under a blue light, it may be worth checking with rose bengal staining as this can sometimes be more sensitive. This is a painful condition, so appropriate analgesia is important. Topical antivirals such as idoxuridine, trifluridine, and cidofovir can be helpful if available, potentially combined with topical interferon, though these require multiple times per day dosing and can be very costly. Additional treatment with hyaluronate/eye lubricant is also useful. Systemic antiviral drugs such as famciclovir may be helpful if available.

e) This kitten requires supportive therapy, e.g. IV fluids and intensive nursing care, e.g. regular gentle facial cleaning, nebulisation with saline, mucolytics, and warming of foods (cats usually will not eat what they cannot smell). Eye lubricants are indicated. Appetite stimulants may be useful, but parenteral nutrition, e.g. a nasogastric, oesophagostomy, or percutaneous endoscopic gastrostomy (PEG) tube might be necessary. Pain relief (usually NSAIDs if hydration can be maintained) and empirical antimicrobials are indicated. While doxycycline may be a better empirical choice due to activity against *Chlamydophila felis*, *Bordetella bronchiseptica*, *Mycoplasma* spp., and other primary respiratory pathogens (Lappin et al. 2017), oral doxycycline hydrochloride may not be ideal in kittens due to the small tablet sizes, making these hard to divide, and the risk of oesophageal strictures or gastrointestinal upsets (Lappin et al. 2017). If administered, doxycycline tablets or capsules should be given coated with a lubricating food, followed by an oral bolus of water, or at least a small amount of food (Lappin et al. 2017). The latter may be a challenge in cats with appetite suppression secondary to upper respiratory tract congestion and/or pyrexia. In contrast, amoxycillin is an acceptable first-line antimicrobial choice where secondary bacterial infection is suspected. This may be available as a licensed, palatable liquid that tends to be better tolerated in kittens. Euthanasia should be considered in severely affected kittens.

REFERENCES

ASV (Association of Shelter Veterinarians) *Guidelines for Standards of Care in Animal Shelters*, 2nd edition (2022). Available at: www.aspcapro.org/resource/asv-guidelines-shelter-checklists.

Cole, J. (2017) In cats infected with feline herpesvirus type-1 (FHV-1) does treatment with famciclovir result in a reduction of respiratory and ocular clinical signs? *Veterinary Evidence* 2(3). doi: 10.18849/ve.v2i3.105.

Lappin, M. R., Blondeay, J., Boothe, D. et al. (2017) Antimicrobial use guidelines for treatment of respiratory tract disease in dogs and cats. (Antimicrobial Guidelines Working Group of the International Society for Companion Animal Infectious Diseases). *Journal of Veterinary Internal Medicine* 31(2):279–294. doi: 10.1111/jvim.14627.

Squires, R. A., Crawford, C., Marcondes, M. & Whitley, N. (2024) 2024 guidelines for the vaccination of dogs and cats – compiled by the Vaccination Guidelines Group (VGG) of the World Small Animal Veterinary Association (WSAVA). *Journal of Small Animal Practice* 65(5):277–316. doi: 10.1111/jsap.13718.

Thomasy, S. M. & Maggs, D. J. (2016) A review of antiviral drugs and other compounds with activity against feline herpesvirus type 1. *Veterinary Ophthalmology* 19(Suppl. 1):119–130. doi: 10.1111/vop.12375.

4.12 Dusty, 6-yo ME Golden Retriever: annual vaccination

a) The environmental impacts of a veterinary practice fall into three main categories:

1. **Greenhouse gas emissions, especially carbon emissions**
   These comprise three so-called scopes:
   - Scope 1 – emissions produced on-site, e.g. gas heating/appliances, anaesthetic gases
   - Scope 2 – electricity purchased from the grid
   - Scope 3 – emissions associated with the operation of the business, due to the purchase of products and services, e.g. waste management, medical consumables and chemicals, employee transport

2. **Waste production and chemical use**
   This contributes to environmental degradation and carbon emissions, e.g. from transporting and processing/recycling waste.

3. **Resource consumption**
   This can be direct, e.g. water, and indirect, such as resources required to produce drugs and consumables, e.g. plastic is made from oil.

b) The reasons for, and benefits of, taking action include the following:
   Responsibility of the veterinary profession to protect animal health and welfare
   - Climate change is impacting all animals, e.g. via heat stress due to increased frequency of very hot days (causing morbidity and mortality in pets, sporting/working animals, farm animals, and wildlife, as well as reduced productivity in farm animals), the

impacts of wildfires and floods, and changes in the distribution of vector-borne and parasitic disease (Figure A4.12). To help address this, veterinary teams need to contribute to both climate change mitigation (reduction of emissions) and adaptation (increasing resilience to climate change impacts)

- Environmental degradation damages habitats, threatening biodiversity and increasing the risk and rate of animal extinctions. Veterinary teams can play an active part in reducing this by modifying their consumption and waste management

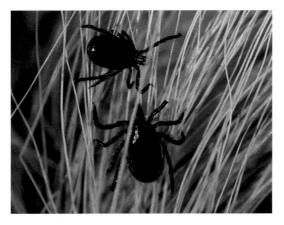

Figure A4.12 *Ixodes ricinus* (also known as the castor bean tick, deer tick, or sheep tick) is a vector of Lyme disease (*Borrelia* spp.), *Rickettsia* spp., tick-borne encephalitis virus, *Anaplasma phagocytophilum*, and *Babesia* spp.

Showing leadership: environmental stewardship is a shared responsibility
- As scientifically trained, respected professionals, veterinarians and their teams have an important role to play in modelling constructive action.

Financial savings
- For example, through on-site solar energy production and improving efficiencies, e.g. in waste management.

Increased client and staff loyalty
- This allows alignment with community expectations, as with Dusty's owner, Wilson.

Improved veterinary team culture and purpose
- This can result in potential mental health and wellbeing benefits.

c) To be successful, the first step is to create a culture of sustainability in the practice. It is very challenging for individuals to implement change without the support of management and the rest of the veterinary team. The following is a list of practical things that motivated veterinary teams can do to make a meaningful impact.

- **Reduce carbon emissions**, particularly those under the direct control of the practice (scopes 1 and 2). To begin with, assess current emissions and identify ways to reduce these. This can be as simple as examining current practices and implementing greener options, e.g. eliminate gas appliances, install solar panels. More comprehensive carbon audits and strategies for moving towards 'net zero' carbon emissions can also be pursued, ideally with the help of consultants. In either scenario, recording and reporting emissions is important for creating a culture of continuous improvement.
- **Re-evaluating anaesthetic protocols** and implementing low-flow anaesthesia and, where possible, partial and total IV anaesthesia are other ways for veterinary practices to reduce scope 1 emissions.
- **Improving waste separation and recycling practices**. This involves both behavioural changes (including staff training) and practical changes, e.g. positioning recycling bins near the point of use. Recycling of medical plastics is challenging, though new technologies are increasingly becoming available.

Awareness and adoption of emerging opportunities is key. Making use of other Rs, e.g. reusing/repurposing, reducing, refusing, is also helpful.

- **Improving efficiency** in water and energy use.
- **Reducing chemical use** and choosing green alternatives.
- **Procurement**: making environmental credentials an important part of all purchasing decisions.
- **Education**: making use of freely available resources and training courses to improve understanding of the reasons and techniques for improving sustainability.
- **Advocacy**: veterinary practices can exert influence as consumers by asking suppliers about their sustainability credentials. They can also promote their own sustainability initiatives and educate their clients about the animal welfare implications of climate change and environmental degradation.

REFERENCES

Stephen, C. & Duncan, C. (2023) *Climate Change and Animal Health*. Boca Raton, FL: CRC Press.

Stephen, C. & Soos, C. (2021) The implications of climate change for veterinary services. *Revue Scientifique et Technique* **40**(2):421–30. doi: 10.20506/rst.40.2.3234.

Vet Sustain (2023) Resources. Available at: https://vetsustain.org/resources.

Veterinarians for Climate Action (2023) Climate Care Program. Available at: www.vfca.org.au/climatecare.

Watson, J. A., Klupiec, C., Bindloss, J. & Morin, M. (2023) The path to net zero carbon emissions for veterinary practice. *Frontiers in Veterinary Science* **10**:1240765. doi: 10.3389/fvets.2023.1240765.

4.13 Kane, 14-yo MN Labrador: booster vaccination

a) You've noticed that Kane has trouble rising and ambulating in the clinic and seems uncomfortable at rest. Questions should focus on assessing Kane's QOL at home. It would be useful to ask the following:

- How long has Kane had difficulty with his mobility?
- Has Kane received any treatment and, if so, has it helped?
- What is Kane's daily routine?
- What proportion of the day does he spend sleeping?
- Is he still excited about walks, and people arriving home?
- Can he get up and lie down easily at home?
- Has he had any difficulty getting outside to toilet and maintaining hygiene?
- Are there any signs of confusion/cognitive decline (dementia)/restlessness at night/changes in behaviour?

You are also asking the above questions to better determine the owner's commitment to Kane's care and what their priorities/capabilities are.

b) Based on what you have witnessed, there are concerns about Kane's mobility and his level of pain. Owners often struggle to identify signs of pain, often confusing pain with ageing. If the owner has booked in for a vaccination, they may not be aware of the extent and severity of Kane's signs. It may be useful to point out Kane's muscle atrophy (muscle condition scoring can assist; see *https://wsava.org/wp-content/uploads/2020/01/Muscle-Condition-Score-Chart-for-Dogs.pdf*) and draw attention to the difficulty Kane has when getting up and down and moving about. Performing a full physical examination and then explaining your findings in terms of the probable impact on Kane's QOL is important. Once you have described all your findings, gently explain to the owners that they are signs of pain. If you have other concerns after discussing his daily routine, also bring these up with the owner. Many people don't realise that subtle changes are signs of larger issues such as cognitive decline. Pointing them out and using more familiar terminology such as 'dementia' can help them to understand. Easy-to use online scoring systems may aid the discussion (such as the DISHAA tool from the Purina Institute: *www.purinainstitute.com/sites/default/files/2021-04/DISHAA-Assessment-Tool.pdf*). Explain what you are concerned about in relatable terms such as 'aching', 'exhaustion', 'confusion', 'stress'. It is important to explain to the owner that, although Kane is eating, this is not in itself an indication that he has a good QOL. Dogs with cognitive decline, and certain breeds such as Labradors, will often continue to eat no matter how much they are struggling.

c) Diagnostic tests may help localise the source of Kane's pain (e.g. radiographs may reveal old injuries, arthritic changes associated with elbow dysplasia, or concurrent conditions such as hip dysplasia). Imaging may also be appropriate to investigate other causes of musculoskeletal pain such as bony neoplasia. Multimodal analgesia may involve the use of a combination of pharmaceutical and non-pharmaceutical measures. This could include NSAIDs, corticosteroids, monoclonal antibodies targeting nerve growth factor (bedinvetmab), pentosan, paracetamol, anxiolytics, amantadine, gabapentin or pregabalin, or cannabidiol (CBD) oil (Monteiro et al. 2023). Non-pharmaceutical measures include hydrotherapy, massage therapy, acupuncture, laser therapy, and environmental modification. A CBC, biochemistry panel, and urinalysis can also be helpful in ruling out potential contraindications for some types of analgesics such as NSAIDs.

d) Any plan needs to be considerate of the owner's capabilities in terms of their time, physical ability, finances, and emotional capacity. A clear, non-judgemental conversation should be had to determine whether the owners are going to be able to adhere to recommendations and treatments prescribed. Potential limiting factors include the owner's ability to give medication and transport Kane for follow-up appointments/injections. Discussion of home visits either with the clinic or a mobile vet could be appropriate here. Finances and the owner's willingness to 'intervene' or 'put him through much at his age' may come into play. Such discussions should include a frank assessment of Kane's pain; often a pain-relief trial is required for owners to fully appreciate the decline in their pet's wellbeing. It is important to discuss pain scoring tools with owners and to perform assessments with the owners in the consultation rooms. This ensures that owners can then perform accurate assessments in the home moving forward. There may be options to work within budgetary constraints, such as writing scripts instead of dispensing some medications. Alternatively, if the owner is informed of potential risks, an empirical treatment trial with analgesics may be undertaken without prior diagnostic tests.

> Tactfully bringing up the topic of euthanasia depends on 'paving the way' through history-taking, physical exam, and discussion of next steps. The discussion then flows more naturally. Many owners are relieved to have the veterinarian raise the topic in this way.

e) Although bringing up euthanasia can feel uncomfortable and it is hard to know how owners will respond, introducing the topic into the conversation is often up to the vet. Do not rely on the owners to do this. Bringing up euthanasia can be difficult if you have not laid the foundations by discussing Kane's current condition and QOL. The use of validated or unvalidated QOL scoring tools can be useful in evaluating and monitoring Kane's condition. If Kane's QOL is poor or declining, steps should be taken to improve it. Euthanasia may ultimately be the best treatment option to ensure that Kane is not suffering. This very much depends on the findings of Kane's clinical exam, discussion with the owner, and the results of any follow-up diagnostic tests. Bringing up the topic of euthanasia indicates to the owner that Kane's QOL is a concern, and that this may not be an unreasonable or inappropriate option. It also gives the owner permission to discuss their thoughts about euthanasia with you and plan ahead, hopefully allowing them to make the decision on a good day, rather than waiting until Kane experiences his worst.

REFERENCE

Monteiro, B. P., Lascelles, B. D. X., Murrell, J. et al. (2023) 2022 WSAVA guidelines for the recognition, assessment and treatment of pain. *Journal of Small Animal Practice* **64**(4):177–254. doi: 10.1111/jsap.13566.

4.14 Rusty, 2-yo ME Dachshund: vaccination

a) Key differentials are orchitis, epididymitis, and possible scrotal infection, which may be caused by agents including *Brucella canis* (common in hunting dogs), Leishmaniasis, Rocky Mountain spotted fever, and fungal disease (Gregory 2022). Testicular neoplasia is common in entire dogs. The most frequent tumours are interstitial cell tumours, seminomas, Sertoli cell tumours, and mixed tumours (Grieco et al. 2008). Testicular trauma can be associated with haematomas.

b) The spermatic cord contains the testicular artery and vein (the pampiniform plexus), which branch off the abdominal aorta and caudal vena cava, respectively. It also contains the ductus deferens, which connects the testicle to the prostatic urethra, and its associated artery and vein. Finally, it contains the testicular lymph vessels and testicular autonomic nerve plexus. Torsion of the spermatic cord is associated with testicular ischaemia, hypoxia, inflammation, thrombosis, fibrin clotting, and damage to germ cells, leading to acute pain and potentially infertility (Raisi & Davoodi 2022).

c) Testicular masses may be associated with infection, which can extend to the prostate via the vas deferens. Rectal examination is needed to assess the prostate, which, if infected, may be enlarged and/or painful. If infection is suspected, ultrasonography of the testes and prostate and, where required, aspiration, cytology, and culture may be required to identify the pathogens involved.

d) Spermatic cord torsion is more frequently reported in undescended cryptorchid and/or neoplastic testes (Raisi & Davoodi 2022). Cryptorchidism is associated with an increased risk of neoplasia. As in this case, in descended testes, the right testicle is more likely to torse than the left. Spermatic cord torsion in cryptorchid dogs is one potential cause of acute abdomen and shock.

e) Scrotal testicular torsion may be associated with pain on scrotal palpation, reduced appetite, stiff hindlimbs, an abnormal gait, and lethargy or malaise. Cryptorchid testicular torsion is more likely to be associated with abdominal pain or tenderness, vomiting, diarrhoea, haematuria, dysuria, pyrexia, and alopecia, as well as an abnormal gait and lethargy or malaise. In some cases, the condition is asymptomatic (Raisi & Davoodi 2022).

f) Bilateral orchiectomy, as there is a high risk of torsion of the unaffected testicle if left behind.

> Cryptorchid testicular torsion can present as an 'acute abdomen', with signs of pain, progressing to shock and collapse in severe cases.

REFERENCES

Gregory, S. P. (2022) Penile and Testicular Emergencies. In: Aronson, L. R. (ed.) *Small Animal Surgical Emergencies*. Wiley Online Library. doi: 10.1002/9781119658634.ch49.

Grieco, V., Riccardi, E., Greppi, G. F. et al. (2008) Canine testicular tumours: a study on 232 dogs. *Journal of Comparative Pathology* **138**(2–3):86–99. doi: 10.1016/j.jcpa.2007.11.002.

Raisi, A. & Davoodi, F. (2022) Testicular torsions in veterinary medicine. *Veterinary Research Communications* **46**(2):303–313. doi: 10.1007/s11259-021-09873-5.

4.15 Shadow, 2-yo ME DSH: O thinks leg is broken

a) Analgesia is indicated immediately due to the expression of pain in the patient, evidenced by vocalisation when touching the non-weight-bearing limb and mild tachycardia. The tacky MMs with no skin tent supports a subjective finding of 5–6% dehydration (see Case 2.3). With this degree of dehydration, and the level of pain shown, an opioid such as methadone or buprenorphine would be the most appropriate choice of analgesic. Addition of an NSAID can be considered once Shadow's hydration status has normalised.

The most effective way to rectify the dehydration is to provide IV fluid therapy. Given that Shadow is not demonstrating signs of cardiovascular shock, a crystalloid fluid (e.g. Hartmann's) would be the most appropriate choice. However, Shadow's cardiovascular status should be monitored carefully following administration of potent opioid analgesia, as signs of shock may be unmasked. The brain can modulate pain transmission through descending pathways (particularly at the spinal level), creating what is called stress-induced analgesia. This phenomenon allows the cat (in this instance) to run away from the accident despite his injuries and the stress response may mask signs of shock. By giving a high dose of opioid analgesia and taking over pain management, any residual stress-induced response may be 'switched off', resulting in some cardiovascular deterioration and potential signs of shock, which may require adjustment of fluid therapy.

b) A DV view of the pelvis and proximal hindlimbs is shown. Typically, a VD projection is used in pelvic radiography; however, due to the traumatic nature of Shadow's injuries, it was safer and more comfortable for him to be positioned in sternal recumbency. From the portion of the abdomen visible, the bladder is full and intact, and the abdominal wall appears intact. The spinal column appears within normal limits. The right femoral head is completely luxated cranially from the acetabulum. The remainder of the pelvis appears normal. The left hindlimb appears normal. The right hindlimb is laterally rotated, creating an area of decreased soft tissue opacity medial to the stifle where the musculature is abnormally positioned. No fractures are evident. The volume of soft tissue mass on the right and left hindlimbs is subjectively equal, suggesting that the luxation is acute as no muscle wastage, which takes time to develop, is evident. Two testes are visible.

> The bladder is full so Shadow should be monitored for normal urination during stabilisation as neurological bladder injury is always a possibility with hindlimb trauma.

c) The right hindlimb lameness is due to complete luxation of the right coxofemoral (hip) joint. Given the scuffed nails on clinical examination, the cause is probably trauma, most likely a road traffic accident. An orthogonal view of the pelvis is required to fully determine the direction of the luxation. However, the majority of femoral head luxations in cats are craniodorsal.

d) There are no obvious fractures of the femoral head, neck, acetabulum, or distal affected limb; therefore, closed reduction is a suitable option. In patients suitable for anaesthesia, closed reduction is most likely to be successful if it occurs within 48 hours of injury, before there is considerable contraction of the musculature. Successful reduction should be followed with 2–3 weeks of strict cage rest to allow scar tissue to form and stabilise the joint. An Ehmer sling is not recommended for use in cats due to reported lack of benefit and risk of soft tissue complications.

The method to perform closed reduction is dependent on the direction of the luxation. In the case of craniodorsal luxation, the technique is as follows:

- The anaesthetised cat should be positioned in lateral recumbency with the affected limb uppermost
- The cat's body should be gently secured on the table by an assistant to provide countertraction
- The femur should be externally rotated to prevent the femoral head impeding reduction
- At the same time, distal-caudal traction is applied to the femur until the head aligns with the acetabulum
- Once alignment is achieved, the femur should be internally rotated and gentle pressure applied at the greater trochanter to push the head back into position
- The limb should then be gently manoeuvred through a normal 'bicycle' range of motion to check for correct positioning and immediate re-displacement

e) If closed reduction fails or is not achievable, or in cases for which it is contraindicated (e.g. concomitant fractures), surgical options can be offered. These include open reduction methods and salvage procedures. There are a range of open reduction methods reported (e.g. transarticular pinning, iliofemoral suture, modified Knowles toggle). There is currently no strong evidence to select one method over another. Selection should be based on surgeon experience, equipment available, and patient/client factors such as cost and compliance.

Femoral head and neck excision is a viable salvage procedure in cats and can result in a rapid return to function if performed correctly. The procedure involves no implant and less specialised equipment, making it a more affordable alternative than most open reduction methods, which can involve multiple procedures. Physiotherapy is recommended to promote an optimal outcome; this requires both patient and client adherence, plus the potential cost of engaging a licensed veterinary physiotherapist. Most cats will heal successfully without physiotherapy however, so lack of physiotherapy should not deter this approach. Total hip replacement is an alternative salvage procedure that is now available for cats; however, this is likely to require referral and involves a significant cost difference to the client compared with all other methods. Another alternative would be amputation if, for some reason, excision arthroplasty was not viable.

See also Case 1.13.

REFERENCES

Dugdale, A. H., Beaumont, G., Bradbrook, C. & Gurney, M. (2020). *Veterinary Anaesthesia: Principles to Practice*. Hoboken, NJ: Wiley-Blackwell.

Meeson R. L. & Strickland, R. (2021) Traumatic joint luxations in cats: reduce, repair, replace, remove. *Journal of Feline Medicine and Surgery* **23**(1):17–32. doi: 10.1177/1098612X20979508.

4.16 Peter, 6-mo ME Cross-breed: health check

a) The following factors will impact your recommendation:
   - Overall health of the dog and their ability to withstand anaesthesia and surgery (e.g. ASA score)
   - Ownership of the dog
   - Owner's intentions for the dog
   - Signalment of the dog

The first is self-explanatory.

The second is about ensuring that indiscriminate breeding will not take place. Dogs that are being fostered from a humane organisation generally are gonadectomised before adoption. For dogs with a dedicated owner, the owner should be included in the decision, with decisions about whether or not to perform gonadectomy and timing of the procedure made on a case-by-case basis.

Some owners will require an explanation of the irreversibility of gonadectomy procedures and of the costs and risks of breeding dogs. For those dogs intended for companionship only, findings about an increase in reactivity in both female and male dogs after gonadectomy should be discussed. This may be exacerbated in some breeds or in dogs with a prior history of reactivity or aggression. Conversely, some male dogs will be much more tractable as companions after castration. There is no truth in the myth that female dogs are somehow 'better behaved' after having a litter or that dogs 'become lazy' after gonadectomy.

> **Known finding**: potential increased risk of reactivity after gonadectomy in some dogs.
> **Myth**: gonadectomy makes working females lazy or 'calms down' difficult behaviours.

Conditions reported to be more common after gonadectomy that are not affected by signalment include obesity, orthopaedic disorders, and some neoplastic disorders. Obesity is likely to be due to a decrease in metabolic rate after gonadectomy. In large-breed dogs, physes of the long bones may not close until well after 1 year of age, such that they reach adult height and weight at a later age then small-breed dogs. A common orthopaedic condition reported to be associated with gonadectomy in dogs is anterior (cranial) cruciate ligament (ACL/CCL) injury (Figure A4.16a,b), and the increased risk is apparently separate from the risk for obesity. Exact cause and

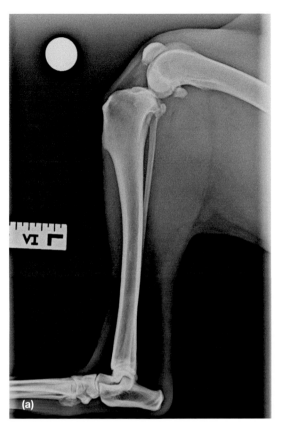 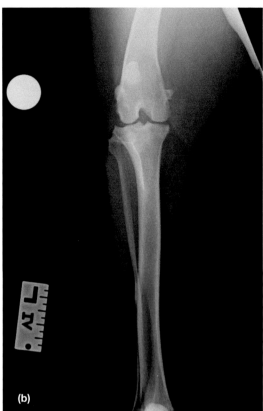

Figure A4.16a,b Cruciate ligament disease may be associated with early gonadectomy in large-breed dogs.

effect have not been identified, but there may be some merit in waiting until skeletal maturity is complete before performing gonadectomy. Recommendations will also vary with the sex of the dog. Mammary neoplasia is a very common tumour in female dogs that is malignant in about 50% of cases; the risk of occurrence can be decreased by spaying female dogs earlier in life (see below). In male dogs, prostatic neoplasia, either primary adenocarcinoma or infiltrative transitional cell carcinoma, is more common in castrated than in intact male dogs. There are other cancers that are reported to be more common after gonadectomy in both females and males, such as osteosarcoma, hemangiosarcoma, lymphosarcoma (with breed predisposition also evident), and mast cell tumours. Cause and effect for these tumours have not been identified.

b) The first thing to consider is not just timing of the surgery, but also what surgery will be performed. OVH is the standard in many countries, but there is little literature to support this, as ovariectomy will achieve the same goals and may be less invasive and associated with quicker post-surgical recovery. There is current interest in hysterectomy only, sometimes colloquially called an 'ovary-sparing spay', based on studies demonstrating greater longevity and other benefits in female dogs that retained their ovaries later into their lives. Most of the research that has been done to date has evaluated OVH.

The most common disorders reported to have a decreased incidence after OVH are mammary neoplasia and pyometra. Incidence of mammary neoplasia later in life is greatly decreased by spaying earlier in life, with the greatest benefit if spaying is performed before the first oestrus and a decreasing benefit seen thereafter. Pyometra is extremely common in aged dogs and there is obvious benefit in spaying dogs before uterine pathology develops. Disorders reported to be increased after OVH in dogs include obesity, urinary incontinence, ACL injury, and the cancers described previously. Obesity is common after OVH and can be managed through dietary and exercise modification. Urinary incontinence is most commonly due to USMI, formerly called oestrogen-responsive urinary incontinence. This is more common in dogs weighing >20 kg, can be minimised by not spaying dogs before 5 months of age, and is easily managed medically in most cases. The various neoplastic conditions other than mammary neoplasia are uncommon; even though risk increases with OVH, they are still uncommon overall.

> To see the greatest benefit (decreased mammary neoplasia later in life, minimising incidence of urinary incontinence, potentially minimising risk of orthopaedic disease), small-breed bitches should be spayed after 5 months of age but before their first heat, or at about 6 months of age. Larger-breed bitches should be spayed nearer the time of skeletal maturity but before they have had more than one or two oestrous cycles, at about 12–18 months of age.

c) Castration in male dogs prevents non-neoplastic prostate disease that is testosterone-dependent (benign prostatic hypertrophy/hyperplasia [BPH]) and testicular neoplasia. These disorders are common and are easily diagnosed and treated by castration when they develop. Disorders that may be more common after castration in male dogs include obesity and the orthopaedic and neoplastic conditions previously described. Obesity can be controlled by diet and exercise.

> Because castration early in life is not associated with benefits similar to those seen in female dogs, there is no reason to castrate dogs early in life unless they are being permitted to breed indiscriminately or are exhibiting reproductive behaviours (mounting, urine-marking, roaming) that are distressing to the owner.

WSAVA reproduction control guidelines are available online (*https://wsava.org/wp-content/uploads/2024/05/J-of-Small-Animal-Practice-2024-Romagnoli-WSAVA-guidelines-for-the-control-of-reproduction-in-dogs-and-cats.pdf*).

REFERENCES

Hart, L. A., Hart, B. L. & Thigpen, A. P. (2023) Decision-making on recommended age of spay/neuter for a specific dog. General principles and cultural complexities. *Veterinary Clinics of North America: Small Animal* **53**(5):1209–1221. doi: 10.1016/j.cvsm.2023.05.005.

Houlihan, K. E. (2017) A literature review on the welfare implications of gonadectomy of dogs. *Journal of the American Veterinary Medical Association* **250**(10):1155–1166. doi: 10.2460/javma.250.10.1155.

Root Kustritz, M. V., Slater, M. R., Weedon, G. R. & Bushby, P. A. (2017) Determining optimal age for gonadectomy in the dog: a critical review of the literature to guide decision making. *Clinical Theriogenology* **9**(2):167–211. doi: 10.5555/20173199995.

4.17 On way in – see immediately: dog collapsed on walk

a) This ECG demonstrates a type of ventricular tachycardia called torsades de pointes. It can be recognised by the characteristic cyclic increasing and decreasing amplitude. This is an arrest rhythm.

b) The high CO_2 levels on the capnograph suggest that the arrest has occurred very recently. Chest compressions should immediately be initiated at a rate of 100–120 bpm, with ventilation every 6 seconds. If a defibrillator is available, it could be utilised in this case; otherwise, a bolus of 2 mg/kg of lidocaine may help. You can review the most recently published Reassessment Campaign on Veterinary Resuscitation (RECOVER) guidelines online (*https://recoverinitiative. org/2024-guidelines/*).

c) There is no set duration for resuscitation to continue; however, if no response is seen within the first 15 minutes, then the likelihood of survival decreases significantly. The decision to stop cardiopulmonary resuscitation (CPR) is never easy and should be made as a group if everyone agrees that the patient is not responding to treatment. Remember that the proportion of dogs surviving cardiac arrest in veterinary medicine is <5%, while the proportion of dogs and cats undergoing CPR that survive to hospital discharge is also <5% (Dazio et al. 2023, Hoehne et al. 2023). These results are with the best-equipped intensive care unit (ICU) teams, so try to take this into account in the post-arrest review. Survival rates are reported to be lower in animals that arrest outside the hospital environment (Hofmeister et al. 2009).

> Survival to discharge of dogs and cats undergoing CPR with fully dedicated ICU teams is typically <5%. In emergency referral hospitals, survival rates range from 5% to 7% for dogs and from 1% to 19% for cats (Burkitt-Creedon et al. 2024).

REFERENCES

Burkitt-Creedon, J. M., Boller, M., Fletcher, D. J. et al.(2024) 2024 RECOVER Guidelines: updated treatment recommendations for CPR in dogs and cats. *Journal of Veterinary Emergency and Critical Care* **34**:104–123. doi: 10.1111/vec.13391.

Dazio, V. E. R., Gay, J. M. & Hoehne, S. N. (2023) Cardiopulmonary resuscitation outcomes of dogs and cats at a veterinary teaching hospital before and after publication of the RECOVER guidelines. *Journal of Small Animal Practice* **64**(4):270–279. doi: 10.1111/jsap.13582.

Hoehne, S. N., Balakrishnan, A., Silverstein, D. C., Pigott, A. M. et al. (2023) Reassessment Campaign on Veterinary Resuscitation (RECOVER) initiative small animal CPR registry report 2016–2021. *Journal of Veterinary Emergency and Critical Care* **33**(2):143–155. doi: 10.1111/vec.13273.

Hofmeister, E. H., Brainard, B. M., Egger, C. M. & Kang, S. (2009) Prognostic indicators for dogs and cats with cardiopulmonary arrest treated by cardiopulmonary cerebral resuscitation at a university teaching hospital. *Journal of the American Veterinary Medical Association* **235**(1):50–57. doi: 10.2460/javma.235.1.50.

4.18 Cleo, 4-yo FN Cocker Spaniel: drinking & urinating lots

a) Cleo's blood work exhibits most, but not all, of the features typical of canine hypoadrenocorticism (Addison's disease). This is an uncommon endocrine disorder most often caused by immune-mediated destruction of the adrenal glands (Klein &

Peterson 2010, Guzmán Ramos et al. 2022). The following changes in Cleo's blood work are suggestive of this disease:

- The absence of a stress leukogram (neutrophilia, lymphopaenia, monocytosis, eosinopaenia) in a clinically unwell dog
- The presence of a moderate-marked lymphocytosis
- Mild hypocholesterolaemia and marked hyponatraemia and hypochloraemia

Note that other changes commonly seen in Addisonian patients (hyperkalaemia, azotaemia, and hypoglycaemia) are not present in Cleo's results.

b) Hypoadrenocorticism is diagnosed with an adrenocorticotropic hormone (ACTH) stimulation test. This test involves taking a serum blood sample for a baseline cortisol, injecting 5 µg/kg of Synacthen (synthetic ACTH) and then taking another serum blood sample 1 hour later. If the dog's post-ACTH cortisol level is <55 nmol/L, the diagnosis of hypoadrenocorticism is confirmed. Some practitioners will run a baseline cortisol as a **rule-out** test, because a baseline cortisol level of >55 nmol/L allows hypoadrenocorticism to be excluded from a list of differential diagnoses. However, it is important to note that a baseline cortisol level of <55 nmol/L does not confirm hypoadrenocorticism – it simply indicates that the disease is possible, and a full ACTH stimulation test is needed for confirmation. Another point of note is that, while this test is the gold standard for hypoadrenocorticism diagnosis, it should not be used for monitoring. Instead, monitoring is largely based on resolution of clinical signs, regular electrolyte checks, and/or CBC if suboptimal control is suspected.

c) The prognosis for hypoadrenocorticism, with appropriate medication and regular monitoring, is excellent (Van Lanen &

Sande 2014). Highlighting this point early in the discussion can allay some of the owner's anxiety about their dog's illness and allow them to focus more fully on subsequent information. It should be emphasised to Cleo's owner that Cleo can have a normal lifespan with this disease, but that it does involve lifelong treatment (including daily oral medication), monitoring for clinical signs of under- or over-supplementation at home, and regular physical examination and blood-work monitoring. It is also important to reinforce to the owner that a well-controlled Addisonian dog should be clinically normal at home. The use of steroids in treatment can lead some owners to believe that the typical signs of glucocorticoid excess (polyphagia, polyuria, polydipsia, and excessive weight gain) are to be expected and tolerated, but this is not the case; if these occur, doses most likely need to be reduced. Undiagnosed or delayed diagnosis of hypoadrenocorticism is associated with mortality due to severe electrolyte derangements (hyperkalaemia, hyponatraemia), dehydration, and hypovolaemic shock (Guzmán Ramos et al. 2022).

d) Typical hypoadrenocorticism requires supplementation of both mineralocorticoids and glucocorticoids, while atypical hypoadrenocorticoid dogs have normal electrolytes and require supplementation with glucocorticoids only. Mineralocorticoids can be supplemented either by giving desoxycorticosterone pivalate (DOCP) by injection approximately once every 25 days (dose and interval of injections can be altered based on serial electrolyte monitoring), or by administering fludrocortisone tablets twice daily. Dogs receiving DOCP injections almost always require separate glucocorticoid supplementation in the form of either cortisone acetate or prednisolone – the former is preferred as it is more physiologic.

This is typically given either once or twice daily, and the dose is increased (usually doubled) in times of stress or illness (to mimic the increased cortisol levels that the adrenal glands of a healthy dog would produce in these situations). Fludrocortisone tablets provide enough glucocorticoid activity for ~50% of dogs (Lathan & Thompson 2018), while the remainder of patients require additional glucocorticoid supplementation as above.

e) Hypoadrenocorticism has been dubbed 'the Great Pretender', as it is known for vague clinical signs that can wax and wane, and for mimicking a number of other conditions, particularly gastrointestinal disease. Electrolyte derangements (hyperkalaemia, hyponatraemia, hypochloraemia) are also seen in dogs with severe gastrointestinal disease (including parasitic infestation, such as whipworm), renal and hepatic disease, congestive heart failure, severe metabolic or respiratory acidosis, and tissue damage (Guzmán Ramos et al. 2022).

> It is suggested that an ACTH stimulation test should be considered in any dog with a history of chronic, recurrent gastrointestinal signs prior to performing invasive tests such as exploratory surgery or gastrointestinal biopsies (Guzmán Ramos et al. 2022).

Increased urea, creatinine, and phosphate can occur secondary to hypovolaemia and dehydration (pre-renal azotaemia), while aldosterone deficiency and sodium losses can lead to a low USG, mimicking renal insufficiency. The onset of signs can be slow and insidious, e.g. gradual weight loss that may not be noticed by the owner. Affected animals do not typically present with a pathognomonic set of clinical signs.

f) Cleo's primary presenting signs were polyuria and polydipsia – these have been reported in only 17–25% of dogs with hypoadrenocorticism (Klein & Peterson 2010). They are, in fact, much more commonly present in the 'opposite' illness, i.e. hyperadrenocorticism, and in other diseases such as diabetes mellitus and renal disease. Conversely, vomiting occurs in 68–75% of patients (Klein & Peterson 2010), yet Cleo's owners reported only one vomit in her recent history. Hyperkalaemia occurs in up to 95% of dogs with primary hypoadrenocorticism, and hence many also have decreased myocardial excitability and slowed conduction resulting in bradycardia (Klein & Peterson 2010). Cleo's normal serum potassium meant her heart rate was unremarkable, two factors which had the potential to confuse or delay the diagnosis. In addition, initial symptomatic treatment such as IV fluid resuscitation may correct electrolyte derangements that might otherwise flag the need for further investigation (Guzmán Ramos et al. 2022). Ultimately, hypoadrenocorticism should be a differential diagnosis for dogs with severe illness and electrolyte derangements, as well as for those with chronic waxing and waning signs of illness, even in the absence of electrolyte derangements.

REFERENCES

Guzmán Ramos, P. J., Bennaim, M., Shiel, R. E. & Mooney, C. T. (2022) Diagnosis of canine spontaneous hypoadrenocorticism. *Canine Medicine and Genetics* **9**(1):6. doi: 10.1186/s40575-022-00119-4.

Klein, S. C. & Peterson, M. E. (2010) Canine hypoadrenocorticism: part I. *Canadian Veterinary Journal* **51**(1):63–69.

Lathan, P. & Thompson, A. L. (2018) Management of hypoadrenocorticism (Addison's disease) in dogs. *Veterinary Medicine (Auckl)* **9**:1–10. doi: 10.2147/vmrr.S125617.

Van Lanen, K. & Sande, A. (2014) Canine hypoadrenocorticism: pathogenesis, diagnosis, and treatment. *Topics in Companion Animal Medicine* **29**(4):88–95. doi: 10.1053/j.tcam.2014.10.001.

4.19 Seamus, 7-yo MN DSH: vomiting ++

a) Primary gastrointestinal causes include gastrointestinal foreign body, intussusception, neoplasia, abscess, granuloma or haematoma, mesenteric volvulus, and/or torsion. Extra GIT causes include a pancreatic mass lesion (neoplasia or abscess), peritonitis, and lymphadenitis.

b) The image shows an ultrasound cross-section of an ileocolic intussusception illustrating the internal loop (the intussuscipiens) within the outer loop. The hyperechoic material is intussuscepted fat/mesentery that is pulled in with the bowel loop. Intussusceptions occur when one area of the GIT telescopes into the lumen of an adjacent area. A typical transverse view of an intussusception can demonstrate an 'onion ring' or 'target-like' mass (Patsikas et al. 2003) made of concentric rings with a hypoechoic centre. Other diagnostic images of intussusceptions are shown in Figure A4.19a–d.

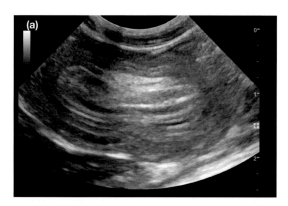

Figure A4.19a Longitudinal view of Seamus's intussusception.

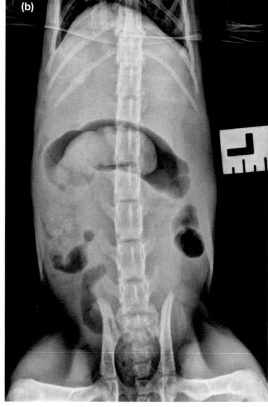

Figure A4.19b VD radiograph of a kitten with an ileocolic intussusception heading into the transverse colon. There is a gravel sign (mineral debris) in the intestine approaching the obstruction.

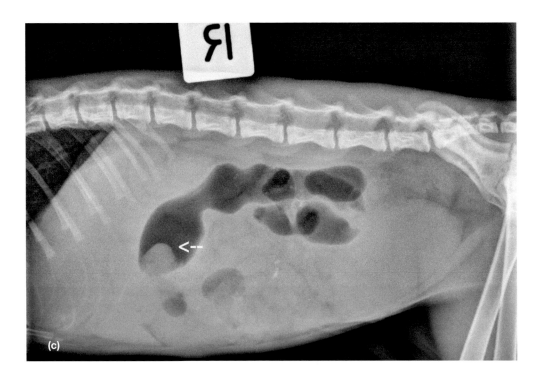

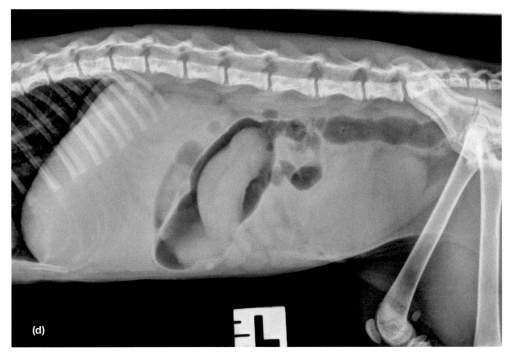

Figure A4.19c,d Right lateral (c) and left lateral (d) radiographs of a kitten with an ileocolic intussusception heading into the transverse colon.

c) Surgery is the recommended treatment; medical management of intussusception is rarely successful. The patient should first be stabilised by collecting blood to assess and address any electrolyte or acid–base abnormalities, followed by administration of IV fluids to provide haemodynamic support, and symptomatic treatment for pain and nausea. Surgical management requires an exploratory laparotomy to locate the intussusception and attempt to manually reduce it. Manual reduction is often not possible because fibrinous adhesions prevent the telescoped bowel from being manipulated back into normal position (Radlinsky & Fossum 2018). When manual reduction cannot be performed, resection and anastomosis of the intussuscepted bowel is required. In cats, jejuno-jejunal intussusception is most common (Burkitt et al. 2009). Like dogs, intussusception at the ileocolic junction also occurs in cats. Seamus's intussusception was located at the ileocolic junction and required resection and anastomosis.

d) Unlike dogs, among whom young animals are over-represented in intussusception cases (Larose et al. 2020), the age distribution of intussusception in cats appears to be bimodal (Burkitt et al. 2009). Most intussusceptions in cats <1 year of age are idiopathic, with common predisposing factors including infectious enteritis, linear and non-linear foreign body, recent abdominal surgery, periparturient, or severe non-gastrointestinal disease (Doherty et al. 2000). Intussusceptions in cats aged >6 years are more likely to be secondary to lymphoma or inflammatory bowel disease (Burkitt et al. 2009). The owner should be questioned about Seamus's diet and overall health to determine if his history is consistent with possible inflammatory bowel disease or intestinal neoplasia. More than half the cats with intussusception have a recent history of diarrhoea (Burkitt et al. 2009). Surgical biopsies should be taken at the time of surgical correction of the intussusception to investigate underlying gastrointestinal disease. On questioning, it was discovered that Seamus had experienced intermittent diarrhoea in the preceding 5 years. Biopsy results revealed non-specific inflammation consistent with inflammatory bowel disease. Following recovery from surgery, he was given a single cobalamin injection. He was treated with prednisolone (1 mg/kg PO q24h), but weaned off after several months and maintained on a prescription low-residue hydrolysed diet.

REFERENCES

Burkitt, J. M., Drobatz, K. J., Saunders, H. M. & Washabau, R. J. (2009) Signalment, history, and outcome of cats with gastrointestinal tract intussusception: 20 cases (1986–2000). *Journal of the American Veterinary Medical Association* **234**(6):771–776. doi: 10.2460/javma.234.6.771.

Doherty, D., Welsh E. M. & Kirby, B. M. (2000) Intestinal intussusception in five postparturient queens. *Veterinary Record* **146**(21):614–616. doi: 10.1136/vr.146.21.614.

Radlinsky, M. & Fossum, T. W. (2018). Chapter 18: Surgery of the Digestive System. In: Fossum, T. W. (ed.) *Small Animal Surgery*, 5th edition. Philadelphia, PA: Elsevier, pp. 331–511.

Larose, P. C., Singh, A., Giuffrida, M. A. et al. (2020) Clinical findings and outcomes of 153 dogs surgically treated for intestinal intussusceptions. *Veterinary Surgery* **49**(5):870–878. doi: 10.1111/vsu.13442.

Patsikas, M., Papazoglou, L., Papaioannou, N. et al. (2003) Ultrasonographic findings of intestinal intussusception in seven cats. *Journal of Feline Medicine and Surgery* **5**(6):335–343. doi: 10.1016/S1098-612X(03)00066-4.

4.20 Home time

The UK's National Health Service (NHS) has created a going-home checklist for healthcare professionals (*https://qi.elft.nhs.uk/collection/developing-a-strategy-and-change-ideas-working-well-handy-guide/*). This is a mindful activity to help people switch their attention to home, and effectively rest and recharge. It involves taking a moment to do the following:

1. Think about **one difficult thing** that occurred during the working day. You might want to imagine placing that difficult thing into a bubble that you can imagine blowing away, or onto a leaf that you can place into a flowing stream and imagine it drifting away. Let it go!

2. Consider **three things that went well** during the working day. They may be things you or another team member did. It may help to write these down.

3. **Check on your colleagues** before you leave. Ask if they are okay. If not, what is needed immediately? What can be done later to address issues (e.g. having a meeting to ensure cover is available to allow breaks)?

4. **Perform an internal inventory** of yourself. Are *you* okay? If not, what do you need immediately? What do you need to follow up (e.g. handing over a case that you feel uneasy about for a colleague to follow up, scheduling an appointment with a physiotherapist for musculoskeletal pain, making an appointment to discuss concerns with your manager).

5. **Consciously switch your attention to home**. What are your plans for resting, relaxing, and recharging? Are you looking forward to a meal? A run? Time with family? Walking the dog? Catching up with a friend? It can be useful to have a ritual or practice such as listening to a podcast or music, observing the natural world, or (if not walking or operating a vehicle) reading or watching something unrelated to work during the trip home.

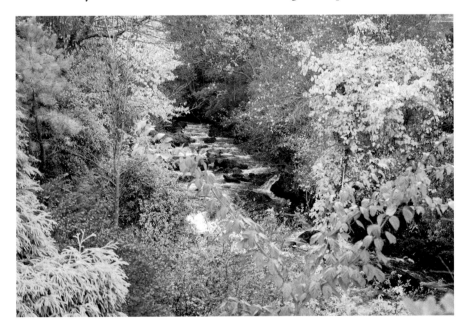

Figure A4.20 **Observing the natural world can help consciously switch your attention to home. Many people find imagining placing each disruptive thought on to a leaf and then visualising this being taken away by flowing water a useful wind-down ritual.**

TODAY'S CASE LIST

5.1 Roxie, 8-yo FE Husky: lethargic and reduced appetite

5.2 Mittens, 12-wo ME DLH: owner stood on him

5.3 Bubba, 3-yo MN American Pit Bull Terrier: still vomiting

5.4 Malibu, 10-wo FE DSH: vaccination

5.5 Max, 4-yo MN DSH: dental

5.6 Sandie, 13-yo MN DSH: making strange noises at night

5.7 Amber, 3.5-yo FN Rottweiler: aggressive to other dogs

5.8 Cat colony on farm – request for TNR

5.9 Enalor, 9-wo FE Scottish Fold: health check

5.10 Gerbera, 3-yo FN Dachshund: sore paws, not eaten breakfast

5.11 Joey, 6-mo ME Griffon Bruxellois: itchy ears

5.12 Greg, 3-yo ME Mixed Breed: breathing strangely

5.13 Scruff, 13-yo MN Jack Russell Terrier: blood from mouth

5.14 Walk-in: wants to surrender 3 cats due to toxo

5.15 Will, 6-yo MN DSH: blocked again

5.16 Jackie, 7-yo MN Mixed Breed: lump in mouth

5.17 Rufus, 14-mo ME Mixed Breed: had a fit

5.18 Clementine, 12-yo FN DSH: vet authorise prescription

5.19 Otis, 4-yo MN Cocker Spaniel: ears

5.20 Ember, 7 yo FN DSH: quieter than normal, constipated?

5.21 Yuuki, 6-yo FE Chihuahua cross: UTI?

5.22 Ten Statements Test

5.23 Sleep

Recipe: 'Cheesecake' challenge

DOI: 10.1201/9781003278306-5

5.1 Roxie, 8-yo FE Husky: lethargic and reduced appetite

Roxie presents due to general malaise and decreased appetite. She has no history of current medication, travel, or scavenging. She is fully vaccinated and appropriately protected against endo- and ectoparasites. On clinical examination, Roxie is quiet, alert, and responsive. She is panting with an HR of 120 and regular rhythm. She resents any abdominal palpation and has a rectal temperature of 39.7 °C.

You perform an oral examination and observe Roxie's buccal mucosa (Figure 5.1a).

a) Describe the abnormality in gross pathological terms.
b) What term is used to categorise this finding?

c) From the differential diagnoses that cause this finding, which should be considered the most likely in this case, at this stage?

There are no other significant findings on clinical examination. To narrow your differential diagnoses, you get permission to take a blood sample. You examine a blood smear under the microscope while waiting for the machine results (Figure 5.1b).

d) Evaluate the smear and comment on any abnormalities, linking them to your differential diagnoses.
e) What additional checks should be performed on the smear to verify these findings?

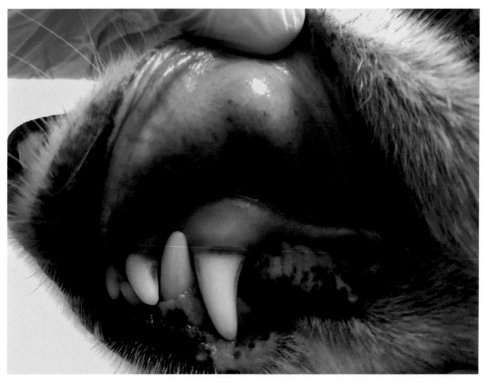

Figure 5.1a Roxie's left buccal mucosa. There are small red 'blotches' across the labial mucosa, seen especially above the canine tooth in this image.

You discuss your findings and suspicions so far with the owner. The owner is insistent that Roxie is not put through too many tests, as they do not think it is fair on her. However, after discussion you both decide that, as imaging is non-invasive, some more information will help decision-making.

An abdominal ultrasound (Figure 5.1c) shows a moderately severe diffuse hepatomegaly, with rounded liver margins and caudal extension of the liver beyond the costal arch.

f) Describe the appearance of the liver parenchyma in Figure 5.1c and discuss how it impacts your list of differential diagnoses.
g) Evaluate options for Roxie and her owner at this stage.

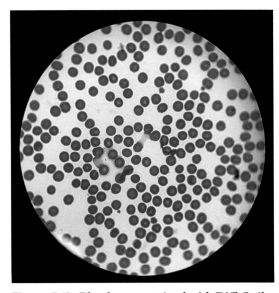

Figure 5.1b **Blood smear stained with Diff-Quik ×100.**

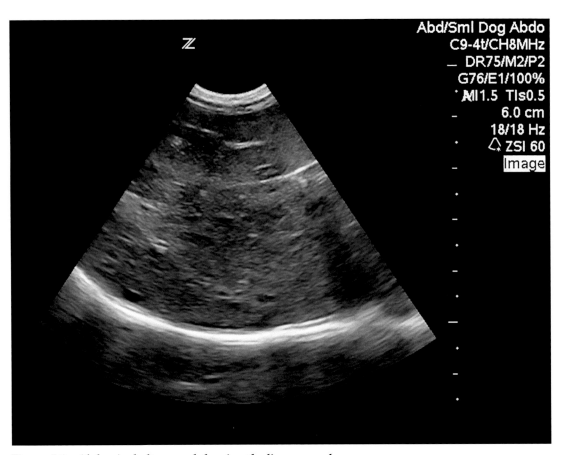

Figure 5.1c **Abdominal ultrasound showing the liver parenchyma.**

5.2 Mittens, 12-wo ME DLH: owner stood on him

Mittens, weighing 1.4 kg, was injured when his owner tripped over him on some steps. You suspect a possible pelvic fracture, and wish to perform radiography, but Mittens is very wriggly. You perform a complete physical examination and feel that Mittens is otherwise healthy. You decide to sedate Mittens with a combination of medetomidine and methadone IM or SC.

a) You wish to administer a combination of 20 µg/kg of medetomidine (you have access to medetomidine with a concentration of 1 mg/mL) and 0.3 mg/kg of methadone (you have access to methadone with a concentration of 10 mg/mL). What is the total volume you would need to administer?

b) You have 1-mL, 3-mL, and 5-mL syringes available (Figure 5.2). Which would you use and why?

c) The accuracy of veterinary team members in drawing up medications has been shown to decrease as the target volume decreases.

When you have a very small injection volume to deliver, what simple thing can you do to ensure that the full dose is received?

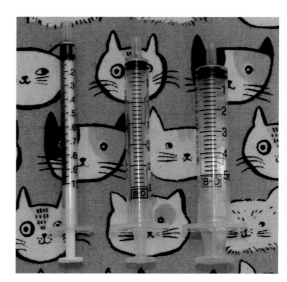

Figure 5.2 **Commonly available syringes in 1-mL, 3-mL, and 5-mL sizes.**

5.3 Bubba, 3-yo MN American Pit Bull Terrier: still vomiting

Bubba (Figure 5.3a) has a 3-week history of occasional vomiting and episodic scant diarrhoea, which sometimes contains traces of blood and mucus. These symptoms started after partial ingestion of a rope toy. It is difficult to tell if the bland diet, anti-emetics, and probiotics that Bubba has been receiving are helping, as the symptoms are so intermittent. He can go 2 or 3 days with no symptoms at all. A colleague took some blood (CBC and biochemistry) 1 week ago, which revealed a mild neutrophilia and no other abnormalities. Bubba can be challenging to examine as he is very wriggly and tends to roll onto his back.

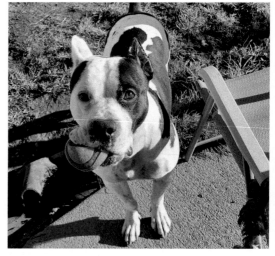

Figure 5.3a **Bubba has been showing mild but persistent symptoms for 3 weeks.**

Physical examination today reveals the following:

- BCS 6/9
- Weight loss of 0.5 kg over the last 3 weeks
- Bright and alert
- Temp: 37.5 °C
- MMs pink and CRT <3 s
- HR 120 bpm, no murmurs
- RR 30
- Mild periodontal disease
- Possible abdominal boarding/splinting/pain on palpation, or just wriggly?

You admit Bubba for sedation and X-rays (Figure 5.3b).

a) Describe the radiographic findings.
b) List some potential differential diagnoses.
c) Do the radiographic findings explain Bubba's presenting problem?
d) Is it time for exploratory coeliotomy? What are the alternatives?
e) During discussion with the owner about next steps, it emerges that Bubba was rehomed through a rescue organisation. Bubba was without testicles on admission to the rescue facility, which surprised staff for a young dog that had been found roaming. Does this inform your differential list at all?

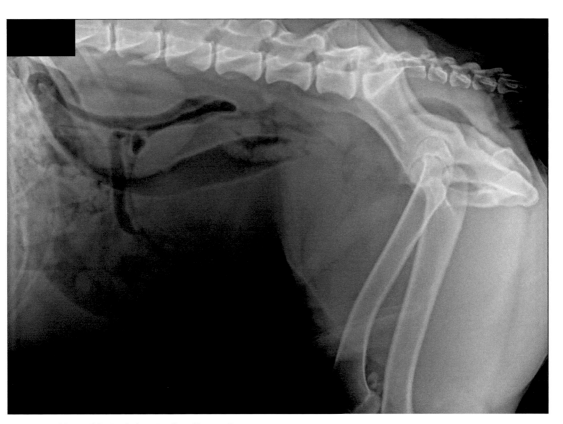

Figure 5.3b **Bubba's abdominal radiograph.**

5.4 Malibu, 10-wo FE DSH: vaccination

Malibu presented this morning for routine vaccinations. She was purchased from a friend of the owner 1 week ago. Malibu's owners have had cats before but always allowed them outdoor access. This time, they want to keep Malibu indoors for her safety and to protect the wildlife around their home. They have asked for guidance on keeping a cat indoors and what they should do to ensure that Malibu is happy. You have become familiar with the Five Domains Model (Figure 5.4b) to assess animal welfare and want to use it to help structure client communication in this case.

a) From studying Figure 5.4b, how might we use the Five Domains Model to evaluate the potential for positive welfare and animal happiness?
b) What do you think is meant by 'animal agency'?
c) How can we apply the Five Domains Model to discuss ways of providing Malibu with opportunities to exercise agency while being kept indoors?

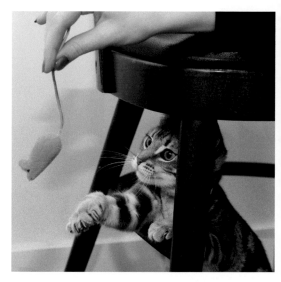

Figure 5.4a Malibu is going to be an indoor-only cat.

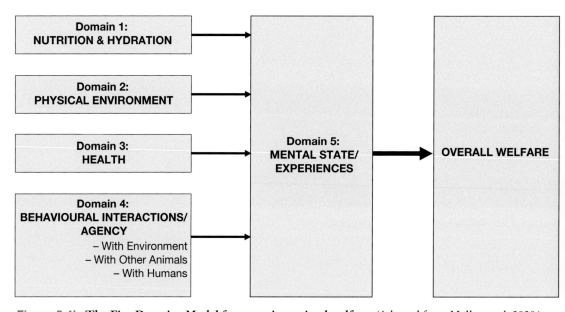

Figure 5.4b The Five Domains Model for assessing animal welfare. (Adapted from Mellor et al. 2020.)

5.5 Max, 4-yo MN DSH: dental

You are called to the dental room. A 3.6-kg cat is under general anaesthesia using isoflurane in oxygen delivered by a T-piece breathing system. The capnograph is shown in Figure 5.5.

a) What is the abnormality displayed in red in Figure 5.5?
b) How would you resolve this?

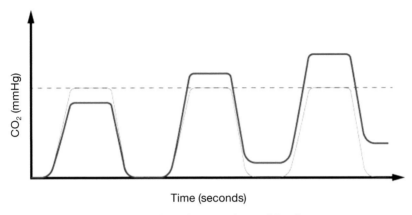

Figure 5.5 **Max's capnograph while anaesthetised for dentistry.**

5.6 Sandie, 13-yo MN DSH: making strange noises at night

You examine Sandie, who has lost 0.5 kg since she was last weighed 1 year ago. Her owner has complained of 'blood-curdling' wailing noises from Sandie in the middle of the night. You take several measurements of Sandie's BP in the clinic and suspect that the high readings are genuine.

a) What are some common behaviours and clinical signs that may alert you to hypertension in cats?

b) What factors should you consider when measuring systolic BP in cats?
c) What is 'low', 'normal' or 'high' for a cat when measuring BP, what is the associated risk of target organ damage for each category, and what would you do if you took readings in these ranges?
d) What are the differential diagnoses for an older cat with increased vocalisation, hypertension, and weight loss?

5.7 Amber, 3.5-yo FN Rottweiler: aggressive to other dogs

Amber's owner complains that Amber has been lunging at and occasionally biting other dogs, on- and off-lead. She is also showing some possessive aggression over toys and has a long-standing habit of jumping up and mouthing her lead. She has a tendency to chase joggers and wildlife.

a) What three or four general background questions will you ask of Amber's owners? *Check your responses against the answers before moving on.*

From your initial questions, it is found that a second Rottweiler, Amber's companion, was

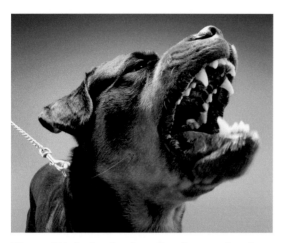

Figure 5.7 Amber has been lunging at other dogs and sometimes biting them.

lost to bone cancer a year earlier. Amber's diet consists of proprietary kibble supplemented with cooked chicken. She is the owners' fifth Rottweiler and is said to be the most 'strong-willed' they have owned. She attended puppy classes run by a veterinary nurse at the practice, positive reward-based follow-on classes up to the age of 18 months, and, latterly, outdoor remedial classes for 'reactive dogs'. Training has been mainly carried out by her female owner, Jill. Amber appeared to become 'bored' with training at around 15 months of age, such that she now no longer follows direction and 'won't do anything she's told'. This change may have started following spaying at 13 months old. Amber is described as a very 'lazy' dog at home and often has to be encouraged to move into the kitchen for food. Since puppyhood, she has displayed intermittent lameness on her left hind leg, particularly after getting up from rest.

b) What three or four specific questions will you ask regarding the aggressive episodes?
Check your responses against the answers before moving on.

You find that, when exercised at home, Amber's owners now use a Halti headcollar, a harness,

and a double-ended training lead in attempts to control her. In class, Amber wears her flat collar only. Two specific incidents have occurred while exercising off-lead. In each case, Amber met other dogs at unexpectedly close quarters and inflicted minor injuries, with her owners subsequently paying for the veterinary treatment of the injured dogs. When on the lead, Amber frequently lunges at other dogs and Jill is now unwilling to walk her owing to her concern that Amber may pull her over. If another dog runs at Amber, however, she tries to retreat behind her owner. Lead-mouthing has progressed to her grabbing Jill's arm instead if she stops to talk to someone on a walk and also nipping the male owner, Jack, when he is getting her out of the back of the car. She can also growl at him if she is in possession of toys. Amber performed perfectly for her training tests in class, including sitting and staying while Jill stopped and talked to a stooge person. The outdoor class, comprising only reactive dogs, is led by a male trainer and Amber is managing to cope in this context, to the extent of being able to walk past the other dogs while off-lead (instead of lunging or attacking as she has done in public). Despite Jill carrying out most class training, Amber is more responsive to Jack at home. Food rewards are routinely used in training, but Amber is often not interested.

c) Are there any health concerns that may be impacting Amber's behaviour and why?
d) How may early success in training have altered the owners' expectations of Amber?
e) Why might Amber behave so differently in different contexts?
f) How can a dog's decisions be influenced?
g) How may Amber's interest in food be increased so that it can be used as a more effective reward?
h) How may consistency of control be achieved across contexts?

5.8 Cat colony on farm – request for TNR

You have recently visited a farm that has a rapidly expanding colony of cats. The farmer has asked whether 'trap–neuter–return' (TNR) could help get the colony under control. The farmer is willing to feed and monitor the cats once neutered, as they consider them useful on the farm, but wishes the population to be stabilised and does not want any more new kittens. The cats will be brought to the practice for neutering in batches in the coming weeks.

a) What equipment list would be needed to perform this TNR work?
b) What advice would you give the farmer in terms of trapping the cats?
c) What are the considerations a veterinary practice would need to bear in mind before performing any TNR work?
d) How will you safely examine the cats?
e) What should you do if you find a serious health concern while examining a cat?
f) Which surgical approach should you consider for spaying colony cats?
g) How do you approach neutering lactating queens?

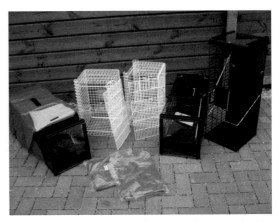

Figure 5.8 A selection of cages and traps suitable for TNR.

h) How would you approach a cryptorchid kitten for neutering?
i) Are any additional surgical procedures required for colony cats?
j) How long should colony cats be left to recover after surgery?
k) Should any further routine veterinary care be performed on a colony cat?

5.9 Enalor, 9-wo FE Scottish Fold: health check

Enalor has been brought to the clinic for her first health check by her new owners who have never had a cat before. They are very keen to do everything required to ensure that Enalor has the best start in life. Enalor came from a breeder who has an established indoor breeding colony of Scottish Folds. The breeder's cats do well at shows and all their cats are fully vaccinated. Nevertheless, as part of the consultation, the new owners would like you to test Enalor for feline immunodeficiency virus (FIV) and feline leukaemia virus (FeLV) because they have read that this is recommended.

a) What do you think is the expected prevalence of FIV and FeLV in an indoor breeding cattery as described above, and therefore the pre-test probability of these diseases in Enalor? Answer in words rather than numbers! *Check the answer to a) before answering b)*.

b) Diagnostic sensitivity and specificity are relevant measures in commonly used point-of-care tests for diseases such as FIV and FeLV. For example, two tests that could be used on Enalor might be described as follows:
  • An FIV test with a sensitivity of 100% and specificity of 64% (Westman et al. 2019)

- An FeLV test with a sensitivity of 91% and specificity of 98% (Westman et al. 2019)

What do the terms diagnostic sensitivity (*Se*) and diagnostic specificity (*Sp*) mean?

c) Diagnostic sensitivity (*Se*) and specificity (*Sp*) are test characteristics in animals of *known* disease status. They are not test *performance* characteristics in animals of *unknown* disease status. Why is this important in real-world situations?

Given the nature of diagnostic sensitivity and specificity, the predictive value of positive and negative test results is very useful. In clinical practice, there are online calculators for predictive value that avoid the need for calculations (e.g. *https://shiny.vet.unimelb.edu.au/epi/epi.predvals/*). For this example using Enalor, the actual equations and calculations are shown below.

If the test result is negative, the probability (*P*) that it is a true negative (*TN*), i.e. the negative predictive value (*NPV*), can be calculated (*FN*, false negative; *PreP*, pre-test probability; *Se*, diagnostic sensitivity; *Sp*, diagnostic specificity):

$$NPV = \frac{Probability\ true\ negative}{Probability\ negative\ test\ result}$$

$$= \frac{P(TN)}{P(TN + FN)}$$

$$= \frac{(1 - PreP) \times Sp}{((1 - PreP) \times Sp) + (PreP \times (1 - Se))}$$

If the test result is positive, the probability that it is a true positive (*TP*), i.e. positive predictive value (*PPV*) can be calculated:

$$PPV = \frac{Probability\ true\ positive}{Probability\ positive\ test\ result}$$

$$= \frac{P(TP)}{P(TP + FP)}$$

$$= \frac{PreP \times Se}{((PreP \times Se) + (1 - PreP \times (1 - Sp))}$$

The predictive values of negative and positive test results for FIV and FeLV in Enalor, given the pre-test probabilities assigned above and the test characteristics, are given in Table 5.9. Positive test results in Enalor are only 3% and 48% likely to be true positives for FIV and FeLV, respectively, i.e. they are more likely (97% and 52%) to be false positives.

Table 5.9 Predictive values for FIV and FeLV test results in Enalor

DISEASE	PRE-TEST PROBABILITY	POST-TEST PROBABILITY	
		NEGATIVE PREDICTIVE VALUE	POSITIVE PREDICTIVE VALUE
FIV	0.01	1	0.03
FeLV	0.02	1	0.48

d) Should you conduct these tests on Enalor in this situation?

e) What congenital disease involving the musculoskeletal system is this breed predisposed to?

5.10 Gerbera, 3-yo FN Dachshund: sore paws, not eaten breakfast

Gerbera typically has a ravenous appetite. Her vaccinations and individually risk-assessed parasite control programme (ecto- and endoparasites) are up to date. She has no history of vomiting or diarrhoea, or trauma. She has a history of licking her paws regularly, and the owners had been giving her a medicated foot bath every 2 weeks. Recently that regime has slipped, as they have just had a baby. Today Gerbera did not want to go on her walk. The owner reports that her feet look terrible, but insists that they did not look like this yesterday. Gerbera is on a supermarket commercial dry diet and is fed occasional table scraps. She readily takes treats when offered in the consultation room.

Physical examination findings:

- Demeanour: BAR
- BCS: 3.5/5 (weight 6.2 kg)
- MMs pink, CRT <2 s, HR = 124 bpm with no murmurs or pulse deficits
- Grade 2/4 tartar accumulation on molars and canines
- Lung fields clear
- On palpation, the abdomen is soft and compliant with no mass effect, fluid wave, or boarding/splinting
- Both front paws (Figure 5.10a,b) and one hind paw have significant inflammation of the pedal skin including the interdigital skin, with marked erythema and purulent discharge. Gerbera tries to withdraw her feet when you examine them. The nails and footpads appear grossly normal. No cysts, nodules, or foreign bodies are visible.

- An impression smear of the lesion on one of the feet reveals many rods, but no inflammatory cells or fungal hyphae.
- Temp: 38.6 °C.

It has been argued that, like otitis externa, pododermatitis is associated with primary, predisposing, and perpetuating factors (Bajwa 2023).

a) Is the infection likely to be primary in this case? If yes, what agent do you suspect? If no, what is the most likely primary cause?
b) Can you identify or think of any predisposing factors in Gerbera's case?
c) Based on the physical examination findings, why do you think Gerbera is not eating?
d) Would you use systemic antimicrobials? Why or why not?
e) When would you recheck Gerbera?

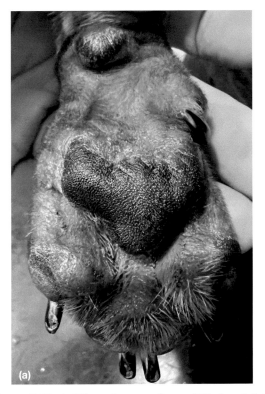 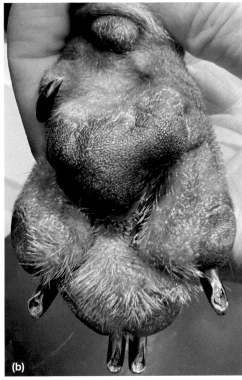

Figure 5.10a,b The palmar surfaces of Gerbera's left and right forepaws at the time of presentation.

5.11 Joey, 6-mo ME Griffon Bruxellois: itchy ears

Joey (Figure 5.11a) is presented with itchy ears. He was adopted from a breeder 3 days ago and the owner has noticed that there are some small scabs on Joey's ear tips. Joey resents otoscopy, but you are able to collect otic discharge via an ear swab. It is reddish to brown in colour, with distinct 'chunks' of ceruminous material. You smear this on a slide and view it unstained under the microscope at low power and see several mites (Figure 5.11b).

a) What types of mite typically cause pruritus in dogs and cats?
b) What type of mite is this, and what signs does it cause?
c) What are the goals of treatment in this case?
d) What congenital diseases involving the skull is this breed predisposed to?

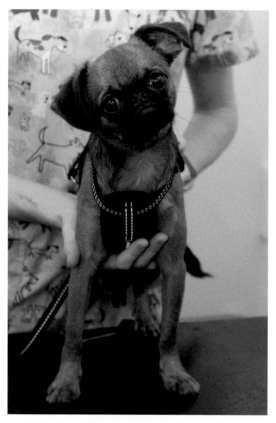

Figure 5.11a **Joey on presentation.**

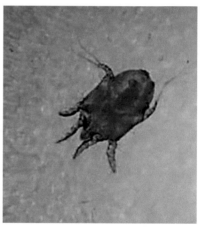

Figure 5.11b **One of the mites seen on Joey's ear swab.**

5.12 Greg, 3-yo ME Mixed Breed: breathing strangely

Greg presents as an emergency. He was 'completely fine' until he was taken for a walk this morning. The owner reports Greg disappeared for around 20 minutes. When Greg returned, he seemed anxious and the owner 'didn't like the look of his breathing'. The owner phoned the practice and was advised to bring Greg in immediately.

Physical findings:

- BCS: 3/5
- Demeanour: quiet, alert, responsive, but seems very anxious
- Tachypnoea/panting with an abdominal component to breathing

- Pale, possibly slightly blue or grey, MMs; CRT <2 s
- Lung sounds reduced, particularly dorsally
- Abdominal palpation causes increased RR and effort
- There is some grazing of Greg's paw pads and some of his nails are scuffed/bleeding
- Temp: 38.3 °C

a) Describe the radiographic findings (Figure 5.12).
b) What are the possible causes of this condition?
c) What are the potential immediate sequelae of this condition, if not treated?
d) What steps would you take to stabilise this patient?

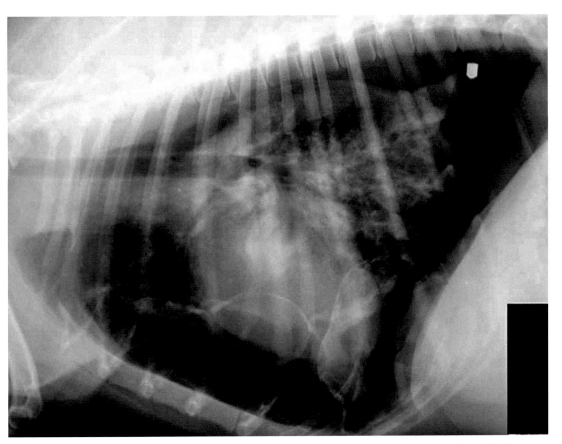

Figure 5.12 Lateral radiograph of Greg's thorax. The pellet was known to be an incidental finding.

5.13 Scruff, 13-yo MN Jack Russell Terrier: blood from mouth

Scruff has presented after his owner noticed blood in the water bowl. His eating has been more 'careful' than normal for the last 3 weeks, but other than this he seems himself. You note weight loss of 0.9 kg, compared with his last visit to the clinic 2 years ago.

Figure 5.13a shows what you see on examination of Scruff's mouth. The right submandibular lymph node is enlarged; the left is normal. Tooth 104 appears to be loose.

Scruff's owner has recently been made redundant and is suffering severe financial

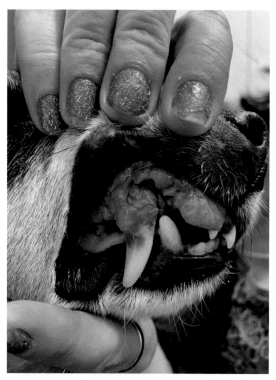

Figure 5.13a Scruff's mouth on examination. The owner was unaware.

hardship. She is primarily interested in his prognosis.

a) Describe the abnormality.
b) What is your overall assessment of Scruff's prognosis, based on history and clinical exam only?

On further conversation with the owner, it seems Scruff's welfare is reasonable. He is doing most of the things he has always done, albeit a bit slower, which the owner has attributed to age. In your consulting room he is quietly attentive and wags his tail when spoken to.

c) What management options could you offer Scruff's owner right now, without any further diagnostics? Are there any ethical/welfare concerns?
d) You decide to use some of the practice's 'angel fund' to obtain more information about Scruff's problem without cost to the

owner. Referral to a dentist/oral surgeon would use up more money than you have available, so you decide to biopsy the mass and remove tooth 104 (Figure 5.13b). You also take the opportunity to scale and polish the rest of Scruff's teeth. Once free of a heavy deposit of calculus, you notice some gingival recession on 108, but the rest of the teeth are in fair condition for an old terrier. The contralateral 204 has a probing depth of 4 mm. You also perform an uncharged-for fine-needle aspiration biopsy of the mandibular lymph node. In-house cytological examination reveals marked neutrophilic inflammation. Do these observations affect your thinking/prognosis?

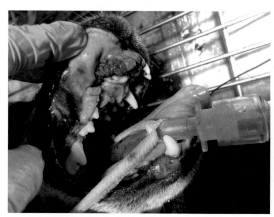

Figure 5.13b Scruff's mouth after biopsy and extraction of tooth 104.

You send Scruff home with amoxycillin-clavulanic acid and meloxicam pending biopsy results. The pathology report arrives in time for Scruff's recheck a week later (see box).

Pathology report

Poorly differentiated oral SCC with osteolysis, with multifocal, chronic, moderate necrosuppurative and lymphoplasmacytic osteomyelitis with intralesional bacteria, likely related to surface ulceration and exposure of bone to oral contaminants.

---

e) The owner reports that Scruff has been much livelier than before and that his water bowl is now clear of blood. He is eating well and even playing with his favourite toy. What are the main points to put across to the owner at this stage?

f) What treatment and advice will you offer going forward? How often should Scruff be rechecked, bearing in mind the owner's financial predicament? Is there any other way you could support the owner to ensure that Scruff does not slip beneath the radar and experience poor welfare prior to euthanasia?

5.14 Walk-in: wants to surrender 3 cats due to toxo

A distraught woman in her early 30s presents with three 10-year-old domestic shorthair cats (Figure 5.14). The cats appear bright and healthy on physical examination and are up to date with appropriate vaccinations and wormers, so you are surprised when she tearfully tells you she wants to surrender them. You enquire further and she mentions that she is pregnancy planning and her obstetrician has informed her that cats can transmit toxoplasmosis, causing fetal abnormalities and necessitating abortion.

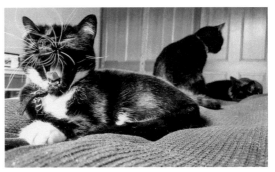

Figure 5.14 **The three 10-year-old domestic shorthair cats presented for surrender because of fears of contracting toxoplasmosis.**

a) What is the causative agent of toxoplasmosis and how are cats implicated in transmission?

b) What are the three main routes of transmission to humans?

c) Who is at risk of contracting clinical toxoplasmosis?

d) What diagnostic tests would you use to determine if your client's cats pose a risk to their owner?

e) What clinical signs would you expect in cats who have recently acquired toxoplasmosis?

f) What advice would you provide your client to help manage her fear of contracting toxoplasmosis?

g) Should veterinary team members who are considering starting a family be concerned about handling cats?

5.15 Will, 6-yo MN DSH: blocked again

You are working sole-charge when Will is presented as an emergency (Figure 5.15). He has been constantly attempting to pass urine overnight, without success. This is the third time he has presented for urinary tract obstruction in 6 weeks. Will has been on a prescription urinary diet for 5 weeks.

Physical examination findings:

- Demeanour: BAR
- BCS: 4.5/5 (Will weighs 7.9 kg)
- MMs pink, CRT <2 s
- Abdominal palpation: Will's bladder is rock-hard, about the size of a small orange, and cannot be expressed manually. Will cries when it is palpated
- HR: 168 bpm

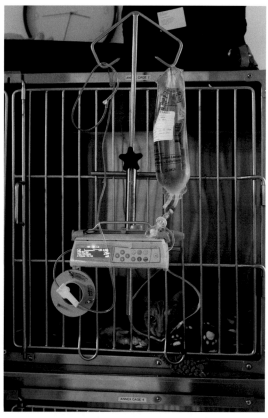

Figure 5.15 Will re-presents for urinary obstruction for the third time in 6 weeks.

- RR: Will is distressed by the examination and occasionally pants
- Urogenital examination: the prepuce and penis are inflamed. The tip of Will's penis is purple-coloured. The prepuce is swollen

The owner tells you that she is running out of funds and, although she does not like the idea, thinks it may be in Will's best interests to have a perineal urethrostomy. The records from the previous visit indicate that your senior colleague – an experienced surgeon – offered to perform this procedure on Will's previous admission. This colleague is currently on leave for 2 weeks.

a) What are the most common causes of urinary tract obstruction in cats?
b) What steps would you take to stabilise Will?
c) What factors would prompt you to refer this case?
d) What factors would prompt you to manage this case in the practice?
e) What are the potential complications of perineal urethrostomy and how are they avoided?

5.16 Jackie, 7-yo MN Mixed Breed: lump in mouth

Jackie presents for a lump in the mouth. On physical examination, you notice a mass associated with the left mandible. When you palpate the mass inside the mouth, it is soft and fluctuant, but, beneath the mandible, it feels hard. It is not painful on palpation. Jackie appears to be missing his left mandibular first premolar (305). Jackie is otherwise healthy. You admit him for anaesthesia and intra-oral radiographs (Figure 5.16).

a) What is the most likely condition in this case?
b) What are the possible causes?
c) What is the recommended treatment for this condition?

d) Aside from intra-oral radiographs, what other tests should you perform?

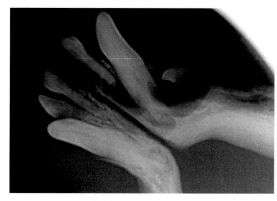

Figure 5.16 Jackie's intra-oral radiograph of the area of mandibular swelling.

5.17 Rufus, 14-mo ME Mixed Breed: had a fit

Rufus is rushed to your practice after having had a 'fit'. Rufus has had two similar episodes in the last 2 months and his owners were asked to make a video if it occurred again. Figure 5.17 shows a still from their video. You suspect that Rufus could be suffering from epileptic seizures.

a) What questions do you ask the owner to help you better understand the nature of the episodes and increase your confidence that Rufus is suffering from seizures?
b) What investigations would you recommend?
c) No abnormality was found after your investigations. What is the most likely cause for the seizures?
d) Should you consider referral for advanced imaging?
e) Which treatment would you recommend?

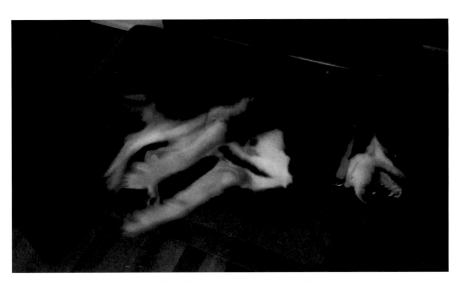

Figure 5.17 **A still from a video that the owners have taken.**

5.18 Clementine, 12-yo FN DSH: vet authorise prescription

Clementine suffers from presumed idiopathic epilepsy. Since her diagnosis 2 years ago, she has been treated with phenobarbital tablets (3 mg/kg, or half of a 30-mg tablet q12h). Jill, her owner, has requested an additional script. According to your calculations, she should have run out of the medication 3 weeks ago if dosing correctly (Figure 5.18a,b).

a) What are the potential impacts of poor adherence to the recommended treatment regime in this case?
b) List as many risk factors as you can for poor compliance or poor adherence to a recommended treatment regime.
c) Describe strategies you can use to improve client adherence.

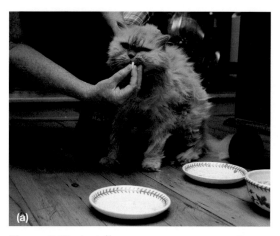
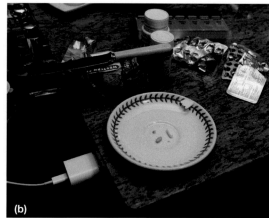

Figure 5.18a,b Adherence to treatment regimes can be challenging for owners. For example, it can be difficult to tablet some animals, and it may be difficult for owners to remember to give medications. Mr Bits, pictured here, is easier to medicate if pills are smeared in a small amount of butter.

5.19 Otis, 4-yo MN Cocker Spaniel: ears

Otis presents with a 2-month history of head shaking, with malodorous ears. The owners have not had a chance to get to the vet, having welcomed a newborn baby into their home 3 weeks ago, a sibling to their 2-year-old child. They attended the practice for the same problem about 6 months ago, and had some topical otic medication left over, which they used for a few days before it ran out. They report that Otis is head-shy, and it takes both of them to hold him for his medication. They have financial constraints and would prefer if you could dispense the largest possible bottle of ear medication so that they can use this at home in the future as needed.

Physical examination findings:

- BCS: 3.5/5
- Dental disease: grade 2/4
- Otis barely tolerates otoscopy. The vertical canals of both ears are erythematous, ulcerated, oedematous, malodorous, and stenotic. The view is obscured by a large amount of hair in the canals
- A swab of the ear collects tenacious, dark-brown-coloured slimy material, which is smeared on a slide and stained with Diff-Quik. Cytological examination reveals a large number of neutrophils, and rods (Figure 5.19a,b)

a) Why is recurrent otitis externa so frustrating?
b) How would you describe this clinical presentation of otitis externa, and what agent do you suspect is involved?
c) Should you perform C&S prior to treatment?
d) What are the goals of treatment?
e) List as many predisposing, primary, and perpetuating triggers for canine otitis externa as you can.

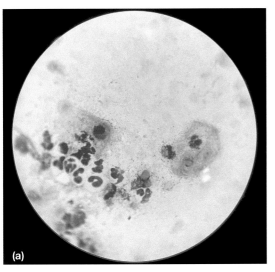 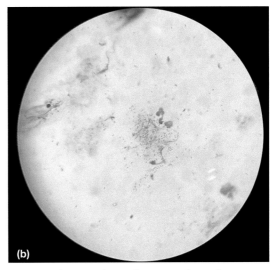

Figure 5.19a,b **Diff-Quik-stained smears from Otis's ear canals, revealing a large number of neutrophils and rods (100× magnification, oil immersion).**

5.20 Ember, 7 yo FN DSH: quieter than normal, constipated?

Ember (Figure 5.20a) has a 2–3 day history of lethargy. Her appetite has been reduced for a week and in the last 24 hours she has not eaten anything. She has vomited twice this morning (frothy bile). She has been an indoor cat since acquired from the local rescue 6 years ago, is up to date on worming and vaccines, is fed a dry diet, and is prone to constipation. The owner reports that she has been cleaning her perineal area a lot. The owner requests some of the laxative product Ember is normally prescribed.

Clinical examination findings:

- Weight: 3.5 kg, BCS 5/9
- HR 150, matching pulses, RR 16
- MMs pale pink, CRT 3 s, slightly tacky
- Hydration borderline, about 5% dehydrated
- Rectal temp: 37.1 °C
- Abdomen doughy, no pain, but a tubular abdominal mass is palpated

a) You persuade the owner to agree to an X-ray (Figure 5.20b). Interpret the radiograph.
b) What are your next steps?

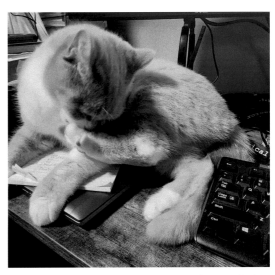

Figure 5.20a **Ember on your consultation desk.**

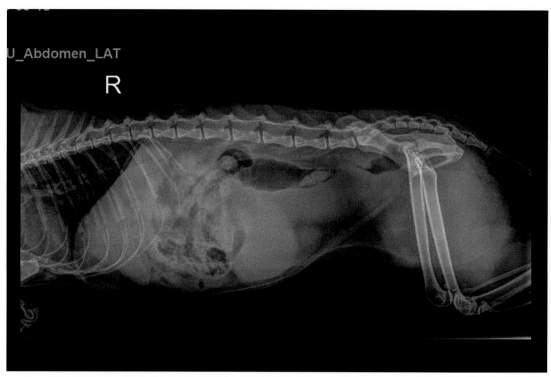

U_Abdomen_LAT

R

Figure 5.20b Ember's right lateral abdominal radiograph.

5.21 Yuuki, 6-yo FE Chihuahua cross: UTI?

The last appointment of the day, at 6.30 p.m., is Yuuki, presented for a suspected UTI. The owners have observed what they believe to be urine drops in places where Yuuki has been sitting the last few days. Yuuki's appetite has been normal, but she has been drinking and urinating more frequently than usual. Her owners report that her last heat was 'probably a month or two ago'.

Physical examination:

- Demeanour: bright, alert (nervous and occasionally snappy), responsive
- BCS: 4/5
- MMs pink, CRT <2 s
- Mouth and teeth: grade 1/4 periodontal disease
- HR = 164, no murmurs, pulse-quality good
- Abdominal palpation: difficult due to

Yuuki's girth and temperament. You cannot palpate a fluid wave or mass effect, but you cannot rule it out
- Temp: 39.1 °C.
- Yuuki's vulva is enlarged and there is a small amount of what appears to be purulent discharge from her vagina

A quick abdominal ultrasound reveals grossly enlarged, fluid-filled uterine horns. Indeed, at surgery, a diagnosis of closed cervix pyometra is confirmed (Figure 5.21).

As you finish the linea alba suture line, the phrase 'never let the sun set on a pyometra' comes to mind. This is an example of a clinical pearl. Clinical pearls are defined as '...small bits of free-standing and self-contained clinically relevant information, based on experience or observation' (Lorin et al. 2008). They tend to be constructed in a pithy, memorable way and tend to be shared widely throughout the profession, including in veterinary schools. Clinical pearls provide a distillation of clinical experience, and – in some cases – guidance where there is no evidence base.

a) List any clinical pearls you have encountered. Ask your colleagues (especially the older ones!).
b) What are the limitations of clinical pearls?
c) What is the basis of the clinical pearl regarding pyometra?
d) Can you think of contextual factors that might contradict this particular clinical pearl?

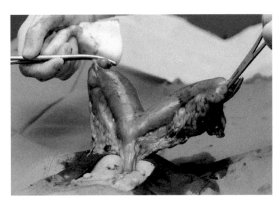

Figure 5.21 **Closed pyometra was confirmed at surgery.**

5.22 Ten Statements Test

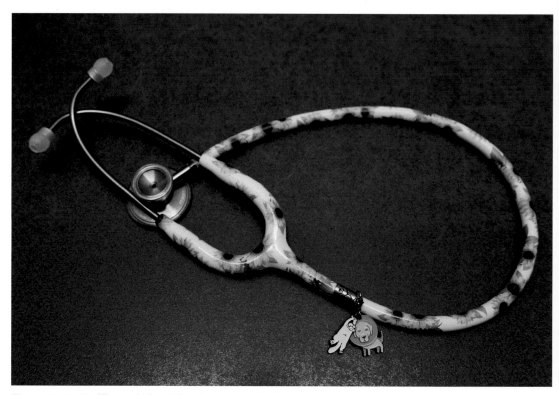

Figure 5.22 Wellbeing behind the stethoscope is important.

Two ways to conceptualise wellbeing are as **hedonic**, i.e. pertaining to the experience of positive affective states such as pleasure and joy (Clise et al. 2021), and as **eudaimonic**, i.e. wellbeing derived from engagement, a sense that one's work is meaningful and deeply fulfilling (Cake et al. 2015).

While veterinary team members often talk about their work as a source of meaning, the hedonic aspects – everyday sources of pleasure, joy, and positive feelings, 'glimmers' – can be overlooked. It can be helpful to remember sources of pleasure in veterinary work. Clise et al. (2021) used a Ten Statements Test for this purpose. This simple exercise can be done individually or as a group, though you should be mindful that team members may not wish

Exercise

- Complete the following sentence 10 times, with 10 different responses:
  I derive pleasure from my work when ...
- Be specific in your responses
- Write the responses from your perspective, not that of someone else
- Write the responses in the order in which they occur to you, not order of priority

Some team members may prefer to draw their responses.

Reviewing this list can provide insights into aspects of work you enjoy most, or highlight interests you might wish to pursue further.

The 'answer' to this item contains the editors' responses.

to share responses, or may respond differently if they anticipate that their responses will be shared. The benefit of sharing responses, however, is that hearing what others enjoy can remind us of aspects of work that we enjoy that don't necessarily spring to mind immediately.

5.23 Sleep

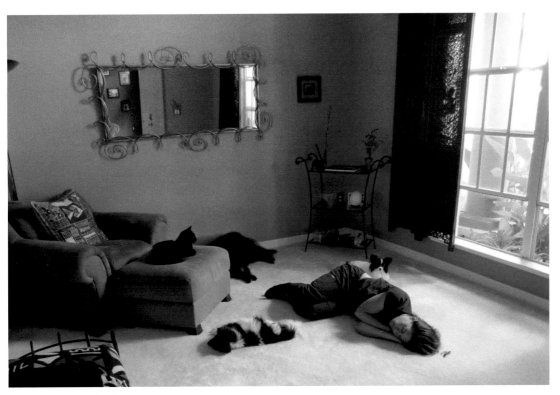

Figure 5.23a **The doctor is out.**

You work the occasional overnight shift in an emergency veterinary centre to earn additional income. You are finally driving home, having spent the last 16 hours fully 'switched on' during the busy emergency shift. You spent significant time talking to colleagues, animal owners, and referring veterinarians, ensuring a smooth patient handover. You jump in the car, wind down the window, take a deep breath of fresh air, put on upbeat music, and start the drive towards home, occasionally pinching your arm or leg to keep yourself alert when you feel your awareness drifting. Only two blocks from your house, your head nods forwards heavily and a speed hump catches you by surprise, reminding you just how dangerous sleep deficiency can be.

a) What do you think are the causes and impacts of sleep deficiency?
b) Try to list some physical, cognitive, and emotional symptoms of sleep deficiency.
c) Have you heard of sleep hygiene? Can you describe what this is? What steps might you take to improve the quality and quantity of sleep you get?

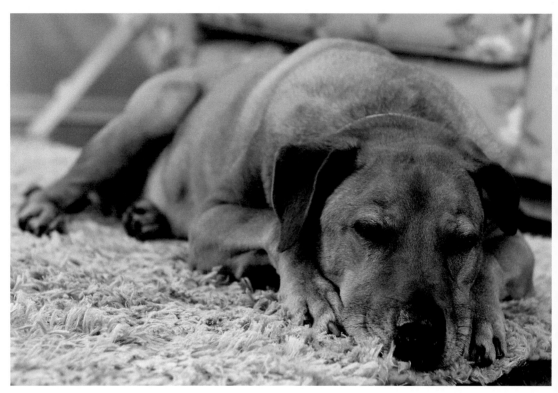

Figure 5.23b **Let sleeping dogs lie.**

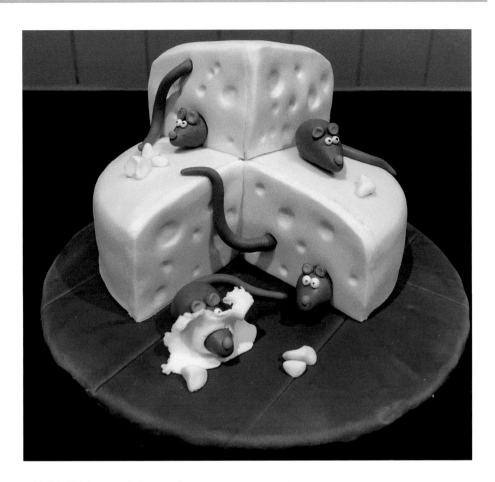

'CHEESECAKE' CHALLENGE

For 'extreme bakers' … from the kitchen of Dr Jude Bradbury.

Ingredients

- Round, baked cake (filled or unfilled, depending on preference)
- Apricot jam or edible glue
- Fondant icing (either pre-coloured or you can colour them yourself):
  - ~100 g white icing, ~100 g grey icing, 2 g pink icing
  - The amounts of yellow and brown icing will vary depending on the size of your cake. For a 10-inch diameter filled cake, you will need ~900 g yellow and ~300 g brown icing
- Black food colouring
- Cornflour

Equipment

- Wooden board or drum cake board at least 1 inch wider than the cake diameter
- Sharp knife
- Ruler
- Rolling pin
- Boning tool (or equivalent)
- Small food paintbrush
- Cocktail sticks
- Baking paper or turntable
- Palette knife

Methods

Base

You can place the cake on a wooden board or, if you prefer, you can decorate a cake board to achieve a similar effect.

1. Warm the brown icing before using a cocktail stick to drag thin lines of black colouring through (Figure 1).

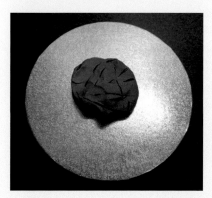

Figure 1

2. Gently stretch and fold the icing to distort the colouring, creating streaks. Do not overwork the icing as this will blend the colours, creating a darker brown.
3. Roll out the icing on top of the cake board into a circular shape until it overlaps the sides.
4. Press the sides down firmly then flip the board over and use a sharp knife around the bottom of the board to remove any excess (Figure 2).

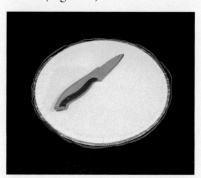

Figure 2

5. Flip the board upright and use a ruler to indent the icing to create a wooden plank effect (Figure 3).

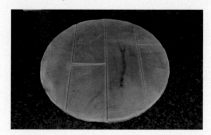

Figure 3

Cake

This style of decoration requires only a single cake, but allows you to create height and space to include a scene without the added baking time and expense.

1. Place your baked cake on a piece of baking paper slightly wider than its diameter. This will allow you to turn/move the cake without the need for a turntable.
2. Using a ruler, measure the height (× 2) and diameter of your cake to calculate the amount and width of icing you will need to roll.
3. Dust your work surface with cornflour, then roll your yellow icing to the correct size. Top tip: to keep the round shape, place one end of your rolling pin near the centre and roll the other end around in an arc (as if using a mathematical compass) (Figures 4 and 5).

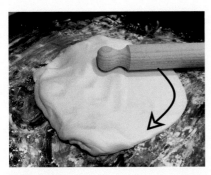

Figure 4

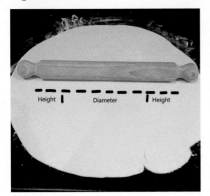

Figure 5

4. Loosen the icing from the worktop using a palette knife, place the rolling pin across the middle, and fold the icing over it in half (Figure 6).

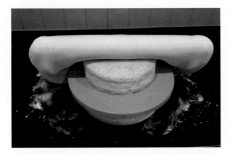

Figure 6

5. Cover the outside of your cake in a very thin layer of apricot jam or edible glue using a brush, then align your rolled icing with one side of the cake (leaving 2.5 cm excess on the worktop) and use the rolling pin to roll the icing away from you so it drapes over the cake. Adjust gently to ensure all sides of the cake will become covered (Figure 7).

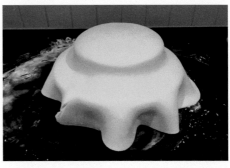

Figure 7

6. With clean, dry, warm hands smooth the top of the case first, slowly working to the edges. Turn the cake periodically as you work from the edges and down the sides to smooth the icing. You will see some pleating; having warm hands and slowly and evenly working around the cake will move these pleats down until they are part of the excess icing at the bottom.

7. Using a sharp knife cut off any excess icing from the bottom (Figure 8), then smooth again with warm hands. Place the excess icing under a cover or in an airtight container to use again shortly.

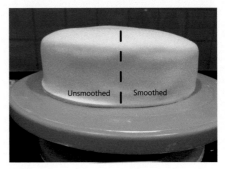

Figure 8

8. Cut a quarter out of the cake using a sharp knife. Using the palette knife, carefully pull this section away and set aside (Figure 9).

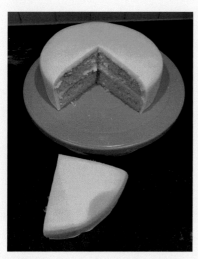

Figure 9

9. Paint an 'L' shape of jam or edible glue on the cake board in the position you would like to place your cake. Using the palette knife or your hands, gently slide the larger piece of the cake (three-quarters) off the baking paper onto the desired area of the cake board and lightly press into place (Figure 10).

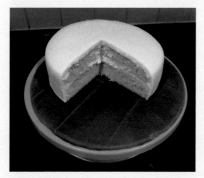

Figure 10

10. Paint a triangle of jam or edible glue on top of the three-quarters portion of cake where you would like to place the cut-out quarter. Using the palette knife for support, gently place the quarter on top and lightly press to secure (Figure 11). If you are using a large or heavy cake, you may want to place a section of cake card and a supporting rod under the quarter.

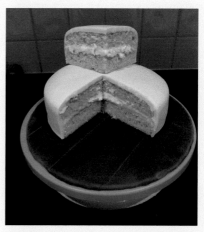

Figure 11

11. Measure the four exposed areas of cake to calculate what size rectangles of icing you will need.

12. Take your excess yellow icing from earlier and add approximately 50–100 g of white icing. Work the icing with your hands, kneading and stretching until the colours blend fully.

13. Roll out the lighter yellow icing and cut the four sizes of rectangles required. Fix them to the exposed areas of cake after painting the areas with jam or edible glue to get them to stick (Figure 12). You may need to use a sharp knife to round off any edges, followed by smoothing with a warm finger.

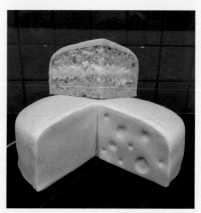

Figure 12

14. Using a boning tool, create circular or oval indentations of varying sizes in the rectangles while the icing is still warm and pliable.

15. With any remaining yellow icing, make small triangular wedges or thin slices suitable for mice to eat to help create your scene.

Mice

The number and size of mice you make will vary depending on the size of your cake, but use the picture as a guide to create the right scale.

1. **Full body:** roll the grey icing into a smooth ball in your palm, then using one or two fingers roll one edge back and forth to create a cone (nose) on one side. On the rounded side, use the boning tool to create a small indentation where you would like to secure the tail. On the tapered cone side, place a very small indentation where you would like to secure the nose. Paint the underside of the body with jam or edible glue before positioning on the cake (Figure 13).

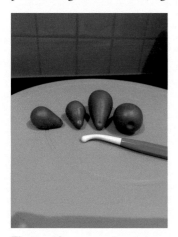

Figure 13

2. **Head only:** as for relevant parts of full body, just smaller. Paint the rounded aspect with jam or edible glue and secure the head into one of your larger indentations on the cake. You may find it best to do this after attaching the eyes/ears/nose.

3. **Tails:** roll a small amount of grey icing in your palm to smooth any lines, then use your fingers to roll it out into a string. Once it is an appropriate diameter, continue rolling one end to taper to a tip. The other end can then be cut as needed to create the desired length. Secure the tail base to the indentation on the mouse body or into an indentation on the cake using jam or edible glue. You may also need to paint the underside of the tail to stop it sliding around.

4. **Eyes:** create two round white balls of approximately 2 mm and glue to the desired head region. Using a cocktail stick, dot the centre of each eye with black food colouring.

5. **Nose:** create a pink round ball the same size as your mouse eyes and secure to the small indentation on the tip of the head with jam or edible glue (Figures 14 and 15).

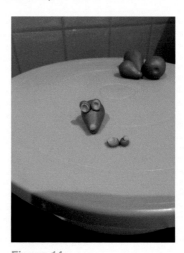

Figure 14

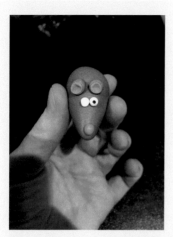

Figure 15

6. **Ears:** create two round grey balls of approximately 2 mm and place about 0.5 mm of pink icing on each one. Using the boning tool, push the pink icing into the grey ball to create a cave on one side. Flatten the area below the pink indentation slightly and secure to the desired position on the head using jam or edible glue.

7. **Scenery:** have your mice engage in the scene by adding your wedges/slices of 'cheese' made earlier, again securing them in place with jam or edible glue (Figure 16).

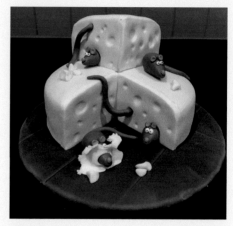

Figure 16

8. Admire your creation! (Or seek the refuge of a dark, quiet room.)

ANSWERS

FRIDAY

281

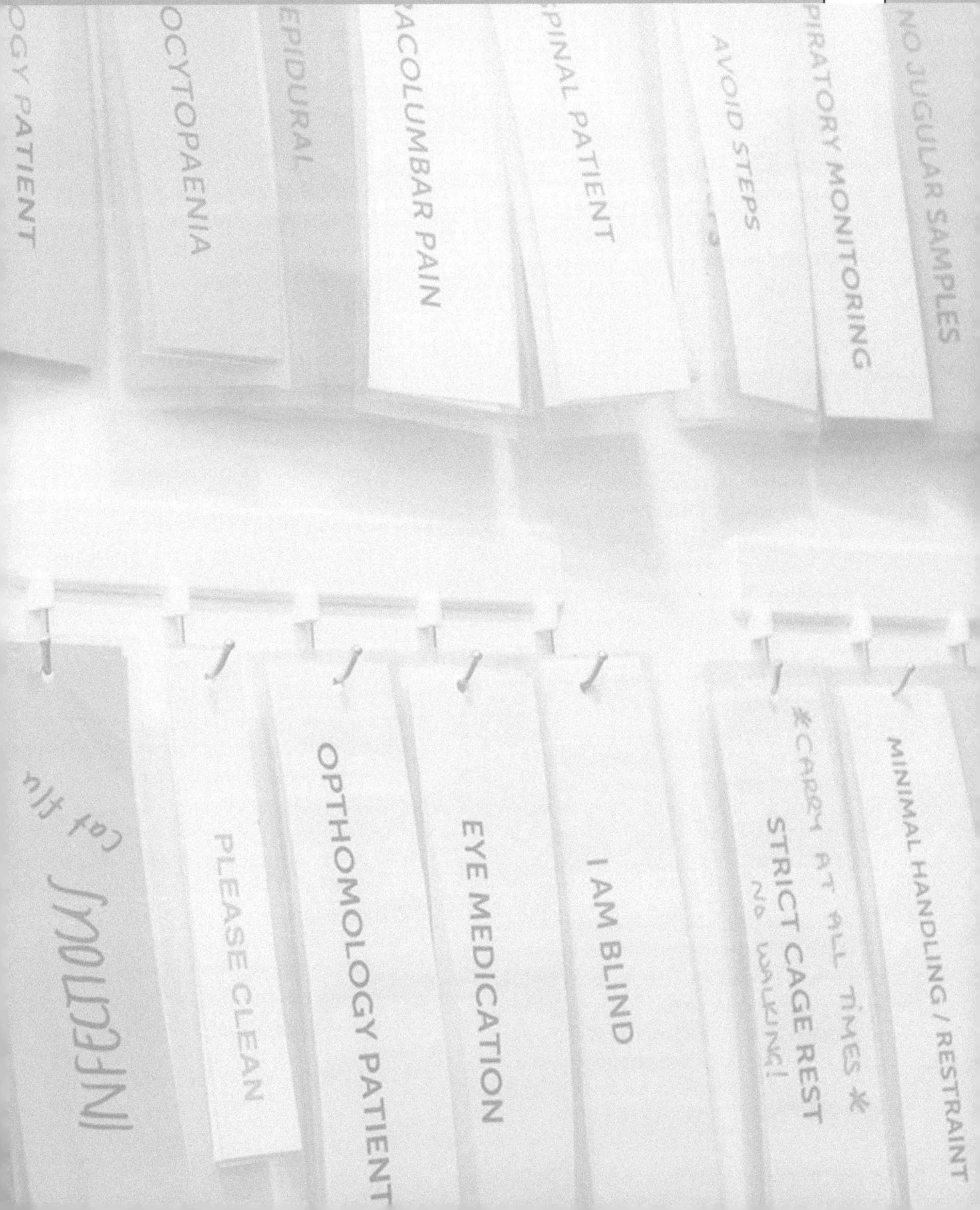

5.1 Roxie, 8-yo FE Husky: lethargic and reduced appetite

a) When accurately describing gross pathological lesions, the following details should be included where relevant:

- Location
- Distribution
- Size and extent
- Shape
- Demarcation
- Contour
- Colour
- Texture

In Roxie's case, there are red, irregular, well-demarcated, smooth, multifocal lesions measuring 1–2 mm in diameter on the buccal mucosa.

b) Petechiae (the haemorrhagic lesions are 1–2 mm in size). Larger (3–5 mm), more blotchy haemorrhages would be termed ecchymoses.

c) The presence of petechiae indicates a primary haemostatic disorder. Petechiae are indicative of thrombocytopenia, thrombocytopathia, or (rarely) a vasculopathy. A retrospective study of thrombocytopenia cases at referral hospitals in the UK developed five disease categories, which can be used as a helpful framework for differential diagnoses in Roxie's case (Table A5.1).

> Thrombocytopenia can be primary (idiopathic) or secondary. Clinicians should seek to exclude secondary causes as far as possible before making a diagnosis of primary IMTP.

d) Assuming this image is a representative average, moderate thrombocytopenia is present as there are four platelets (plt) in the single high-power field (hpf), which equates to approximately 60,000 plt/µL (4 × 15,000). A normal platelet count is 8–15 plt/hpf. Both low numbers of platelets and dysfunction of platelets contribute to petechiation. No white blood cells are seen, which could indicate decreased production (e.g. bone marrow disease) or increased consumption (e.g. sepsis).

e) Platelet clumping can occur and result in a relative thrombocytopenia. The edges of the smear should be checked to determine if any clumping is present, and the total platelet count interpreted accordingly. Due to the relatively large size and weight of white blood cells, these cells often move to the sides of a smear during preparation. While the absolute number of white blood cells cannot be determined from the smear, the presence of white blood cells can be evaluated in general, and a percentage distribution of the different white cell types can be determined. In addition, any other features that may be relevant can be noted, e.g. presence of toxic neutrophils associated with inflammation and infection.

f) There is a diffuse nodular appearance to the liver with small (1–2 cm) hypoechoic nodules disseminated throughout the parenchyma. In addition to the nodules, there are several small anechoic cysts. These findings are abnormal but are not pathognomonic for any disease, meaning further investigation is required to reach a definitive diagnosis. It is possible that Roxie has thrombocytopenia secondary to hepatic disease, e.g. neoplasia.

g) No definitive diagnosis has been reached at this point. Further diagnostic investigation could include liver fine-needle aspirates (FNAs) or a biopsy to assess the changes seen on ultrasound at a cellular level. The risk of bleeding needs to be addressed as a priority in this case due to the thrombocytopenia. Liver biopsies are contraindicated in dogs with platelet counts of <80,000/µL and so are not a suitable

Table A5.1 Differential diagnosis categories for thrombocytopenia referring to Roxie's case (adapted from Martín-Ambrosio Francés et al. 2023)

DIFFERENTIAL DIAGNOSIS CATEGORY	CLINICAL REASONING
Primary immune-mediated thrombocytopenia (IMTP)	Given the age of the patient and presenting signs, primary IMTP should be considered likely
Secondary thrombocytopenia	
Neoplastic disease	
• Lymphoma • Sarcoma • Leukaemia • Carcinoma • Mast cell tumour • Other	Given the age of the patient and presenting signs, neoplasia should be strongly considered
Infection	
• Bacterial (e.g. leptospirosis)/rickettsial • Parasitic • Protozoal • Viral • Fungal • Sepsis • Other	• Given that there is no history of travel and Roxie's vaccines and parasite control are well maintained, many infectious disease differentials are unlikely • Bacterial infection and progression to sepsis should be considered
Inflammation	
• Pancreatitis • Primary IMHA • Chronic enteropathy • Meningomyelitis • Other	• Resistance to abdominal palpation could indicate pain in that area, raising clinical suspicion of pancreatitis and possibly chronic enteropathy • Lack of pallor/jaundice in the MMs makes primary IMHA less likely • Lack of neurological signs makes meningomyelitis unlikely
Miscellaneous disorders	

• Drugs/toxins (including vaccine reaction)
• Chemotherapy
• Other
  – Renal, e.g. cutaneous and renal glomerular vasculopathy
  – Hepatobiliary
  – Gastrointestinal, e.g. acute haemorrhagic diarrhoea syndrome
	• Roxie has no history of chemotherapy, recent drug therapy, or potential exposure to toxins, making these differentials unlikely
	• Other miscellaneous disorders include a wide range of options, some of which fit with the history and clinical findings and could be considered

option for Roxie at this time. FNAs have a lower risk of causing bleeding than biopsies and are more suitable here, although close monitoring post-sampling would be advised. FNAs are less invasive than a biopsy, which may be preferable to the client; however, they are also less reliable in providing a definitive diagnosis. In one study of 97 cases of FNAs, cytological findings agreed with the histopathological diagnosis in only 30% of dogs (Wang et al. 2004). Cytology has been shown to be most effective in the diagnosis of diffuse vacuolar change or neoplastic disease, with variable sensitivity demonstrated for inflammatory liver disease. The risk–benefit balance of further diagnostic tests should be discussed with the client to reach a shared decision.

Alternatively, the option for treatment without a definitive diagnosis can be considered. The challenge here is the potential to make the patient's condition worse due to contraindicated medication, e.g. corticosteroids for assumed primary immune-mediated disease or neoplastic disease when the cause is actually infectious. Lastly, there is the option of treating Roxie symptomatically, e.g. with analgesics for pain, and monitoring the progression of her signs before undertaking further diagnostics or treatments. The benefit of such a 'wait and see' approach is that further symptoms could arise or progress that then guide further investigations. This must be weighed against the risk of progression of a disease that may have been treatable, or more easily treated, with more aggressive or early intervention.

Ultimately, the course of action depends on the client's resources, wishes, and informed shared decision-making and consent between vet and client, after you have communicated the possibilities in an understandable way and highlighted any welfare and wellbeing implications for Roxie. Every client's context is different and what may be right for one client and patient may not be right for another. This is a frequent scenario in general practice.

REFERENCES

Martín-Ambrosio Francés, M., Seth, M., Sharman, M. et al. (2023) Causes of thrombocytopenia in dogs in the United Kingdom: a retrospective study of 762 cases. *Veterinary Medicine & Science* **9**(4):1495–1507. doi: 10.1002/vms3.1091.

Villiers, E. & Ristić, J. (2016) *BSAVA Manual of Canine and Feline Clinical Pathology*. Cheltenham: British Small Animal Veterinary Association.

Wang, K. Y., Panciera, D. L., Al-Rukibat, R. K. & Radi, Z. A. (2004) Accuracy of ultrasound-guided fine-needle aspiration of the liver and cytologic findings in dogs and cats: 97 cases (1990–2000). *Journal of the American Veterinary Medical Association* **224**(1):75–78. doi: 10.2460/javma.2004.224.75.

5.2 Mittens, 12-wo ME DLH: owner stood on him

a) The dose is calculated by multiplying the weight of the patient by the dose per kg. This is a 1.4-kg cat, so the calculation is 20 μg × 1.4 kg = 28 μg (or 0.028 mg), i.e. 28 μg of medetomidine is needed.

Medetomidine is 1 mg/mL (= 1000 μg/mL):

$$28 \text{ μg} \times (1 \text{ mL}/1000 \text{ μg}) = 0.028 \text{ mL}$$

Because of the small volume, this could be rounded up to 0.03 mL. So the volume of medetomidine required is 0.03 mL.

For a methadone dose of 0.3 mg/kg in a 1.4-kg cat:

$$0.3 \times 1.4 = 0.42 \text{ mg}$$

Methadone is 10 mg/mL:

$$0.42 \text{ mg} \times (1 \text{ mL}/10 \text{ mg}) = 0.042 \text{ mL}$$

In this case, the volume would be rounded down to 0.04 mL.

Thus, the total volume to be injected is:

$$0.03 \text{ mL medetomidine} + 0.04 \text{ mL}$$
$$\text{methadone} = 0.07 \text{ mL}$$

You would also want to draw up the reversal agent, atipamezole, at the same time in a separate syringe. Atipamezole is 5 mg/mL (= 5000 μg/mL). The dose in micrograms is 2.5 times that of the medetomidine hydrochloride dose (or five times that if dexmedetomidine hydrochloride had been used).

For our patient, we used 28 μg, so

$$28 \times 2.5 = 70 \text{ μg}$$
$$70 \text{ μg} \times (1 \text{ mL}/5000 \text{ μg}) = 0.014 \text{ mL}$$

In this case, the volume would be rounded up to 0.015 mL. The label says that the reversal agent should equate to half of the volume of medetomidine injected, so you can do a quick sense-check of your calculation here: 0.015 mL is half of 0.03 mL, which was the volume of medetomidine you drew up.

b) To reduce the risk of error, select the syringe with a volume as close as you can to the desired volume to be administered. Ideally, the volume you draw up should be more than 20% of the measured syringe capacity (Jordan et al. 2021). Therefore, if using a 1-mL syringe, ideally the volume you draw up should be at least 0.2 mL. In this case, the 1-mL syringe is the smallest you have available, even if the volume being drawn up is <0.2 mL.

> U-100 insulin syringes can be useful for accurately drawing up very small volumes. The small, thin insulin needle, with no hub volume, allows for more precise measurement. This works with products of low viscosity only. U-40 syringes are not suitable as the markings do not correspond.

c) In a study, very large percentage errors were seen when target volumes of <0.04 mL were drawn up in syringes (Cambruzzi et al. 2023). You can dilute medication with sterile water for injection, particularly where the volume to be injected is <0.2 mL, as it is in this case. This produces a larger injection volume, which can be easier to administer and will ensure that the full dose is received.

REFERENCES

Cambruzzi, M., Knowles, T. & MacFarlane, P. (2023) Accuracy of drawing up liquid medications by veterinary anaesthetists and nurses. *Veterinary Anaesthesia and Analgesia* **50**(6):502–506. doi: 10.1016/j.vaa.2023.09.002.

Jordan, M. A., Choksi, D., Lombard, K. & Patton, L. R. (2021) Development of guidelines for accurate measurement of small volume parenteral products using syringes. *Hospital Pharmacy* **56**:165–171. doi: 10.1177/0018578719873869.

5.3 Bubba, 3-yo MN American Pit Bull Terrier: still vomiting

a) The X-ray shows two opaque, round, caudal abdominal structures, one of which appears to be the bladder. Palpation of the abdomen under sedation confirmed the bladder as one of the two masses when urine was voided.

> Sedation may be required for meaningful abdominal palpation, especially in medium- and large-breed dogs that are tensing their abdominal muscles. It can be impossible to feel anything if a larger dog strongly 'boards' or 'splints' their muscles.

b) Top differentials for the mass lesion are enlarged prostate gland, lymph node, paraprostatic cyst, enlarged cryptorchid testicle, or neoplasia of mesenteric or splenic origin.

c) Not entirely. A mass has been identified, but it is still unclear what has been causing Bubba's gastrointestinal signs. His gastrointestinal signs could still be caused by the after-effects of known foreign body ingestion, but could also be caused by abdominal pressure, discomfort, or pain associated with the mass. Physical derangements caused by a necrotic/torsed mass might also be responsible for Bubba's signs, although his blood results a week ago were fairly unremarkable.

d) Repeat blood tests could be useful, and a rectal exam should definitely be performed. Exploratory coeliotomy is a logical step and entirely appropriate in the general practice setting. Consideration of the different eventualities and preparation for these would be helpful, as in all surgery. Equally valid would be further imaging, such as ultrasonography and/or CT scan. The former may well be available in the general practice context, but the latter is likely to require referral. At this point, the next steps should be discussed with the owner and informed consent obtained.

e) This means that retained testicle(s) figure more strongly in the differential list. And this was, in fact, the source of Bubba's mass, which turned out to be a torsed testicular neoplasm in an abdominally retained testicle. It was most likely a Sertoli cell tumour. A second testicle was found partially descended high up in the inguinal region, which would have been difficult to palpate in the conscious, wriggly Bubba.

Both testicles were successfully removed and Bubba made an uneventful recovery. His vague gastrointestinal symptoms resolved after surgery and were attributed to the testicular torsion and associated 'subacute abdomen'.

> The temperament or behaviour of the veterinary patient can affect the thoroughness of clinical examination. If you are unable to complete a portion of the exam for these reasons, it should be noted in the clinical record. Carrying out the missed portion under sedation, or trying again at another time, or using another approach, minimises the risk of missing something.

5.4 Malibu, 10-wo FE DSH: vaccination

a) The Five Domains Model evaluates an animal's mental state (Mellor et al. 2020). Mental state represents an animal's overall mental experiences or 'feelings' (Domain 5). Evidence across the first four domains is collated towards an overall picture of whether an animal is experiencing positive or negative welfare. For example, if an animal is very hungry because they do not have access to sufficient food (Domain 1), they are unlikely to feel happy (Domain 5) because their overall balance of mental experiences is negative. However, if they have access to sufficient food and water (Domain 1), are physically comfortable (Domain 2), and are in good health (Domain 3), they are much more likely to want to engage in rewarding behavioural interactions (Domain 4) and feel happy (Domain 5). The Five Domains Model provides a structure to think broadly about ways of ensuring animals have opportunities to experience overall positive welfare

or happiness, while identifying ways of mitigating negative mental experiences.

b) Agency is the capacity of animals to engage in voluntary, self-generated, and goal-directed behaviour that they are motivated to perform. These behaviours can be motivated by positive mental experiences (e.g. maternal bonding) or negative mental experiences (e.g. avoiding predation). Choice, control, and challenge are all features of agency. A choice between two or more options allows animals to exercise agency. When animals can consistently and predictably make choices, they have a sense of control. Complex (but not too tricky) interactions and novelty can challenge animals and encourage problem-solving.

c) A full 'five domains' assessment should be performed and discussed with Malibu's owner because an indoor-only lifestyle could impact Domains 1–3 (e.g. relative overfeeding leading to obesity and joint disease, resulting in pain and debility).

However, Domain 4 is where animal agency is considered, and provides the best way of framing our discussion of providing Malibu with opportunities to exercise agency while being kept indoors. Domain 4 (behavioural interactions) is subdivided into interactions with the environment, other animals, and people. This helps us consider opportunities for agency within each sub-category:

i) For interactions with **the environment**, you might like to consider the house size and design features (e.g. escape areas, vertical environment, varied spaces), resource distribution (e.g. location of food bowls, litter tray[s] and bedding), presence of environmental enrichment opportunities (e.g. food puzzles, toys designed for individual cat play preferences)

ii) For interactions with **other animals**, you can consider the presence of other cats in the household or external environment and whether they are in the same social group (i.e. do they display affiliative behaviours such as allogrooming and allorubbing), neuter status, presence of other species (e.g dogs), and Malibu's reactions during such interactions

iii) You can explore **the owner's** interactions with Malibu (e.g. frequency/time frame, time spent engaging in playful interactions, reward-based training, time of day interactions occur), owner experience, owner attitude, Malibu's demeanour towards the owner, and evidence of effective learning/training

Overall, these details should provide us with plenty of information about the opportunities Malibu has to exercise agency (via choice, control, and challenge) and experience positive welfare. The model can be useful in the general practice context as a means of structuring useful client discussion and bringing them to an understanding of, in this case, a cat's behavioural and welfare needs but can, of course, be used with any animal.

REFERENCE

Mellor, D. J., Beausoleil, N. J., Littlewood, K. E. et al. (2020) The 2020 Five Domains Model: including human–animal interactions in assessments of animal welfare. *Animals* **10**(10):1870. doi: 10.3390/ani10101870.

5.5 Max, 4-yo MN DSH: dental

a) The patient is rebreathing expired gas. This is demonstrated by the inspiratory plateau gradually climbing in a step-wise manner. The dotted horizontal line shows the normal end tidal CO_2. Rebreathing expired CO_2 will make the patient become hypercapnic. This will increase the sympathetic tone and cause peripheral vasodilation. If the situation persists long enough and the CO_2 climbs high enough, it will cause central nervous system (CNS) depression and death.

b) The fresh gas flow should be increased. With the T-piece or Bain breathing system, the reservoir bag is in the waste part of the circuit. The bag's function is not the same as with systems such as the Lack, and will contain exhaled gas (the reservoir bag in a Lack system contains fresh gas from the machine). Because of this, the gas flow with T-piece/Bain must be sufficient to meet the patient's peak inspiratory flow, otherwise gas will be pulled back from the expiratory circuit, causing rebreathing. The fresh gas flow settings when using a T-piece or Bain circuit must therefore be 2–3 times the minute volume. For the Lack, the flow rate need only match the patient's minute volume. For Max, we would work out the correct flow rate as follows:

3.6-kg cat breathing an estimated 20 breaths per minute

Tidal volume = 10 mL/kg = 36 mL

Minute volume = tidal volume × breathing rate = 36 × 20 = 720 mL/min

Minimum flow rate for Max on a T-piece:

2.5 × 720 = 1800 mL/min = 1.8 L/min

The higher fresh gas flows make T-pieces uneconomical to use for larger patients. There is also a sustainability argument against them for the same reason.

5.6 Sandie, 13-yo MN DSH: making strange noises at night

a) Hypertensive cats will vocalise and do strange things, with some owners reporting concerns that their cat has 'dementia' or cognitive decline. Hypertensive encephalopathy can manifest as brain oedema with increased intracranial pressure, causing vocalisation, head pressing, change of behaviour, aggression (due to pain), disorientation, ataxia, and seizures. Target organ damage can lead to sudden-onset blindness, and owners may notice haemorrhage in the eyes. Clinical signs may reflect underlying disease, e.g. CKD may be associated with PU/PD; polyphagia and vomiting may be associated with hyperthyroidism.

b) Cats are prone to 'situational hypertension' (Acierno et al. 2018). 'Situational hypertension' (known as 'white coat syndrome' in humans) is high blood pressure arising from fear, anxiety, or distress as a result of being in a clinical setting, so ensuring that the cat is as calm as possible and in surroundings that are as quiet and stress-free as possible will help avoid this artefact. Administering gabapentin 60–90 minutes before measurement in stressed cats can help obtain more accurate measurements. Ideally, familiarising yourself with the use of a Doppler machine on anaesthetised patients prior to trying on an awake cat can ensure a better technique. Oscillometric devices rely on a very still patient for accurate results – hard to do on a cat.

c) Table A5.6 categorises severity of hypertension and associated risk of future target organ damage. Systolic BP readings of <119 mmHg in conscious cats and <90 mmHg in anaesthetised cats indicate hypotension.

Table A5.6 **American College of Veterinary Internal Medicine (ACVIM) classification for severity of hypertension and risk of target organ damage (Acierno et al. 2018)**

CATEGORY	SYSTOLIC BP (mmHg)	RISK OF FUTURE TARGET ORGAN DAMAGE
Normotensive	<140	Minimal
Pre hypertensive	140–159	Mild
Hypertension	160–179	Moderate
Severe hypertension	>180	High

Most healthy cats have systolic BP of 120–140 mmHg as measured by Doppler. Pre-hypertensive cats should be monitored regularly and assessed for a potential target organ damage or an underlying condition such as CKD. Cats with BP of >160 mmHg should have repeat measurements at least two times in 8 weeks. If readings are still >160 mmHg, or there is evidence of target organ damage, anti-hypertensive therapy should be instituted. If readings are >180 mmHg, anti-hypertensive therapy should be commenced and the cat rechecked within 14 days, or sooner in the case of any deterioration.

d) Hypertension, hyperaldosteronism, kidney disease, cardiac disease, arthritis, and hyperthyroidism are important differentials in older cats with weight loss, high BP, and uncharacteristic vocalisation. Hypertension may be primary or idiopathic, or may be a sequelae of hyperthyroidism or, less commonly, hyperaldosteronism (Conn's syndrome). Cats with hyperthyroidism may be at increased risk of situational hypertension (Stammeleer et al. 2024). Cats with kidney disease can have a systolic BP of >300 mmHg (Sparkes et al. 2022), while hyperthyroid cats often have a BP of ≤180 mmHg (Stammeleer et al. 2024).

Cats presenting with visual deficits, hyphaema, blindness, retinal swelling, and detachment may be suffering from hypertensive retinopathy. Cats with azotaemia, proteinuria, or CKD should be screened for hypertension. Azotaemia is found in almost three-quarters of cats with hypertension, while 19–65% of cats with CKD are hypertensive (Taylor et al. 2017).

Any cat with a heart murmur or gallop rhythm may be hypertensive (the heart is affected in 70% of hypertensive cats). It is important to measure systolic BP in older cats if a new heart murmur is detected.

Some cats will vocalise more at night because there are less distractions. It is prudent to ensure that their environment is set up for them to rest comfortably, pain is ruled out, and hypertension excluded. Night vocalisation may occur due to visual, auditory, or olfactory contact with stray or neighbouring cats or wildlife. Blocking or restricting access to area where this may occur, e.g. the use of shutters or opaque screens, may help.

REFERENCES

Acierno, M. J., Brown, S., Coleman, A. E. et al. (2018) ACVIM consensus statement: guidelines for the identification, evaluation, and management of systemic hypertension in dogs and cats. *Journal of Veterinary Internal Medicine* **32**(6):1803–1822. doi: 10.1111/jvim.15331.

Sparkes, A., Garelli-Paar, C., Blondel, T. & Guillot, E. (2022) 'The Mercury Challenge': feline systolic blood pressure in primary care practice – a European survey. *Journal of Feline Medicine and Surgery*, **24**:e310–e323. doi: 10.1177/1098612x221105844.

Stammeleer, L., Xifra, P., Serrano, S. I. et al (2024) Blood pressure in hyperthyroid cats before and after radioiodine treatment. *Journal of Veterinary Internal Medicine* **38**(3):1359–1369. doi: 10.1111/jvim.17032.

Taylor, S. S., Sparkes, A. H., Briscoe, K. et al. (2017) ISFM consensus guidelines on the diagnosis and management of hypertension in cats. *Journal of Feline Medicine and Surgery* **19**(3):288–303. doi: 10.1177/1098612X17693500.

5.7 Amber, 3.5-yo FN Rottweiler: aggressive to other dogs

a) The following are some suitable initial questions to ask of Amber's owners:
- What is the household and family set-up? Are there any other pets? What was Amber's relationship like with the dog they lost most recently?
- What is Amber's general health/daily routine/exercise/diet/feeding times?
- What is Amber's training history? Carried out by whom?
- When did her aggression start? Has this changed in nature or severity?

b) Suitable specific questions to ask include the following:
- What control measures are being used? How have these altered Amber's behaviour?
- Where and how severe were the bites inflicted on the other dogs?
- To whom is possessive aggression directed?
- With whom is she most compliant?

c) Despite the clinical note on Amber's records of hindquarter lameness at 6 months of age, no investigation seems to have been carried out. She should have a full examination under general anaesthetic together with X-rays of her hips, spine, and both stifles to eliminate any orthopaedic problem that may be causing pain and discomfort. While metabolic disease is unlikely at her age and systemic disease unlikely in her condition, she should be screened with a CBC, biochemistry panel including T4, and urinalysis to detect underlying disease that may drive behaviour.

d) Owners tend not to appreciate that dogs are context-specific learners and assume that if progress has been made in one context, it will automatically extend to others. Amber's owners are likely to be frustrated by her apparently regressive steps and this will be reflected in their relationship with her. They may feel they have failed and be frustrated after all the work they have put in, but they must be prepared to go back to 'lure and reward' as if she were a puppy to remind her of how worthwhile it is to do as they ask. Training classes often give the impression that dogs should be rewarded when they are being good and when they are doing well, whereas in real life, Amber must be amply rewarded according to the level of difficulty of the task ahead of her, rather than just how well she has behaved when she may be about to behave her worst. In other words, owners must try to be predictive and reward *before* Amber lunges, jumps up, and mouths the lead or spots a rabbit to chase. They must also rehearse when life is easy at home, in preparation for the difficulties that present themselves in public.

e) Amber is looking at all three contexts (home, being walked in public, training classes) in entirely different lights; therefore, what she feels she needs to do in each context varies accordingly. At home, she is left to her own decisions to do as she pleases; outside the house and in the park, she is compliant until something more pressing to chase or lunge at grabs her attention; and in class, she does what the trainer instructs her owner to tell her to do. However, the trainer is not with her in the park. There are two major differences between Amber's training and real life. The presence of the trainer and absence of a headcollar predicts dogs she has already met before and is tolerant of, whereas the presence of the Halti and harness and absence of the trainer have come to mean she may meet other strange dogs to which she may have to react. As many features as possible must be transferred between contexts and as many of the same cues as possible should appear in her home life, training, and walks outside the house. Thus the edges are blurred between home life, training, and walks outside, making the guidance she needs more consistent across all three contexts. Until Amber is equally responsive to her owners at home as in training, then no progress will be made in the park.

f) A 'training methods' diagram (see Figure A2.2 in Chapter 2) may be used to remind owners of the ways in which a dog's behaviour can be altered. A stern voice from Jack and the trainer may at times 'work' as Amber wants to avoid the implicit threat, so she complies in order to stop it. However, it can evidently have the opposite effect when Amber will not drop a toy for Jack, but turns away and growls at him instead. By threatening a dog into obedience, one does not indicate the behaviour one wants from the dog, one simply sends the message that the current behaviour, if continued, may cause a threat to be realised. Thus, all the balls are left in the dog's court as to how to respond, which may confuse the dog. On the other hand, using positive rewards tells dogs which specific behaviour we value, and rewards them for performing these. If a stern command is effective, Amber should be given a piece of chicken, thus combining positive punishment (the stern command that worked) with positive reward (the chicken).

g) At present, Amber is not particularly interested in doing anything for food as all her favourites are already put in her bowl – in other words, she gets the rewards 'for free'. Slightly less in her bowl, and fewer or no favourites, will ensure that she is kept a little hungry, which will make her more receptive to reward-based training. She should not be given 'treats' just because she is loved but she should be asked to do something first, e.g. to sit. Amber's owners already know that she will jump in the car willingly for chicken, which she will not do simply on command. This need to be rewarded for jumping may be a reflection of Amber's associated orthopaedic pain. Once that is ruled out, the owners should aim to progress to giving chicken *after* Amber has jumped in the car, rather than using it to lure her into the car.

h) Amber should not be let off the lead at all for the moment in view of the risk she poses to others, even by accident. It is essential for Jill to regain confidence in walking Amber and remain in control, which the current reactive dog classes are not achieving. Although Amber is doing reasonably well in being walked off-lead past the dogs she is now familiar with, this is not helping her or the owners deal with unknown dogs at close quarters on the street or in the park. Her Halti, double-ended training lead and body harness that are needed on a walk must be used in the house and garden, and all the standard tasks she performed in puppy class must be rehearsed over again while wearing these devices at home. Seeing them should

not mean she is always going for a walk. Instead, they should put her, as well as the owners, into a 'training' frame of mind. Any bag containing, and therefore predicting, food should be clearly visible to Amber during training. It is far better for Jill to practise in class with Amber wearing what is needed in public than to be led into a false sense of security in class.

Rehearsal of obedience before it becomes necessary

As she generally causes no problem at home, Amber's owners have not seen the need to rehearse 'obedience'; consequently, Amber sees no reason to do as they ask. Everything she does at home is her own decision, with her owners responding to her needs rather than the other way around. By thinking 'Whose idea is this?' the owners will be reminded to test out how easy it is to change her mind (Amber is thinking of one thing; they would like her to do another), as well as to deliberately ask her to do things routinely throughout the day. Anything Amber wants to do can be turned to their advantage, e.g. if she's standing by the back door to go out or come in or looks as if she is about to get onto the sofa, the owners should ask her to sit first before the door is opened or before she is invited onto the sofa.

Mental versus physical exercise

The owners should not be too concerned about Amber not having the amount of off-lead exercise they would ideally like her to have (especially before potential orthopaedic problems are investigated). It is far better for her to have a successful calm walk on-lead, with plenty of mental stimulation in being asked to do as the owners say, than risk over-aroused failure. Other dogs need not be deliberately avoided, but Amber should be given space by crossing the road or retreating into a driveway when other dogs are about to pass, asking her to follow and rewarding her when she does. The owners must have the belief that dogs do not want to behave as Amber has been doing. This evasive action will give Amber a 'get-out clause' to avoid having to react. Her tendency to seek the owners for comfort if another dog approaches her is an indication that she wants to avoid conflict but, paradoxically, at present Amber sees displaying aggression as the safest way to respond.

Resorting to psychotropic medication to try to 'calm' dogs like Amber carries several risks. Firstly, it may create the illusion of an 'easy fix' with consequently less attention given to behavioural advice, which carries better prospects for long-term improvement or cure. Secondly, behavioural drugs may carry a risk of a paradoxical increase in aggression. For these reasons, full commitment to a professionally constructed and implemented behavioural programme is nearly always the best course of action. Taking dog–dog aggression seriously at the general practice level is vitally important (including early referral if necessary), both for animal welfare reasons and also because intervening in dog conflict is a very common cause of inadvertent bites to people.

REFERENCE

Shepherd, K. (2021) *Demystifying Dog Behaviour for the Veterinarian*. Boca Raton, FL: CRC Press.

5.8 Cat colony on farm – request for TNR

a) It is important that colony cats are not handled directly. Trapping is the most humane way of achieving this. Before any TNR work is performed, a risk assessment should be written. For the majority of TNR work, the following equipment will be required:
   - Traps, either automatic and/or manual
   - Trap transfer restrainers, this can be either transfer baskets or restrainer containers
   - Trap covers
   - Strong-smelling bait such as fish
   - Small paper plates to place the bait on in the trap
   - Water bowls
   - Absorbable pads to place in the transfer baskets
   - Torches (if carrying out trapping in the dark)
   - Pen and paper or device to log information during the trapping process
   - Disposable gloves and other items of PPE that may be required
   - Mobile phone

b) There are several procedures to follow prior to starting the TNR work. The first is to allow a period of acclimatisation for the cats. Most cats will be naturally wary of traps placed in their environment, so it is best to start by feeding near or next to a trap *in situ*. This lowers the perceived threat level of the trap. Once this has been carried out over a 5–7 day period, and the cats are less wary of the trap, the next step is to start placing food inside the unset trap. This can then eventually proceed to setting the trap. This process improves trapping success by 50–60% (Cats Protection 2021). Furthermore, by following this acclimatisation process, we help to avoid trap shyness, which is when cats have a very negative association with traps and become scared on entering them.

Once the cat is securely in the trap, cover the whole trap with a sheet or towel as soon as possible. This helps to keep the cat calm and lowers the risk of injury. Then transfer the cat from the trap to a transfer carrier (which is lined with something absorbent). It is often helpful to have someone to assist at this stage. Once the cat is in the carrier, it should be secured immediately. It is important to note that automatic traps shouldn't be left unattended in public spaces and should be checked regularly. The details of the organisation involved in the trapping should be written on the trap clearly, along with legible contact details.

c) Before performing TNR work, the practice should consider where they will keep all the transfer carriers/restrainer containers. These will require physical space and ideally be kept separate from other inpatients. The practice should also consider whether it can offer the flexibility required for TNR work. It can be very unpredictable in terms of number of cats trapped, male to female ratios, and the time of day the cats are presented to the practice. All these factors should be considered when deciding if TNR work can be facilitated by the practice.

d) Absolutely no attempt should be made to handle these animals manually. An accurate body weight of the cat should be obtained by calculating the weight of the cat and the carrier, minus the weight of the carrier. This will give you the weight of the cat, which can then be used to calculate the dosage for injectable agents to be used for induction. Once the injection has been administered (ideally using a transfer restrainer container), the cat should be placed somewhere quiet, and the container covered with a towel. Only once the cat is

asleep should it be carefully removed from the container and assessed. A full health check should be performed initially.

> To facilitate accurate hands-off weighing, the carriers used for TNR should all be weighed and have this figure attached to them using some sort of waterproof label or tag so that it is not detached/lost.

e) If a serious condition is identified on health check, euthanasia should be considered on welfare grounds. Euthanasia should be considered for the following conditions:
- Suspected malignancy
- Limb fractures or soft tissue disorders requiring major surgery and long recovery periods
- Unwell cat with an infectious disease
- Other serious clinical signs that would require prolonged, repeated treatment and/or would compromise welfare

f) When performing a spay on minimally socialised or colony cats, it is ideal to perform this through the left flank, while the cat is intubated and being maintained on oxygen. The left flank approach enables the surgical site to be assessed from a distance on release of the cat back to its colony. It also offers increased surgical efficiency, a smaller incision, and reduced risk of evisceration. It is worth noting that colony cats with advanced pregnancy are more easily spayed via a midline approach. As the cats are released back to their colony as quickly as possible, it is important that these incisions are as small as possible. Some vets will apply tissue glue to the surgical site as well as absorbable sutures to give an extra layer of protection.

g) If a queen is lactating, she should be trapped, neutered, and returned to site as soon as possible. Unlike bitches, spaying a lactating cat does not prolong lactation so there is no need to delay until weaning.

In addition, kitten mortality has not been shown to increase where lactating queens are neutered. It has been shown that the feeding of kittens in a colony can be shared out among related females, so the kittens are unlikely to starve while separated from the queen (Crowell-Davis 2005). Lactating queens should be neutered via a flank approach, and any anaesthetic agents that are reversible should be reversed. Multimodal analgesia should be administered to ensure continued pain relief. Intraoperative fluid therapy may be indicated.

h) If a cat or kitten is suspected of being cryptorchid on the health check, exploratory surgery should be performed to identify the missing testicle(s). An assessment of the penis for penile barbs is useful, as entire males or cats with any intact testicular material in their body will have these due to the presence of testosterone. The barbs usually develop at 12 weeks of age and are fully present by 5–6 months of age. Once a tom is neutered, the barbs start to disappear within 2 weeks of neutering and are fully regressed by 6–8 weeks post-neutering.

> Penile barbs indicate testosterone and can be used to help identify cryptorchid cats. The barbs disappear within 6–8 weeks of neutering.

i) Ear-tip cuts (Figure A5.8) are frequently performed in TNR programmes to provide a visual indication of neuter status that does not require handling to confirm (as might be the case with an ear tattoo or microchip). This allows easy visual identification of neutered animals from a distance, preventing them from having to be re-trapped. It is performed under the same anaesthesia as the health assessment and neutering. It involves the removal of 10 mm (or 5 mm in small kittens) of the tip of the left ear with a straight and obvious surgical cut. Ear tipping is legal and is not classed as a mutilation in the UK and other legislatures, being an internationally recognised method of showing that the cat has been neutered (Dalrymple et al. 2022).

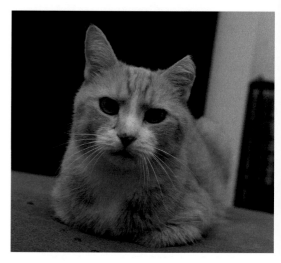

Figure A5.8 Ginge, an ear-tipped ex TNR cat who subsequently transitioned to being a house cat, but this is unusual.

j) Colony cats should not be confined for prolonged periods of time. They should be recovered in cleaned traps or transfer carriers to avoid any additional handling. There should be no signs of bleeding, vomiting, breathing issues, or incomplete recovery from the anaesthetic before leaving the vet practice. Ideally, cats will be released in daylight without being confined overnight. However, if the cats need to stay in overnight to recover, then it is helpful to place water and food bowls in the cage while the cat is still asleep. Once fully recovered, food can be placed in the bowl through the bars, and a watering can or funnel be used to fill the water bowl.

k) If the TNR work is being performed through a charitable service, the charity may have its own policies and procedures regarding preventive healthcare of colony cats. Some charities may advocate for the use of parasite treatment and/or vaccination.

Colony cats are very likely to be harbouring internal and external parasites. If an antiparasitic product is selected, it will need to be a spot-on applied under anaesthetic. Although treatment will be effective for only a limited amount of time, there is an argument that it does help to improve the general health of the cat in the post-operative period.

In terms of vaccination, colony cats can be given a dose of the combined vaccination against feline parvovirus and cat flu at the same time as neutering. There isn't any significant benefit to be gained by administering the FeLV vaccination as only one dose of vaccination will be available to the cat. Studies have shown that even a single dose of feline parvovirus vaccine can be effective (Fischer et al. 2007). In theory, by vaccinating individual cats, the overall health of the colony will improve as the 'herd immunity' is increased.

> TNR approaches are not universally accepted, e.g. the process is debated in Australia, and is considered illegal in many jurisdictions. The programme must be planned carefully to be effective and to safeguard welfare (Tan et al. 2017, Gunther et al. 2022).

REFERENCES

Cats Protection (2021) *The Feral Guide*. Haywards Heath: National Cat Centre.

Crowell-Davis, S. L. (2005) *Understanding Feline Signaling and Social Interactions*. Proceedings of the North American Veterinary Conference, 8–12 January 2005, Orlando, FL.

Dalrymple, A. M., MacDonald, L. J. & Kreisler, R. E. (2022) Ear-tipping practices for identification of cats sterilized in trap–neuter–return programs in the USA. *Journal of Feline Medicine and Surgery* **24**(10):e302–e309. doi: 10.1177/1098612X221105843.

Fischer, S. M., Quest, C. M., Dubovi, E. J. et al. (2007) Response of feral cats to vaccination at the time of neutering. *Journal of the American Veterinary Medical Association* **230**(1):52–58. doi: 10.2460/javma.230.1.52.

Gunther, I., Hawlena, H., Azriel, L. & Klement, E. (2022) Reduction of free-roaming cat population requires high-intensity neutering in spatial contiguity to mitigate compensatory effects. *Proceedings of the National Academy of Sciences USA* **119**(15):e2119000119. doi: 10.1073/pnas.2119000119.

Tan, K., Rand, J. & Morton, J. (2017) Trap–neuter–return activities in urban stray cat colonies in Australia. *Animals (Basel)* **7**(6):46. doi: 10.3390/ani7060046.

5.9 Enalor, 9-wo FE Scottish Fold: health check

a) The short answer is that the expected prevalence of either FIV or FeLV in this cattery will be negligible (probably 0). However, to really understand the value of these tests in Enalor, we need to use numbers. It is not as scary as it first seems!

To do this, we require a starting point. In Australia, among pet cats with outdoor access, the prevalences of FIV and FeLV were found to be 0–4% and 8–20%, respectively (Westman et al. 2019). The prevalence of FIV is likely to be much lower among this breeder's cats who have no outdoor access and do not mix with outdoor cats (Little et al. 2020). We could also expect that the biosecurity of the activities associated with the cattery (e.g. showing cats) is very good, although of course that might not always be the case. An estimated prevalence of FIV and FeLV in this cattery might reasonably be 1% and 2%, respectively, at most. If biosecurity is not so good, you could estimate higher prevalences such as 2% and 4% for FIV and FeLV, respectively.

This is a key point – in clinical practice, prevalence is a **subjective value** that you assign given a starting point and the circumstances (history and clinical signs) of the animal in your examination room. In another example, if the prevalence of parvovirus is 10% in your region, but the 10-week-old puppy on your examination table is unvaccinated, comes from a suburb in which there is currently a parvovirus outbreak, and has severe vomiting and diarrhoea, your estimate is likely to be much higher.

These 'population-level' estimates of disease burden (prevalence, or the proportion of diseased animals in the population) are equivalent to the probability of disease in an individual animal. Probability is measured on a scale from 0 to 1, with 0 signifying that something will not happen (e.g. that an animal will not test positive for a disease) and 1 signifying that something will certainly happen (e.g. that an animal will test positive for a disease). Therefore, my pre-test probabilities of FIV and FeLV in Enalor are 0.01 and 0.02, respectively. My pre-test probability that the puppy has parvovirus is 0.9 because, in my experience, a population of puppies similar to the one on the table would have a parvovirus prevalence of 90%.

b) **Diagnostic sensitivity** (*Se*) is the probability that a test will correctly classify animals with disease.
- For example, if a parvovirus test has a sensitivity of 75%, there is a 75% chance (or 0.75 probability) that it will detect parvovirus in a puppy that has parvovirus (i.e. there is a probability

of 0.25 that the test will return a false-negative result). The FIV test mentioned in part (b) of the question has perfect sensitivity; cats with FIV will always be correctly classified as true positive (i.e. false negatives are not possible).

Diagnostic specificity (*Sp*) is the probability that a test will correctly classify animals without disease.
- For example, if a parvovirus test has a specificity of 80%, there is an 80% chance (or 0.8 probability) that it will identify a puppy without parvovirus as negative (i.e. there is a probability of 0.2 that the test result will be a false positive).

c) Diagnostic test performance is also known as the 'predictive value' of a test result, and this varies on a case-by-case basis according to the pre-test probability (*PreP*) of disease in the individual being tested. In clinical practice, predictive values are really important, but most vets use them without realising and without using numbers. You maximise positive predictive values by increasing the pre-test probability of disease through a comprehensive history and clinical examination so that only diseases that are likely (i.e. those with a high pre-test probability of disease) make the final list. This means that when your test returns a positive result, you are generally confident that it is a true positive (and conversely, you are less likely to trust a negative result; you might conduct another type of test to confirm it). You will question test results less often if the test has good characteristics (i.e. high sensitivity and specificity).

d) If you went through the calculations, you will have found that these tests have no value in Enalor. You already knew this without numbers: you were already 98–99% sure that Enalor would be negative for FIV and FeLV. However, by using numbers you can see that, if a test is positive, the chance that it is a true positive is very low.

The most likely outcome (98–99%!) is that Enalor will test negative, but if she doesn't, you have a difficult situation in which you need to explain to the owners that you don't trust the test result (so why did you do it in the first place?!).

Like any intervention, diagnostic tests should be used judiciously. By conducting a thorough history and clinical examination, you already inherently assign qualitative pre-test probabilities to prioritise your differential diagnosis list and your investigations. It is a small step to convert these to numbers, look up test characteristics, and use an online calculator to calculate the value of using a particular test in numerical terms. This can be very useful when you are questioning a test outcome or using a test with poor test characteristics.

In this example, we have not explored likelihood ratios – they can be misleading because they do not incorporate pre-test probabilities. We have also not explored using multiple tests for one disease (using tests in parallel and in series). These can be useful to manipulate diagnostic sensitivity and specificity, especially in the context of screening apparently healthy animals (inherently low pre-test probabilities) or poor test characteristics (we did touch on it briefly when we suggested that you might conduct another – different – test if you didn't trust the result of the first test).

The case shows just how interesting thinking about diagnostic testing is, and how it can inform decision-making with 'hard data'.

c) All Scottish Fold cats are affected by osteochondrodysplasia, a progressive degenerative joint disorder (Velie et al. 2023). The breed is characterised by forward-folding ears, which is an autosomal dominant trait that affects the development of cartilage. Scottish Fold osteochondrodysplasia (SFOCD) is a chronic, painful syndrome affecting cats homozygous for the fold mutation, as well as heterozygous cats (though potentially to a lesser degree than their homozygous counterparts). It manifests as narrowed joint spaces and irregularly shaped bones, particularly in the limbs. Clinical signs include lameness, reluctance or unwillingness to jump, and a stiff, inflexible tail, with diagnosis generally occurring before the age of 30 months. Affected cats require ongoing pain relief and environmental modifications and should not be bred.

REFERENCES

Little, S., Levy, J., Hartmann, K. et al. (2020) AAFP feline retrovirus testing and management guidelines. *Journal of Feline Medicine and Surgery* **22**(1):5–30. doi: 10.1177/1098612x19895940.

Velie, B. D., Milden, T., Miller, H. & Haase, B. (2023) An estimation of osteochondrodysplasia prevalence in Australian Scottish Fold cats: a retrospective study using VetCompass Data. *BMC Veterinary Research* **19**:252. doi: 10.1186/s12917-023-03811-0.

Westman, M. E., Malik, R. & Norris, J. M. (2019) Diagnosing feline immunodeficiency virus (FIV) and feline leukaemia virus (FeLV) infection: an update for clinicians. *Australian Veterinary Journal* **97**(3):47–55. doi: 10.1111/avj.12781. (Erratum published in *Australian Veterinary Journal* **97**(9):371.)

5.10 Gerbera, 3-yo FN Dachshund: sore paws, not eaten breakfast

a) Primary infections associated with pododermatitis include mycobacteria, dermatophytosis, blastomycosis, fungal mycetoma, and sporotrichosis. Given the appearance of the lesions, the fact that the condition has been well controlled by regular foot bathing, and the presence of rods, the infection is more likely to be secondary in Gerbera's case. Common secondary infections implicated in canine pododermatitis include *Staphylococcus* spp., *Streptococcus* spp., *E. coli*, *Pseudomonas*, *Corynebacterium*, *Enterococcus*, and *Malassezia*. The most likely primary cause – consistent with the ongoing need for foot bathing – is allergic dermatitis (atopy, contact hypersensitivity, or cutaneous food reaction). The fact that multiple feet are involved, and the absence of nodules and draining tracts, suggest that a foreign body or foreign bodies are unlikely. The age of the dog, lack of other clinical signs, and the physical examination findings suggest that endocrine disease such as Cushing's syndrome or hypothyroidism are unlikely. The fact that Gerbera is on excellent parasite control suggests that parasites such as demodex or hookworm can be ruled out (though it is important to double-check with owners that preventive care has been attended to consistently). The vaccine history and absence of nodules or hyperkeratosis suggest that papillomatosis, neoplasia, leishmaniasis, and distemper virus are unlikely causes. The fact that the nails and footpads are normal, the involvement of three out of four limbs (i.e. not all), and the absence of a drug history suggest that autoimmune and immune-mediated diseases are unlikely.

b) Dogs with short, spiky hair, those that are overweight, and those with abnormal weight bearing (many dachshunds have valgus of the limbs) are reported predisposing factors.

c) Given the absence of a history of other gastrointestinal signs such as vomiting and diarrhoea, a lack of abnormalities (including abdominal pain) on abdominal palpation, Gerbera's readiness to take treats in the consultation, and the fact that inappetence has coincided with an acute presentation of the pedal lesions, it is most likely that Gerbera is not eating because she is in pain.

d) While rods are present on a direct impression smear, there are no inflammatory cells, or phagocytosed bacteria. There are no nodules or draining tracts that may indicate deep pyoderma, for which antibiotics are indicated based on C&S. Superficial pyoderma may be successfully treated by addressing primary causes (in this case, allergy was high on the list of suspicion) and topical antimicrobial therapy. In this case, a medicated shampoo containing 2% miconazole and 2% chlorhexidine every 2 or 3 days for 2–4 weeks was recommended. The allergy was treated using an injectable monoclonal anti-interleukin-31 antibody (lokivetmab), paired with a short tapering course of prednisolone (0.5 mg/kg BID [twice daily] PO q12h initially, then q24h, then q48h) to reduce pruritus and inflammation. An alternative may be oclacitinib tablets. Instead of steroids, an NSAID might have been used to relieve pain, but would be less effective in addressing pruritus. Additionally, paracetamol could be considered.

e) It is important to recheck Gerbera soon to ensure (1) that the treatment of the primary and secondary diseases are effective and (2) that she is not deteriorating. If she develops vomiting or diarrhoea, this could suggest that her inappetence reflects gastrointestinal disease that requires investigation, or an adverse drug reaction, rather than a response to pain as initially suspected. In this case, she should be seen as soon as possible. If her feet do not improve within 48 hours (less redness, swelling, and discharge), or if they worsen at any point, she should be rechecked, as this could indicate progression of an underlying infection. If the condition resolves, but recurs following lokivetmab, an elimination diet may be trialled (though it may be introduced while on steroids initially to reduce pruritus). It is important that infections are addressed as persistent infection can become a perpetuating factor.

REFERENCE

Bajwa, J. (2023) Canine pododermatitis: a complex, multifactorial condition. *Canadian Veterinary Journal* **64**(5):489–492.

5.11 Joey, 6-mo ME Griffon Bruxellois: itchy ears

a) *Cheyletiella* spp., *Sarcoptes scabiei*, *Notoedres cati*, *Otodectes cynotis*, and trombiculid mites (e.g. chiggers, harvest mites, red bugs) are the most common culprits.

b) The mite identified is *Otodectes cynotis*, or ear mite. They are Sarcoptiformes and are the same size as *Sarcoptes scabiei*. The pretarsi consist of a sucker attached to a short stalk on the first two pairs of legs of the female and all four pairs of legs on the male (Little & Cortinas 2023). While this mite typically lives in the ears, it can also be found elsewhere on the skin of the dog, particularly the head, back, and tail. It has been found on dogs, cats, ferrets, foxes, and, rarely, humans in close contact with these animals. The life cycle, from eggs to larvae to proto- and deutonymphs to adults, can take about 3 weeks, though may be shortened in warmer, humid conditions (Little & Cortinas 2023). Mites are transmitted between animals via direct contact, though may survive off the host for up to 17 days in favourable conditions. The mite causes intense pruritus (often evidenced by head shaking, aural haematoma[s], and self-trauma to the skin around the face and neck), inflammation of the ear canal, excessive cerumen production, and secondary bacterial and yeast infections. Mites may also cause miliary dermatitis. Affected dogs may be agitated and distressed. Mites may be visualised via otoscopy, but more readily on microscopy.

> Check for mites before fixing and staining slides. Use low power (4× or 10×) and increase the contrast on the microscope by lowering the substage condenser. Mites are often found on or within 'chunks' of cerumen. Infestation in cats is more common than dogs, with *Otodectes cynotis* commonly associated with otitis externa in cats.

c) The goals of treatment are to eliminate mites, minimise pruritus, and treat or prevent the development of secondary infections and chronic changes to the lining of the ear canal – including ceruminous gland hyperplasia – which may predispose to otitis externa. Historically, treatment has involved filling the ear canals with mineral oil (effectively drowning the mites), cleaning the ears with a cerumenolytic agent (removing the mite food supply), and possibly a local application of an acaricide (killing the mites). The limitations of topical treatment alone are the need for extended treatment (up to 3 weeks) to kill all mites and the possibility that mites outside the ear canal will survive. Systemic acaricidal products, such as selamectin and imidacloprid/moxidectin, and isoxazolines, such as fluralaner, afoxolaner, lotilaner, and sarolaner, may provide effective treatment of *Otodectes cynotis* (Carithers et al. 2016, Taenzler et al. 2017, Little & Cortinas 2023), though it is important to check product labels to confirm spectrum of activity. In this case, the patient was treated with an otic preparation containing polymyxin B sulfate, miconazole nitrate, and prednisolone acetate (and licensed for the treatment of otitis externa and skin infections caused by fungi, yeasts, Gram-negative and -positive bacteria, and *Otodectes cynotis*). This helps reduce pruritus and inflammation of the ear canals. Afoxolaner was administered orally. All in-contact animals should be treated.

d) Griffons have high rates of Chiari-like malformation and syringomyelia. Chiari-like malformation describes the herniation of the cerebellum and medulla into or even through the foramen magnum (Freeman et al. 2014). Syringomyelia refers to abnormal cerebrospinal fluid (CSF)-like fluid accumulation within the spinal cord (Freeman et al. 2014). These conditions can lead to spinal pain (particularly in the neck) and neurological deficits, but may not cause clinical signs. Chiari-like malformation and syringomyelia should be considered in differential diagnoses in Griffons presenting with neck or back pain and/or neurological deficits. They also display prognathism (a mandible longer than the maxilla), which can impact dental occlusion and predispose to dental disease.

REFERENCES

Carithers, D., Crawford, J., De Vos, C. et al. (2016) Assessment of afoxolaner efficacy against *Otodectes cynotis* infestations of dogs. *Parasites & Vectors* 9:635. doi: 10.1186/s13071-016-1924-4.

Freeman, A. C., Platt, S. R., Kent, M. et al. (2014) Chiari-like malformation and syringomyelia in American Brussels Griffon dogs. *Journal of Veterinary Internal Medicine* 28(5):1551–1559. doi: 10.1111/jvim.12421.

Little, S. & Cortinas, R. (2023) Mites. In: Sykes, J. E., Rankin, S. C., Papich, M. G. et al. (eds) *Greene's Infectious Diseases of the Dog and Cat*, 5th edition. St Louis, MO: Elsevier.

Taenzler, J., De Vos, C., Roepke, R. K. et al. (2017) Efficacy of fluralaner against *Otodectes cynotis* infestations in dogs and cats. *Parasites & Vectors* 10(1):30. doi: 10.1186/s13071-016-1954-y.

5.12 Greg, 3-yo ME Mixed Breed: breathing strangely

a) The cardiac silhouette is elevated from the sternum, with air between the sternum and cardiac silhouette. The lung lobes are collapsed (atelectasis). The patient has pneumothorax, i.e. accumulation of air or gas within the pleural space. There is a radiodense opacity in the caudodorsal lung fields that is consistent with a metallic ballistic projectile, possibly from an air gun. This was judged an incidental finding. There is a mass effect superimposed on the cardiac silhouette. Lung lesions cannot be ruled out in the presence of this degree of atelectasis (Mooney 2018). Because patients with pneumothorax are at risk of decompensating, this is one situation where a single lateral thoracic view is considered sufficient to make a diagnosis (Mooney 2018). Additional views may be taken once the pneumothorax is treated.

b) Pneumothorax can be acquired or spontaneous. The most common causes of acquired pneumothorax are blunt trauma (e.g. motor vehicle accidents, falls, horse kicks) or penetrating trauma (e.g. gunshot, stabbing, stick injuries, bite wounds). Iatrogenic pneumothorax may be secondary to thoracic wall surgery, thoracocentesis, or barotrauma (e.g. during anaesthesia, where the pop-off valve is left closed) (Mooney 2018). Spontaneous pneumothorax can be primary (e.g. ruptured bullae or blebs) or secondary to lung disease (e.g. pneumonia, granuloma, parasitic infestation such as heartworm, pulmonary thromboembolism, neoplastic disease, or foreign body, e.g. grass-seed migration) (Gilday et al. 2021).

c) Pneumothorax reduces ventilation and oxygenation, as air in the pleural space compresses the lungs and causes loss of the negative pulmonary pressure that keeps the alveoli open (Gilday et al. 2021). As pneumothorax worsens, intrapleural pressure can increase from negative to positive, causing more alveoli to collapse. Pressure is also exerted on the intrathoracic vessels, reducing volume and venous return. When the intrapleural pressure exceeds central venous and pulmonary arterial pressure, cardiogenic shock and hypoxaemia (tension pneumothorax) ensue, and death occurs unless there is rapid intervention (Mooney 2018).

d) Thoracocentesis should be performed immediately to remove free air from the thoracic cavity. This can be performed in sternal recumbency or standing. Sterile technique is used. The centesis should be performed bilaterally by introducing a needle (e.g. a butterfly type) at the level of the costochondral junction between the seventh and ninth intercostal spaces. A large syringe is connected via a three-way tap. Light sedation, e.g. with butorphanol and medetomidine, may be required. The needle should be introduced cranial to the ribs, as the intercostal nerves and vessels are caudal to the ribs. If the patient requires multiple thoracocenteses (e.g. three times in 24 hours), if thoracocentesis fails to relieve dyspnoea, or if tension pneumothorax occurs, indwelling thoracostomy tubes with continuous suction are likely to be needed. Supplementary oxygen (e.g. placement in an oxygen enclosure) may benefit the patient. Analgesia should be provided.

> In critical cases, thoracocentesis may correctly be performed before X-ray. The patient *in extremis* may not tolerate being handled for X-ray. In these situations, when clinical judgement indicates, immediate centesis can be both diagnostic and life-saving.

REFERENCES

Gilday, C., Odunayo, A. & Hespel, A.-M. (2021) Spontaneous pneumothorax: pathophysiology, clinical presentation and diagnosis. *Topics in Companion Animal Medicine* **45**:100563. doi: 10.1016/j.tcam.2021.100563.

Mooney, E. (2018) Pneumothorax. In: Drobatz, K. J., Hopper, K., Rozanski, E. & Silverstein, D. C. (eds) *Textbook of Small Animal Emergency Medicine*. Wiley Online Library. doi: 10.1002/9781119028994.ch44.

5.13 Scruff, 13-yo MN Jack Russell Terrier: blood from mouth

a) There is a proliferative gingival growth at the rostral maxillary area with exposure of the cementum/root of tooth 104 and a strong suggestion of alveolar bone loss or destruction. There is evidence of mild to moderate calculus accumulation on this tooth. There is no nasal discharge at the ipsilateral nostril that might suggest oronasal fistula. There is loss of right upper incisors (probably 102 and 103 or else they are obscured by the gingival tissue).

b) The blood is most likely coming from this proliferative gingival tissue when traumatised. Prognosis is guarded. The reaction looks highly localised, and very severe for periodontal disease; therefore, neoplasia must be suspected. The most common oral tumours in the dog are malignant melanomas, SCCs, and fibrosarcomas, followed by osteosarcomas, acanthomatous ameloblastomas, and peripheral odontogenic fibromas (Sarowitz et al. 2017). SCCs may be tonsillar, which are highly metastatic and likely to recur following treatment, or non-tonsillar, which are less likely to metastasise (Grier & Mayer 2007).

c) This is a severe presentation that could, taken with a QOL assessment, prompt discussion about euthanasia. The owner should be informed that, to definitively treat Scruff's condition, appropriate tumour staging would be needed. This would ideally include CT to check for invasion of surrounding structures, including the nasal cavity and cribriform plate. Following this, if feasible, wide local excision of the mass (while preserving function) could be undertaken (Sarowitz et al. 2017). Alternatively, or additionally, radiation therapy may be recommended. However, Scruff's owner does not have the funds, and it appears that Scruff is coping well at the moment, so palliative care can be considered. This might include antibiotics for infection and almost certainly analgesics, e.g. NSAIDs. There is some evidence that NSAIDs may have anti-tumour effects, e.g. decreasing migration and invasion of some cancer cells (Iturriaga et al. 2017). Alternatively, corticosteroids could be administered. Paracetamol could be administered concurrently with either NSAIDs or corticosteroids for additional analgesia. Welfare concerns centre around probable progression and consequent deterioration in Scruff's overall QOL. At this point, both euthanasia and palliative care can be ethically supported using a contextualised care approach that takes account of Scruff's current signalment, the owner's financial status and wishes, and the probable prognosis.

d) The moderate periodontal disease suggests that there is separate pathology going on at 104, making tumour more likely than severe, local periodontal disease. In particular, 204 has a near normal probing depth in contrast to the massive loss of attachment evident at 104.

e) The main point is to ensure that the owner realises that Scruff has malignant disease that is likely to develop into more serious local problems and may have already metastasised to the regional lymph nodes and beyond. However, it is good news that he has responded to palliative treatment and that his QOL is satisfactory for now.

f) Scruff is likely to need ongoing analgesics or anti-inflammatories and may also require empirical antibiotic treatment. A diet of soft food may be recommended to minimise discomfort when eating. Regular rechecks are advised but, depending on the owner's ability to monitor, these could be reduced to monthly in order to save costs. There is also the possibility of interim telephone/remote consultations. Monitoring Scruff's demeanour, appetite, and weight will also be important and can all be done at home, with revisits if there are any changes.

REFERENCES

Grier, C. K. & Mayer, M. N. (2007) Radiation therapy of canine nontonsillar squamous cell carcinoma. *Canadian Veterinary Journal* **48**(11):1189–1191.

Iturriaga, M. P., Paredes, R., Arias, J. I. & Torres, C. G. (2017) Meloxicam decreases the migration and invasion of CF41.Mg canine mammary carcinoma cells. *Oncological Letters* **14**(2):2198–2206. doi: 10.3892/ol.2017.6400.

Sarowitz, B. N., Davis, G. J. & Kim, S. (2017) Outcome and prognostic factors following curative-intent surgery for oral tumours in dogs: 234 cases (2004 to 2014). *Journal of Small Animal Practice* **58**(3):146–153. doi: 10.1111/jsap.12624.

5.14 Walk-in: wants to surrender 3 cats due to toxo

a) The causative agent of toxoplasmosis is *Toxoplasma gondii*, a protozoan parasite. Cats are the definitive hosts, meaning they are the only species in which the parasite can complete its sexual reproduction, but they are not the sole source of infection to humans (Jones & Dubey 2012, Dubey et al. 2020). Cats primarily become infected by eating prey or undercooked meat containing tissue cysts. Infected cats can shed oocysts in their faeces, which take a minimum of 24 hours to sporulate and become infectious. These oocysts can be highly resilient in the environment and are a source of infection to other animals and humans. Notably, cats typically shed oocysts only once in their lifetime, for about a week from 6–7 days post-infection, often displaying only mild symptoms during this time (Dubey 2001). Most cats become infected early in life once they start hunting prey (Dubey et al. 2020).

b) See Figure A5.14. The three main routes of *T. gondii* transmission to humans are as follows:

1. Ingestion of tissue cysts in undercooked or raw meat and filter feeders such as oysters. This route of transmission is more common in adults (Jones & Dubey 2012)

2. Ingestion of oocysts from contaminated environments and surfaces, such as cat litter, sandpits, soil, water, unwashed fruit and vegetables, or pet fur. This route of transmission is more common in children (Frenkel et al. 1995)

3. Congenital transmission from an infected mother to the fetus during pregnancy. This route of transmission is rare, and clinical disease from congenital transmission is even rarer

c) While anyone can contract toxoplasmosis, the risk of clinical disease is mainly a concern in immunocompromised individuals, such as those with HIV/AIDS, organ transplant recipients, and individuals undergoing chemotherapy (Jones & Dubey 2012). Pregnant women are an important risk group because a primary infection acquired during pregnancy can be transmitted to the fetus, potentially causing severe congenital abnormalities or miscarriage.

Once infected, individuals remain infected for life but are usually asymptomatic unless they become immunocompromised. Importantly, prior infection provides immunity against subsequent infections; thus, pregnant women with past exposure have a significantly lower risk of congenital transmission. It is advisable for pregnant women to discuss serological testing with their obstetrician to determine past exposure and prior immunity.

d) Routine serological testing in cats is not common, and there is no defined antibody titre cut-off (Dubey et al. 2020). However, testing for *T. gondii* antibodies in cats can indicate past exposure and therefore give some indication of infection risk. The two main types of antibodies tested are immunoglobulin M (IgM) and immunoglobulin G (IgG):

- **IgM antibodies.** The presence of IgM antibodies typically indicates a recent or acute infection. IgM is the first antibody

Note that contact with dogs can pose a higher risk than direct contact with cats due to dogs' xenosmophilic behaviour (behaviour driven by a love of foreign smells), such as rolling in cat faeces, potentially facilitating transmission to humans via contact with sporulated oocysts in dogs' fur (Frenkel & Parker 1996).

① CONSUMPTION OF **TISSUE CYSTS** IN UNDERCOOKED MEAT. THIS ROUTE IS MOST COMMON IN ADULTS.

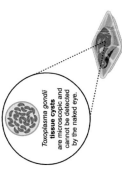

Toxoplasma gondii **tissue cysts** are microscopic and cannot be detected by the naked eye.

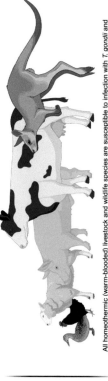

All homeothermic (warm-blooded) livestock and wildlife species are susceptible to infection with *T. gondii* and should be considered a potential source of transmission. Tissue cysts can be inactivated by **freezing meat (<10°C) for a minimum of three days** or **cooking thoroughly (internal temperature >65°C)**.

② INGESTION OF **SPORULATED OOCYSTS** FROM CONTAMINATED ENVIRONMENTS AND SURFACES, SUCH AS CAT LITTER, ANIMAL FUR, SOIL, SAND AND WATER. THIS ROUTE IS MOST COMMON IN CHILDREN.

Cats are the **definitive hosts** of *T. gondii*. They maintain the life cycle via ingestion of tissue cysts in undercooked meat and prey. The tissue cysts contain slow growing **bradyzoites** that emerge and undergo sexual reproduction in the cat.

Cats typically only shed **unsporulated oocysts** once in their lives for about a week 6-7 days after they become infected.

Unsporulated oocysts take a minimum of 24 hours to **sporulate** and become infectious.

Homegrown fruit and vegetables should be thoroughly washed to remove oocysts shed by outdoor cats.

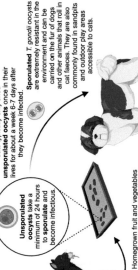

Sporulated *T. gondii* oocysts are extremely resistant in the environment and can be carried on the fur of dogs and other animals that roll in cat faeces. They are also commonly found in sandpits and outdoor play areas accessible to cats.

Filter feeders, such as oysters, can accumulate oocysts from contaminated water sources.

③ CONGENITAL TRANSMISSION OF **TACHYZOITES** FROM A RECENTLY INFECTED MOTHER TO THE FOETUS VIA THE PLACENTA. THE MOTHER MAY BECOME INFECTED DURING PREGNANCY VIA ROUTES ONE OR TWO.

Mothers infected just prior to or during pregnancy can pass the infection onto their unborn child via invasion of rapidly dividing **tachyzoites** across the placenta. It is important to remember that you can only get infected once, and previous infection is protective against congenital transmission.

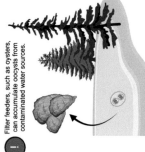

Tachyzoites, shed by infected animals into milk, are inactivated by pasteurisation. This is one of many reasons raw milk and raw milk products including cheese should be avoided during pregnancy.

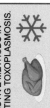
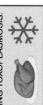

ALTHOUGH THEY ARE THE DEFINITIVE HOSTS OF *T. GONDII*, CATS ARE ONLY ONE SOURCE OF INFECTION. GOOD HAND HYGIENE AND INACTIVATION OF TISSUE CYSTS BY COOKING OR FREEZING ARE THE MOST EFFECTIVE METHODS IN PREVENTING TOXOPLASMOSIS.

Figure A5.14 A schematic representation of the three main routes by which humans can become infected with *T. gondii*, namely (1) consumption of tissue cysts in undercooked meat; (2) ingestion of sporulated oocysts from contaminated environments such as sandpits, vegetable gardens, and dog fur; and (3) congenital transmission of tachyzoites across the placenta. Raw milk and dairy products made from raw milk also present a *T. gondii* tachyzoite transmission risk and should be avoided during pregnancy. Although cats are the definitive hosts of *T. gondii*, oocysts are not the most common source of infection in adults. The most effective form of protection against infection is good hand hygiene and thoroughly cooking or freezing meat prior to eating. (Image created with BioRender.com.)

type to be produced in response to an infection and usually appears within 1–2 weeks after exposure. However, IgM can persist for several months, and, in some cases, false positives can occur. Therefore, the presence of IgM antibodies suggests recent exposure, but is not a reliable indicator of current infection

- **IgG antibodies.** IgG antibodies develop later in the course of infection and usually indicate past exposure or a chronic infection. The presence of IgG antibodies alone, especially in high titres, suggests that the infection occurred in the past, and the individual (or cat, in this case) has most likely developed immunity. A high IgG titre without detectable IgM suggests that the cat has been infected in the past and is less likely to be currently shedding oocysts

Serological tests do not indicate whether a cat is shedding oocysts, which is the primary concern for transmission to humans. Faecal tests for the detection of oocysts are not recommended due to the low frequency and short duration of shedding, making detection challenging (Dubey 2001, Dubey et al. 2020).

e) In otherwise healthy cats, toxoplasmosis is often transient (occurs 1–2 weeks after initial infection) and asymptomatic. However, if clinical signs do occur, they can be non-specific and include fever, lethargy, loss of appetite, and possibly respiratory or gastrointestinal symptoms (Dubey et al. 2020). In some cases, more severe signs such as ocular disease, neurological symptoms, or pneumonia can be observed. Severe clinical toxoplasmosis is extremely rare and usually indicative of another pathological process causing immune compromise such as FIV, FeLV, or feline infectious peritonitis (FIP); neoplasia; and/or chronic administration of certain immunosuppressive drugs, including cyclosporin (Dubey & Carpenter 1993) and oclacitinib (Moore et al. 2022). These cats may resume shedding of unsporulated oocysts, adding to environmental contamination.

f) To alleviate the owner's concerns, advise her on preventive measures:
- Keep the cats indoors to prevent them from hunting and eating infected prey
- Avoid feeding the cats raw or undercooked meat. If feeding them raw meat, owners should be advised to freeze it for at least 3 days prior to thawing and feeding to inactivate tissue cysts
- Practise good hygiene, such as washing hands after handling animals and their waste, and before eating

For pregnant individuals who have not been previously infected with *T. gondii*, it is advisable to avoid cleaning cat litter boxes if possible. If they must clean the litter box, they should do so daily (as oocysts take a minimum of 24 hours to sporulate and become infectious), wear protective gloves, and thoroughly wash their hands afterwards (Jones & Dubey 2012). This reduces the risk of transmission via sporulated oocysts on pet fur or other surfaces. It is important to emphasise to your client that, while cats can shed oocysts, the risk of transmission to adults from direct contact with cats is relatively low compared with other infection sources such as undercooked meat. However, it is generally recommended to avoid introducing new kittens or new cats into a household while pregnancy planning, as they are more likely to shed infectious oocysts than older, well-established cats.

g) Good hygiene practices are protective against toxoplasmosis. Clinicians or anyone planning to start a family should exercise caution but not necessarily avoid handling cats. A Canadian study found that veterinary staff have a lower seropositivity rate for *T. gondii* than the general public, suggesting that professional hygiene practices are effective in preventing transmission (Shuhaiber et al. 2003). These findings support the view that cat ownership or contact is not a significant risk factor for *T. gondii* infection.

REFERENCES

Dubey, J. P. (2001) Oocyst shedding by cats fed isolated bradyzoites and comparison of infectivity of bradyzoites of the VEG strain *Toxoplasma gondii* to cats and mice. *Journal of Parasitology* **87**(1):215–219. doi: 10.1645/0022-3395(2001) 087[0215:OSBCFI]2.0.CO;2.

Dubey, J. P. & Carpenter, J. L. (1993) Histologically confirmed clinical toxoplasmosis in cats – 100 cases (1952–1990). *Journal of the American Veterinary Medical Association* **203**(11):1556–1566.

Dubey, J. P., Cerqueira-Cézar, C. K., Murata, F. H. A. et al. (2020) All about toxoplasmosis in cats: the last decade. *Veterinary Parasitology* **283**:109145. doi: 10.1016/j.vetpar.2020.109145.

Frenkel, J. K. & Parker, B. B. (1996) An apparent role of dogs in the transmission of *Toxoplasma gondii*. The probable importance of xenosmophilia. *Annals of the New York Academy of Sciences* **791**(1):402–407. doi: 10.1111/j.1749-6632.1996.tb53546.x.

Frenkel, J. K., Hassanein, K. M., Hassanein, R. S. et al. (1995) Transmission of *Toxoplasma gondii* in Panama City, Panama: a five-year prospective cohort study of children, cats, rodents, birds, and soil. *American Journal of Tropical Medicine and Hygiene* **53**(5):458–468. doi: 10.4269/ ajtmh.1995.53.458.

Jones, J. L. & Dubey, J. P. (2012) Foodborne toxoplasmosis. *Clinical Infectious Diseases* **55**(6):845–851. doi: 10.1093/cid/cis508.

Moore, A., Burrows, A. K., Malik, R. et al. (2022) Fatal disseminated toxoplasmosis in a feline immunodeficiency virus-positive cat receiving oclacitinib for feline atopic skin syndrome. *Veterinary Dermatology* **33**:435–439. doi: 10.1111/ vde.13097.

Shuhaiber, S., Koren, G., Boskovic, R. et al. (2003) Seroprevalence of *Toxoplasma gondii* infection among veterinary staff in Ontario, Canada (2002): implications for teratogenic risk. *BMC Infectious Diseases* **3**:8. doi: 10.1186/1471-2334-3-8.

5.15 Will, 6-yo MN DSH: blocked again

a) The most common causes of urethral obstruction are urethral plugs, urethral spasm, urolithiasis (calcium oxalate or struvite are most common), strictures, and urethral trauma (Breheny et al. 2022a). Less commonly, blood clots, urinary tract neoplasia, and perineal or intrapelvic lesions or trauma are implicated.

b) Urethral obstruction is an emergency. Treatment depends on the clinical status of the patient. As this is a painful and distressing condition, analgesia is important. An opioid such as methadone can be given at 0.2–0.5 mg/kg initially while IV access is established and blood is drawn. At a minimum, blood work should include PCV/TP to assess hydration, glucose, and electrolytes. If additional blood is available, it is useful to measure ionised calcium (hypocalcaemia can exacerbate the effects of hyperkalaemia; both are commonly found in cats with urethral obstruction) and renal parameters (Breheny et al. 2022a). BP can be measured via Doppler and helps guide fluid therapy. As hypotension is common, NSAIDs should be avoided for now. Some patients may benefit from the administration of a benzodiazepine (such as diazepam or midazolam) for anxiolysis, and ketamine may be suitable in feline patients without cardiac disease to provide sedation prior to general anaesthesia. The use of maropitant may help reduce nausea and visceral pain associated with this condition

(Breheny et al. 2022a). IV fluid resuscitation (Breheny et al. 2022a) with an isotonic crystalloid helps restore renal perfusion and dilute potassium levels. While it contains a small amount of potassium, Hartmann's may help normalise acid–base disturbances more rapidly than saline.

Depending on severity and presence of concurrent hypocalcaemia, hyperkaelamia may require treatment. Medical management of hyperkalaemia may include administration of calcium gluconate, glucose, neutral insulin, terbutaline, or sodium bicarbonate as described in detail elsewhere (Breheny et al. 2022a). It would be useful to take abdominal radiographs, adding contrast if required, to determine the presence and location of uroliths, which may alter the treatment plan (e.g. the presence of uroliths in the bladder may require cystotomy). As a urinary catheter is required for perineal urethrostomy, retrograde urethral catheterisation is recommended. A urine sample should be collected for urinalysis. The catheter (or, prior to this, a syringe attached to a lubricated IV cannula with the stylet removed) is used to pulse-flush the obstruction retrograde into the bladder, and empty the bladder. In anaesthetised cats, prior to preparation of the perineum for aseptic urinary catheter placement, a rectal examination should be performed to assess the intrapelvic urethra, and possibly palpate the cause of obstruction (Breheny et al. 2022b). Decompressive cystocentesis can be performed to relieve pressure on the bladder, but this may need to be repeated and will not address the physical urethral obstruction.

c) Perineal urethrostomy is a procedure that was once commonly performed in general practice, but is now increasingly performed in specialty practice. In a retrospective case series of 74 cats undergoing perineal urethrostomy, all owners felt that their cat's QOL was at least the same post-surgery as before the onset of urinary tract disease (Slater et al. 2020). In this study, most surgery was performed by specialists. All owners rated their cat's QOL as ≥7 on a scale of 1–10, where 10 was excellent, and 75% of owners rated their cat's QOL as 10/10.

The following factors may prompt you to refer the case:

- A belief that **referral is in Will's best interests** (more expedient surgery, the availability of a surgeon more proficient in this procedure, the availability of ancillary staff, the availability of continuous 24-hour care including post-operative monitoring and analgesia)
- The client may wish to seek **the highest standard of care available** and be able to pay for the costs of surgery in a referral facility/have appropriate insurance cover
- The **veterinarian–client relationship is ineffective** (i.e. even if you have the expertise and capacity to perform this procedure, the client lacks confidence or there is conflict about the management of the case) (McKenzie 2024)

Other reasons for referral include an unusual presentation of a common condition, an unusual condition, or the patient has complex comorbidities that require ongoing management.

d) Key reasons for managing Will's case in-house are as follows:

- **Referral is not available** (e.g. there may be no facility nearby, or available facilities may have no immediate capacity. In the latter case, it may also be possible to place a urinary catheter and delay referral for definitive surgery). If referral is not available or is declined, the offer of referral and the client's reasons for declining should be noted in Will's records

- Will's owner is informed of the option of referral and accurate costs, and is aware of the potential risks of not referring the case (e.g. lack of continuous overnight monitoring or intensive care), but **specialty care is not affordable, accessible, or acceptable to the client**. If this is the case, the offer of referral and the client's reasons for declining should be noted in Will's records. The outlay for perineal urethrostomy may be weighed against potential costs for medical management of urethral obstruction, as well as ongoing costs including prescription diets (Slater et al. 2020)
- You and other members of the general practice team **have or can acquire the appropriate knowledge, skills, and equipment** to perform the surgery
- You can provide **appropriate pre-, peri- and post-operative monitoring**
- There is an **effective veterinarian–client relationship**
- This **condition is commonly encountered and treated in veterinary general practice**

e) Potential complications of perineal urethrostomy are common. They include wound breakdown, SC urine leakage, urinary incontinence, UTI, sterile cystitis, peristomal dermatitis, and urethral stricture or obstruction of the stoma (Milgram 2016, Seneviratne et al. 2021). The risk of surgical complications can be minimised through meticulous surgical technique (ensuring that the pelvic attachments of the urethra are cut to mobilise the urethra, allowing adequate dissection to the level of the bulbourethral glands, avoiding excessive resection of tissues dorsal to the penis and damage to the pelvic plexus, careful apposition of the urethral mucosa to the skin, tension-free closure) and prevention of self-trauma (adequate pre-, peri-, and post-operative analgesia, rapid diagnosis and treatment of cystitis, Elizabethan collar placement where required) (Milgram 2016). As with all procedures, the client should be informed about potential complications, including the potential for wound breakdown, urethral stricture, and increased risk of UTI. In addition, perineal urethrostomy does not address the underlying causes of urinary tract obstruction (Slater et al. 2020). Thus, clinical signs such as haematuria, stranguria, pollakiuria, and periuria may persist or recur, and affected cats may require further treatment.

The feline penile urethra is divided into four discrete sections, with increasing internal diameter (Table A5.15). Thus the diameter of the urethra at the level of the bulbourethral glands is almost twice that of the penile urethra. Failure to dissect the urethra cranially to this level leads to a smaller stoma, which is at an increased risk of stricture or obstruction (Milgram 2016). This is a common complication of the procedure.

Table A5.15 **The progressively narrowing internal diameter of the penile urethra of the cat (adapted from Milgram 2016 and Borges et al. 2017)**

ANATOMICAL SECTION	Vesicourethral junction	Pre-prostatic	Prostatic	Post-prostatic urethra at level of bulbourethral glands	Penile
INTERNAL DIAMETER	2.4 mm	2.0 mm	Variable	1.3 mm	0.7 mm

Tips

- Initial unblocking of the urethra may be aided by using an IV cannula (without stylet) attached to a 5-mL syringe of warmed saline for gentle, pulsed retropulsion.
- The distal two-thirds of the urethra cannot be evaluated by ultrasonography. To examine this area, contrast urethrography or rectal examination must be performed (Breheny et al. 2022b).
- A caudal epidural block may facilitate retrograde urethral catheterisation.
- The distal urethra should be gently straightened to facilitate smooth catheter placement.
- The application of topical local anaesthetics (e.g. EMLA cream) to the skin of the perineum prior to suture placement may be of benefit. These should be applied 30 minutes before suture placement (Leask 2021).
- Avoid placing sutures in the prepuce. Rather, place sutures in the perineum adjacent to the prepuce (Figure A5.15a,b).

REFERENCES

Borges, N. C., Pereira-Sampaio, M. A., Pereira, V. A. et al. (2017) Effects of castration on penile extracellular matrix morphology in domestic cats. *Journal of Feline Medicine and Surgery* **19**(12):1261–1266. doi: 10.1177/1098612x16689405.

Breheny, C., Blacklock, K. B. & Gunn-Moore, D. (2022a) Approach to urethral obstruction in cats. Part 1: presentation and stabilisation. *In Practice* **44**(8):372–384.doi: 10.1002/inpr.107.

Breheny, C., Blacklock, K. B. & Gunn-Moore, D. (2022b) Approach to urethral obstruction in cats. Part 2: catheterising and postobstruction management. *In Practice* **44**(8):452–464. doi: 10.1002/inpr.248.

Leask, E. (2021) Efficacy of EMLA™ cream for reducing pain associated with venepuncture in felines. *Veterinary Evidence* **6**(3). doi: 10.18849/ve.v6i3.456.

McKenzie, B. (2024) Do it yourself or send for help? Considering specialty referral from a general practitioner perspective. *Journal of the American Veterinary Medical Association* **262**(5):715–720. doi: 10.2460/javma.23.11.0612.

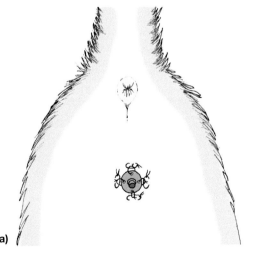
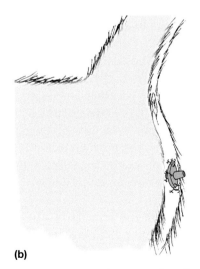

(a) (b)

Figure A5.15a,b **Illustration of how a Slippery Sam urinary catheter can be secured to the skin. Sutures are placed in the perineum at 3, 6, 9 and 12'o clock positions with an exposed loop. Sutures are then placed through the holes in the catheter hub, and these are threaded through the pre-placed skin sutures. To remove and replace the catheter, cut the sutures attached to the catheter hub while leaving skin sutures intact. These can be used to secure a replacement catheter if required.** (Adapted from Breheny et al. 2022b.)

Milgram, J. (2016) Chapter 70: Feline Perineal Urethrostomy. In: Griffon, D. & Hamaide, A. (eds). *Complications in Small Animal Surgery*. Wiley Online Library. doi: 10.1002/9781119421344.ch70.

Seneviratne, M., Stamenova, P. & Lee, K. (2021) Comparison of surgical indications and short- and long-term complications in 56 cats undergoing perineal, transpelvic or prepubic urethrostomy. *Journal of Feline Medicine and Surgery* **23**(6):477–486. doi: 10.1177/1098612x20959032.

Slater, M. R., Pailler, S., Gayle, J. M. M. et al. (2020) Welfare of cats 5–29 months after perineal urethrostomy: 74 cases (2015–2017). *Journal of Feline Medicine and Surgery* **22**(6):582–588. doi: 10.1177/1098612x19867777.

5.16 Jackie, 7-yo MN Mixed Breed: lump in mouth

a) Jackie has a dentigerous cyst (sometimes known as a follicular cyst). These cysts develop in association with the enamel of the crown of an unerupted, usually permanent tooth (D'Astous 2011). The cyst attaches to the tooth at the cemento-enamel junction and encloses the crown of the unerupted tooth. The most commonly affected teeth are the mandibular first premolars, but mandibular and maxillary canine teeth and mandibular third molar teeth are also commonly affected. They are more common in dogs than cats, and more frequent in brachycephalic breeds (Bellei et al. 2019). Dentigerous cysts can grow, damaging surrounding bone and oral structures. Those in the upper dental arcade can invade and obstruct the nasal cavity (Martinez et al. 2023). Differentials for absent teeth (hypodontia) include congenital absence (see Case 1.3), previous extraction, exfoliation, tooth resorption, and crown fracture with root retention (D'Astous 2011).

b) Dentigerous cysts can form due to tooth impaction, which physically obstructs tooth eruption, lack of eruption (leading to embedding of teeth), or iatrogenic damage to the tooth bud during extraction (most commonly extraction of retained deciduous canine teeth), leading to malformation and impaction of the permanent tooth (D'Astous 2011).

c) Treatment requires extraction of the unerupted tooth and removal (enucleation) of the cyst wall. If part of the cyst wall is retained, the cyst may recur (D'Astous 2011). The larger the cyst, the more challenging the surgery. To ensure early detection, intra-oral dental radiographs should be performed in any animal with hypodontia beyond the normal period of tooth eruption (taking into account breed variation) or repeated in animals where an unerupted tooth is not extracted (Figure A5.16).

d) Cytology of the cyst may help diagnose or rule out secondary infection. Histopathology is recommended to rule out neoplasia, which can appear similar on intra-oral radiographs. Histopathology is

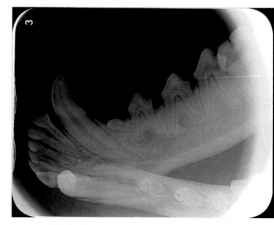

Figure A5.16 Intra-oral radiograph of an unerupted lower left first premolar (305).

important as dentigerous cysts can undergo neoplastic transformation over time.

REFERENCES

Bellei, E., Ferro, S., Zini, E. & Gracis, M. (2019) A clinical, radiographic and histological study of unerupted teeth in dogs and cats: 73 cases (2001–2018). *Frontiers in Veterinary Science* **6**:357. doi: 10.3389/fvets.2019.00357.

D'Astous, J. (2011) An overview of dentigerous cysts in dogs and cats. *Canadian Veterinary Journal* **52**(8):905–907.

Martinez, I., Rich, A., Haseler, J. & Mielke, B. (2023) Complete nasal obstruction caused by a dentigerous cyst in a 4-year-old pug. *Veterinary Record Case Reports* **11**:e538. doi: 10.1002/vrc2.538.

5.17 Rufus, 14-mo ME Mixed Breed: had a fit

a) Key questions are as follows:
- What was Rufus doing during the episode (e.g. falling to the side, paddling)?
- How long did the episode last?
- Any salivation, urination, defaecation?
- Was Rufus conscious?
- Was there any sign prior to the main episode?
- How quickly did Rufus recover from the episodes?
- What were the clinical signs post-seizure (e.g. ataxia, blindness)?

> The history is an extremely important part of the consultation as the description may help you differentiate between other conditions such as syncope or movement disorder. If you have any doubt about the nature of the episode from an owner's verbal description, always consider asking for a video.

b) Perform a general examination and a neurological examination. Then perform a CBC, general biochemistry, electrolyte test, and urinalysis.

> Being able to perform a neurological examination is very important. Differential diagnoses and treatments can be found in the literature, but you will need an accurate neurolocalisation to navigate efficiently and accurately within the literature. Consider spending time performing neurological examinations on normal dogs to improve your skills.

c) The diagnosis for Rufus is idiopathic epilepsy (IE) with a tier 1 confidence level (Bhatti et al. 2015, Di Risio et al. 2015). The criteria for tier 1 confidence level are as follows:
- Two or more unprovoked seizures occurring more than 24 hours apart
- Age of onset: between 6 months and 6 years
- Normal physical and neurological examinations
- Unremarkable urinalysis and routine blood tests

IE is a diagnosis of exclusion. The causes of seizures are usually classified into three groups:
- **Reactive seizures**, secondary to intoxications (e.g. organophosphate, strychnine) or metabolic disorders (e.g. hypoglycaemia, liver disease, electrolyte imbalance)
- **Structural epilepsy**, secondary to a wide range of forebrain disorders, such as inflammatory/infectious, neoplastic, or congenital disorders
- **Idiopathic epilepsy** (or suspected to be of genetic origin)

d) As IE is a diagnosis of exclusion, advanced imaging and CSF analysis could be considered to increase the level of confidence (tier II). However, considering the strong clinical suspicion of IE, advanced imaging is not considered necessary in the first instance. But if Rufus does not respond to anti-epileptic treatment, or if he develops cluster seizures, status epilepticus, or interictal neurological abnormalities, then referral for advanced imaging and CSF analysis is recommended.

e) The decision to initiate treatment with an anti-epileptic drug should be guided by factors such as seizure frequency, seizure severity, severity of post-ictal signs, and owner considerations (e.g. lifestyle and cost). In this case, considering Rufus had three seizures in 2 months, anti-epileptic medications should be considered. First-line treatment is usually phenobarbital (start at 3 mg/kg BID). Phenobarbital dose should be adjusted based on clinical response, side effects, and serum phenobarbital levels. It is recommended to check serum phenobarbital levels 2 weeks after the start of treatment or change of dose, and every 6–12 months thereafter. Other anti-epileptic drugs can also be considered such as imepitoin (not available in all countries), levetiracetam, or potassium bromide.

REFERENCES

Bhatti, S., De Risio, L., Muñana, K. et al. (2015) International Veterinary Epilepsy Task Force consensus proposal: medical treatment of canine epilepsy in Europe. *BMC Veterinary Research* **11**:176. doi: 10.1186/s12917-015-0464-z.

De Risio, L., Bhatti, S., Muñana, K. et al. (2015) International Veterinary Epilepsy Task Force consensus proposal: diagnostic approach to epilepsy in dogs. *BMC Veterinary Research* **11**:148. doi: 10.1186/s12917-015-0462-1.

5.18 Clementine, 12-yo FN DSH: vet authorise prescription

a) Poor adherence may impact the patient, the client, the practice, and the environment, as outlined in Table A5.18.

b) Reasons may include, but are not limited to, the following:
- The costs of prescriptions, medication, and/or veterinary visits
- Practical factors such as lack of time or resources to attend follow-up appointments or collect medication
- Negative perceptions about the medication, including concerns about potential side effects (e.g. polyphagia, weight gain, or sedative effects associated with phenobarbital)
- The medication works, thereby appearing to 'cure' the underlying problem (e.g. Clementine does not have seizures while on medication), and the owner no longer perceives a need for it
- The perception that the medication does not make a difference
- A long time has elapsed since the initial treatment recommendations

Table A5.18 **Potential impacts of poor adherence to medical treatment (adapted from Maddison et al. 2021)**

STAKEHOLDER	POTENTIAL IMPACTS
Clementine (the patient)	• Failure to manage the condition being treated (with possible seizures) • Poor management of chronic disease • Adverse effects associated with withdrawal of medication (such as seizures) • Adverse effects where doses are missed and the owner attempts to catch up
Jill (Clementine's carer)	• Potential increase in costs (e.g. if emergency treatment is required to manage status epilepticus or adverse events) • Reduced confidence in veterinary medicines and/or veterinary recommendations
Others	• Risk of accidental ingestion/overdose from medicines accumulated but not administered • Ecotoxicity if medicines are not disposed of correctly (including inadvertent ingestion by free-roaming or wild animals)

- Forgetfulness
- Lower social or practical support
- Mental health challenges faced by the owner, e.g. depression
- Difficulty administering medication to the patient
- Lack of understanding of the importance of giving medication (Maddison et al. 2021, Taylor et al. 2022)

c) When outlining a treatment regime, explain the rationale for the use of a particular medication or treatment, and the need for following up within a particular time frame. It is important for owners to understand, to the best of their ability, how the medication addresses the treated condition, as well as expected and potential adverse effects. It is also useful to explain impacts of non-adherence, e.g. continued seizures and associated complications. Then:

- Listen to the client. What are their concerns about treatment? What constraints will impact their ability to adhere to the recommendations? The treatment plan should factor in practical constraints and patient temperament. For example, orally medicating an aggressive animal may not be possible. Consider alternative formulations (e.g. liquid or paste instead of tablet), alternative routes of administration (e.g. transdermal preparation), or alternative treatment regimes (e.g. inpatient treatment during medication induction). Check whether the plan is actually workable, e.g. 'Will Clementine let you give her tablets?'
- Where possible, give the first dose in the consultation room or engage nurses to teach owners how to administer medication.
- Where possible, reduce the frequency of medication. In one study, once-daily administration of phenobarbital in cats with presumed IE resulted in remission in 88% of cats, and good seizure control in the remaining 12% (Mojarradi et al. 2023).
- Recommend pairing medication administration with a daily habit, e.g. 'Why not give Clementine the medication when you put the kettle on in the morning?'
- Consider printing a dosing chart (particularly important with tapered doses of medication) or weekly pill box, especially if multiple medications are required.

REFERENCES

Maddison, J., Cannon, M., Davies, R. & Farquhar, R. (2021) Owner compliance in veterinary practice: recommendations from a roundtable discussion. *Companion Animal* **26**(6):S1–S12. doi: 10.12968/coan.2021.0029.

Mojarradi, A., De Decker, S. & Van Meervenne, S. (2023) Once-a-day oral treatment with phenobarbital in cats with presumptive idiopathic epilepsy. *Journal of Feline Medicine and Surgery* **25**(9). doi: 10.1177/1098612x231196806.

Taylor, S., Caney, S., Bessant, C. & Gunn-Moore, D. (2022) Online survey of owners' experiences of medicating their cats at home. *Journal of Feline Medicine and Surgery* **24**(12):1283–1293. doi: 10.1177/1098612X221083752.

5.19 Otis, 4-yo MN Cocker Spaniel: ears

a) Otitis externa is one of the most common clinical presentations in canine patients. One-year prevalence of otitis externa in the UK was 7.3% in 2016 (O'Neill et al. 2021), with the Cocker Spaniel being the second most commonly affected breed (behind the Labrador). Among insured dogs in Australia, otitis externa was the most common diagnosis made (34.12 events per 1000 dog-years at risk in 2016,

34.82 events per 1000 dog-years at risk in 2017) (Wolf et al. 2020). Despite this being a common condition, otitis externa is frustrating because, while topical treatment may appear to resolve the problem in the short term, repeated cycles of inflammation and infection lead to chronic changes of the ear canal (which become perpetuating factors), pain and aversion (leading, in some cases, to incomplete examination and poor adherence to the treatment protocol), and antimicrobial resistance (leading to failure of previously successful treatments) (Nuttall 2023). Adding to the frustration in this case are the delayed presentation of Otis, with the owners hoping that the problem could be resolved by using leftover medication, and a lack of ear cleaning, which means that medication is applied to whatever is sitting in the ear canal (accumulated cerumen, biofilm, epithelial cells, and hair). It is difficult to treat affected dogs comprehensively without multiple sedation events, which increase the costs of veterinary visits. As the condition cannot be definitely cured and is likely to recur, owners may lose faith in veterinary treatment. Simply dispensing more medication is unlikely to resolve Otis's current condition, and is highly likely to increase the risk of further bouts of otitis externa that are resistant to this treatment protocol.

b) This is suppurative otitis, characterised by erythema, ulceration, and a purulent discharge. The tenacious, dark-brown slime is most likely a biofilm. The most commonly implicated agent is *Pseudomonas* spp. This is clinically different from erythroceruminous otitis, which is characterised by erythema and ceruminous to seborrhoeic otic discharge. The most commonly implicated agents are *Malassezia* yeasts and *Staphylococcus* spp.

c) C&S is not very helpful when selecting topical treatment, as the results reflect systemic antimicrobial activity and are poorly predictive of response to topical treatment (Nuttall 2023). Resistance *in vitro* does not equate to poor efficacy *in vivo*, as concentrations of topical medications are higher than those of systemic medications. Furthermore, sensitivity to agents *in vitro* does not reflect performance in the ear, where local factors such as inflammation, stenosis, the presence of biofilm, hair, and/or cerumen, and other predisposing/ primary/perpetuating factors can thwart efficacy (Nuttall 2023).

d) Treatment of otitis externa can be divided into an induction or reactive phase, which addresses immediate inflammation and infection, and a maintenance or proactive phase, which aims to prevent relapses by addressing predisposing, primary, and perpetuating factors (Table A5.19). According to Nuttall (2023), 'failure to move from induction to maintenance will increase the risk of treatment failure and progression to medically irreversible chronic otitis'. This should be explained to owners so that they appreciate the rationale for treatment.

Table A5.19 **Predisposing, primary, and perpetuating factors for otitis externa (adapted from Nuttall 2023)**

PREDISPOSING	PRIMARY	SECONDARY	PERPETUATING

• Conformation/anatomy
  ○ Pendulous pinnae
  ○ Hairy pinnae
  ○ Increased number/
    altered physiology of
    ceruminous glands
    (common in Cocker
    Spaniels)
  ○ Narrow ear canals in
    some breeds (e.g. Shar
    Pei)
• Lifestyle/husbandry
  ○ Swimming
  ○ High ambient
    temperatures/humidity
• Treatment/cleaning
  ○ Plucking of ears
  ○ Excessive cleaning of
    ears (e.g. moisture
    introduced, impaction of
    material, iatrogenic
    damage)
  ○ Dysbiosis/superinfections
	• Parasitic
	  ○ *Otodectes cynotis*
	  ○ Demodicosis
	• Foreign body
	  ○ Grass awn
	  ○ Items used to clean ears
	    (or parts of)
	• Hypersensitivity
	  ○ Atopic dermatitis
	  ○ Adverse food reactions
	  ○ Allergic or irritant contact
	    dermatitis (can be
	    triggered by ear cleaners,
	    active pharmaceutical
	    agents, or vehicles such
	    as propylene glycol)
	• Space-occupying lesions
	  ○ Inflammatory polyps
	  ○ Neoplasia, e.g.
	    ceruminous gland
	    adenoma or
	    adenocarcinoma
	• Endocrinopathy
	  ○ Hyperadrenocorticism
	  ○ Hypothyroidism
	  ○ Hypooestrogenism
	• Immunosuppression
	  ○ Primary
	  ○ Secondary
	    (glucocorticoids,
	    chemotherapy)
		• Yeasts, e.g. *Malassezia* spp.
		• Bacteria, e.g.
		  Staphylococcus spp.,
		  Pseudomonas spp., *Proteus*
		  spp., *Escherichia* spp.,
		  Klebsiella spp.
			• Nodular epidermal and
			  glandular hyperplasia
			  leading to 'cobblestone
			  appearance'
			• Epidermal and dermal
			  hyperplasia and thickening
			• Failure of epithelial
			  migration
			• Ear canal stenosis and
			  occlusion
			• Fibrosis of the skin lining
			  the ear canal
			• Mineralisation of auricular
			  cartilage
			• Otitis media
			• Cystadenomatosis
			• Cholesteatoma formation

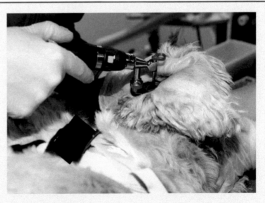

Chronic changes of the skin of the ear are perpetuating factors for otitis externa.

Tips for management of recurrent otitis externa

- All ear infections should be considered secondary, i.e. they are a form of dysbiosis.
- Examine and perform cytology on both ears, as true unilateral otitis externa is uncommon. Sedation may be required to examine and clean ears of affected dogs (Figure A5.19a).
- Perform a complete physical examination, e.g. other areas of skin may be impacted in dogs with atopic dermatitis.
- Identify and address all primary, predisposing, and perpetuating factors

Figure A5.19a Otoscopy on the left ear of a sedated dog.

Continued

and create a plan for both maintenance and managing acute flares.

- Treat pruritus. Antipruritic agents including glucocorticoids, oclacitinib, and lokivetmab can reduce pruritus, though their efficacy may be inhibited in the presence of active infection (Miller et al. 2023).
- Treat pain. Otitis externa is painful, particularly where inflammation is severe, where ulceration is present, or where *Pseudomonas* spp. are involved. It may be prudent to avoid using NSAIDs, as glucocorticoids may be required to reduce inflammation and pruritus. Additionally, paracetamol or gabapentin may be helpful. Long-acting topical agents that are left in the ears may help in such cases by providing a 'treatment holiday', but their increased viscosity can reduce spreadability within the ear canal (Song et al. 2023). They can also cause neurogenic keratoconjunctivitis sicca.

- Explain the anatomy of the canine ear to the owners, as this can help them better understand the pathophysiology of otitis externa and potential challenges to treatment success (Figure A5.19b,c).
- Demonstrate appropriate ear-cleaning technique to owners and encourage them to reward their dogs during or immediately after each ear clean.

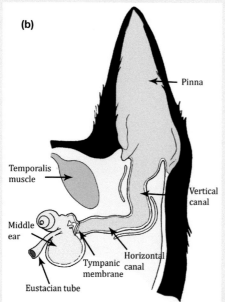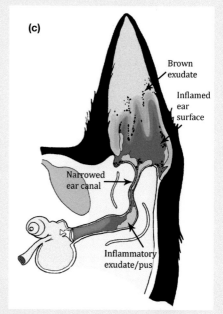

Figure A5.19b,c Schematic diagram of the anatomy of a normal canine ear (b) and an ear with otitis externa (c). Explaining the anatomy – including the L-shape of the ear canal, the vertical and horizontal ear canals, and the middle ear – can be useful in explaining how to apply topical medication, and why otitis externa may recur.

REFERENCES

Miller, J., Simpson, A., Bloom, P. et al. (2023) AAHA management of allergic skin diseases in dogs and cats guidelines. *Journal of the American Animal Hospital Association* **59**(6):255–284. doi: 10.5326/jaaha-ms-7396.

Nuttall, T. (2023) Managing recurrent otitis externa in dogs: what have we learned and what can we do better? *Journal of the American Veterinary Medical Association* **261**(S1):S10–S22. doi: 10.2460/javma.23.01.0002.

O'Neill, D. G., Volk, A. V., Soares, T. et al. (2021) Frequency and predisposing factors for canine otitis externa in the UK – a primary veterinary care epidemiological view. *Canine Medicine and Genetics* **8**(1):7. doi: 10.1186/s40575-021-00106-1.

Song, Y., Abdella, S., Afinjuomo, F. et al. (2023) Physicochemical properties of otic products for canine otitis externa: comparative analysis of marketed products. *BMC Veterinary Research* **19**:39. doi: 10.1186/s12917-023-03596-2.

Wolf, S., Selinger, J., Ward, M. P. et al. (2020) Incidence of presenting complaints and diagnoses in insured Australian dogs. *Australian Veterinary Journal* **98**(7):326–332. doi: 10.1111/avj.12981.

5.20 Ember, 7 yo FN DSH: quieter than normal, constipated?

a) The right lateral view is well exposed and positioned for the abdomen. There is gas in the colon, together with a small amount of faeces. Beneath this is a large, folded tubular soft tissue opacity, which lies between the colon and the bladder (which is small and not clearly visible). This mass displaces the small intestines cranially. This would appear to be an enlarged uterus or part thereof. Ember is however registered as a neutered female. There is no sign of constipation.

b) The next step would be to inform the owner of the findings and enquire about Ember's neuter status. As she was rehomed from a shelter this may be difficult, but it would be useful to see the clinical notes from the neutering surgery in case anything was reported as unusual. Regardless, it would be useful to take bloods for a CBC, especially looking at WBCs, since Ember is now presenting as a pyometra. If the white cell count is raised, this would be highly suggestive. An ultrasound scan will confirm the radiographic findings and might help determine the nature of the findings (e.g. one horn or both affected), although the radiographic findings are themselves sufficient and consent for exploratory laparotomy is a rational next step.

Ember did indeed have a pyometra. It was an open pyometra and Ember's perineal cleaning was attending to the discharge, which was immediately evident when the sedated Ember was palpated at the time of X-ray. On surgery, only one ovary and uterine horn were present (the right side), but she had a scar on her left flank, which suggests a partial spay had been performed, perhaps with difficulty in locating the deep (right) ovary and uterine horn in a young cat when the structure can be small. Ember's surgery proved curative.

> If partial neutering surgeries are performed for any reason (e.g. unilateral cryptorchid or partial spay as in Ember's case), it is very important to note this prominently in the record and to ensure that the client is aware and understands that additional investigation/surgery will be needed to complete the procedure or assess for congenital defects. Segmental uterine aplasia has been reported in female cats and may impact the structure, size, and location of reproductive organs, which may complicate definitive identification during routine neutering (Fawcett et al. 2009). Where normal structures are not identified, and there is no history of prior surgical removal, exploratory laparotomy or abdominal ultrasonography are recommended.

REFERENCE

Fawcett, A., Phillips, A., Sullivan, N. & Allen, G. (2009) Segmental uterine aplasia with ipsilateral renal agenesis in a mixed breed cat. *Australian Veterinary Practitioner* **39**(1):31–33.

5.21 Yuuki, 6-yo FE Chihuahua cross: UTI?

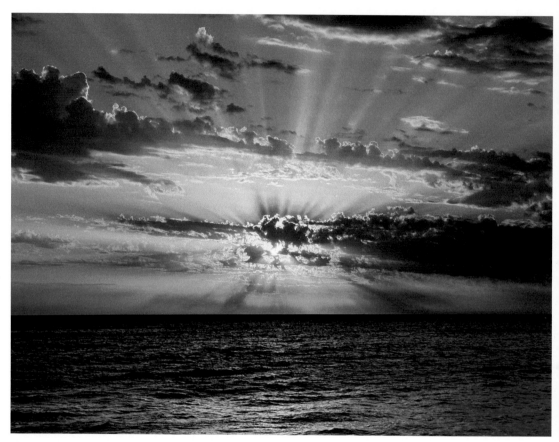

Figure A5.21 The sun setting (on a pyometra somewhere?).

a) Examples include the following phrases:
- *More is missed by not looking than by not knowing* – emphasising the importance of thorough history-taking and physical examination
- *Wounds heal side-to-side, not end-to-end* – suggesting that a larger surgical incision will not delay healing and will improve visibility during surgery
- *When you hear hoofbeats, think of horses, not zebras* – underscoring the need to consider common conditions
- *Better pred than dead* – suggesting that corticosteroids may work when other treatment options fail
- *No good deed goes unpunished* – used to warn that doing 'favours' for clients raises expectations, such that they will subsequently be disappointed and may complain
- *They don't care how much you know until they know how much you care* – emphasising the central importance of empathy and communication
- *A week too early is better than a day too late* – in relation to euthanasia, suggesting that QOL for animals is more important than quantity

Can you think of other examples?

b) Clinical pearls sound appealing, but are usually accepted on trust rather than evidence. They are generalisations that do not apply in all contexts, and in the worst cases may mislead. It has been suggested that clinical pearls come with a warning that 'use of this pearl without analysis and without clinical judgment can be dangerous to your patients and to your intellectual development' (Lorin et al. 2008).

c) This clinical pearl is based on the concern that, if not treated definitively with prompt surgery, pyometra can progress to endotoxaemia, systemic sepsis, and sequelae such as systemic inflammatory response syndrome (SIRS) (Maritato & Benaryeh 2017).

d) One key factor regarding pyometra is whether the cervix is open or closed. Closed-cervix pyometras are more commonly associated with sepsis, and with a poorer condition at presentation, than open-cervix pyometras (Jitpean et al. 2017). Another factor is the overall condition of the patient, who may require stabilisation including IV fluid resuscitation, analgesia, anti-emetics, and systemic antimicrobials prior to being taken to surgery. Another factor is resources and staffing. For example, a client may not be able to afford after-hours surgery. Or there may not be enough staff to perform the surgery safely, and the client declines referral to an after-hours facility. If a dog is bright and clinically well, with an open pyometra, it may often be possible to delay surgery until the following morning with appropriate supportive care.

REFERENCES

Jitpean, S., Ambrosen, A., Emanuelson, U. & Hagman, R. (2017) Closed cervix is associated with more severe illness in dogs with pyometra. *BMC Veterinary Research* **13**:11. doi: 10.1186/s12917-016-0924-0.

Lorin, M. I., Palazzi, D. L., Turner, T. L. & Ward, M. A. (2008) What is a clinical pearl and what is its role in medical education? *Medical Teacher* **30**(9–10):870–874. doi: 10.1080/01421590802144286.

Maritato, K. C. & Benaryeh, B. (2017) The case: the GI obstruction that wasn't. *Clinician's Brief* February 2017, www.cliniciansbrief.com/article/case-gi-obstruction-wasnt.

5.22 Ten Statements Test

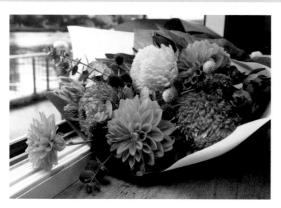

Figure A5.22a 'I am recognised and appreciated by a client.'

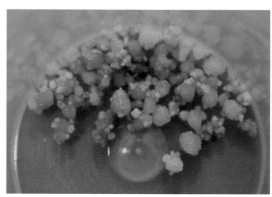

Figure A5.22b 'I remove uroliths by cystotomy.'

I derive pleasure from my work when …

1. A patient who was not eating begins to eat ravenously following treatment
2. An owner sends me a video or photos of an animal who is clearly happy at home, having recovered from illness, injury, or surgery
3. I extract all roots of a multi-rooted tooth without fracturing any
4. I locate and remove a foreign body
5. A fearful patient takes treats or accepts a reward and allows me to perform a procedure with minimal restraint
6. I feel like I've been able to support a client or colleague in making a difficult decision
7. I remove uroliths via cystotomy
8. I perform sedation and euthanasia in an animal, and they die peacefully and without distress in the presence of a loved one
9. I receive acknowledgement of a job well done from a client or colleague
10. I learn something new at a conference or webinar or wet lab and I am able to use this

(AQ)

1. I find a difficult vein and give a smooth injection
2. An animal starts to eat
3. I see the effect of a painkiller I have given
4. I defuse a difficult communication situation
5. I reflect on the animals I have helped in whatever way that day
6. I take a well-positioned X-ray
7. I make an animal comfortable in a cage or kennel
8. I am recognised and appreciated by a client
9. I slow down and remember why I am doing this
10. I read and research about the history of my profession

(AG)

REFERENCES

Cake, M. A., Bell, M. A., Bickley, N. & Bartram, D. J. (2015) The life of meaning: a model of the positive contributions to well-being from veterinary work. *Journal of Veterinary Medical Education* **42**(3):184–193. doi: 10.3138/jvme.1014-097R1.

Clise, M. H., Mathew, S. & McArthur, M. L. (2021) Sources of pleasure in veterinary work: a qualitative study. *Veterinary Record* **188**(11):e54. doi: 10.1002/vetr.54.

5.23 Sleep

a) Primary sleep deficiency can be caused by insomnia, anxiety, or sleep fragmentation (e.g. on-call duties), whereas secondary sleep deficiency is a result of an underlying medical condition (e.g. obstructive sleep apnoea). Sleep deficiency can lead to fatigue, errors, and accidents, and is associated with depression and burnout. A global survey of veterinary anaesthesia personnel (n = 393) reported high levels of poor sleep, fatigue, depressive symptoms, and burnout (Ho et al. 2023). Over half reported insufficient sleep to meet job demands, and almost three-quarters reported mistakes due to work-related fatigue. Concerningly, almost 90% reported driving while fatigued, putting them at risk of motor vehicle accidents. A study of veterinary house officers (n = 303) (Scharf et al. 2022) found that they slept much less when they had clinical responsibilities than when they had time off clinics (6.0 versus 7.5 hours). Longer working hours were negatively correlated with sleep quantity, and perceived sleep quality was worse during on-call periods (Scharf et al. 2022). Most perceived that fatigue negatively impacted technical skills, clinical judgement, and ability to empathise, with the authors concluding that most house officers failed to get enough sleep for optimal cognitive function and health. In a cohort of doctor of veterinary medicine (DVM) students (n = 187), over half reported getting <7 hours of sleep per night, almost 30% had trouble sleeping, and half reported feeling sleepy all day (Royal et al. 2018). Only one in 20 reported excellent sleep quality. A prospective study of veterinary students over a 12-month period (n = 308) reported overall poor sleep quality

and higher than normal daytime sleepiness across the academic year (Nappier et al. 2019). This could negatively impact student learning, morale, and wellbeing.

Our bodies require sleep, just as they need oxygen, food, and water to function. During sleep, the body heals itself and restores its chemical and energy balance. In a driving simulation study, sleep deprivation had a greater impact on driving performance than a breath alcohol reading over the legal limit (Lowrie & Brownlow 2020). Sleep-deprived drivers had slower reaction times and poorer vehicle control than those exposed to alcohol. Coffee did not improve performance in the sleep-deprived – indeed, performance seemed to be worse following exposure to coffee. Sleep deficiency can be short term or chronic, although there is some debate about what constitutes chronic sleep deficiency (De Bruin & Dewald-Kaufmann 2021). Chronic sleep deficiency has been associated with increased risks of obesity and diabetes, and may also impact cardiovascular disease, cognitive function, emotional regulation, general health, and risk of mortality.

b) Possible signs of sleep deficiency are listed in Table A5.23. The signs and symptoms of chronic sleep deficiency vary in nature and severity depending on a myriad of individual and contextual circumstances. Altogether, however, it is known that sleep deprivation to any degree has significant impacts on our personal and professional wellbeing.

c) The term 'sleep hygiene' refers to good habits, behaviours, and environmental factors that can be modified to improve sleep quality and quantity.

Table A5.23 **Examples of signs of sleep deficiency**		
PHYSICAL	**COGNITIVE**	**EMOTIONAL**
• Dark circles under eyes • Yawning • Head-nodding • Inability to keep eyes open/'microsleeps' • Headache • Changes in appetite • Cravings, e.g. for caffeine • Lack of energy to perform routine tasks • Reduced balance/coordination • Hand tremors • Changes in sleep patterns, e.g. falling asleep when not intending to • Muscle aches and pains • Waking up feeling exhausted • Increased risk of chronic conditions, e.g. hypertension, diabetes, hypercholesterolaemia, obesity	• Difficulty concentrating/maintaining attention • Poor/slow decision-making • Difficulty problem-solving • Increased tendency to make errors • Impaired recall • False memories • Reduced awareness/responsiveness • Increased risk of accidents	• Irritability • Increased emotional reactivity • Lack of motivation • Reduced ability to cope • Changes in mood, e.g. feeling depressed, anxious • May also experience paranoia, suicidal ideation • Significant sleep deprivation can induce psychosis, which can change perception of reality, leading to disorganised thoughts and speech, hallucinations, delusions, and distress

HABITS

- Schedule time for rest.
- Restrict daytime naps to 20 minutes or less, so that they don't interfere with regular sleep.
- Create a bedtime ritual, e.g. have a hot bath or shower, enjoy a herbal tea, set up for your morning routine before turning the lights off.
- Where possible, set devices such as smartphones aside 1 hour before going to sleep.
- Wind down and go to bed at around the same time each night – including on weekends.
- Get up at the same time each morning – including on weekends.
- Keep a notebook beside the bed that can be used to write down things you remember or things you are worried about, which can be dealt with when you're awake.
- Use relaxation techniques, such as guided meditation, deep breathing, or progressive muscle relaxation, to help you get to sleep.
- If you cannot sleep for 20 minutes or more, get up and do something relaxing such as reading or listening to music. Then return to bed when you are sleepy. This helps break an association between your bed and worrying about not getting to sleep.

HEALTHY BEHAVIOURS

- Avoid alcohol, sugary beverages, caffeine, nicotine, and stimulants for several hours before bed, and minimise intake of these where possible. Herbal tea such as camomile may help.
- Get regular exercise each day – even a brisk walk for 30 minutes. Avoid exercise for 90 minutes before sleeping.
- Spend some time outdoors each day.
- Eat more fibre and minimise ingestion of saturated fats and carbs before sleep.

ENVIRONMENT

- Invest in a good-quality mattress, pillows, and bedding, and ensure sheets are washed regularly.
- If possible, only use the bedroom for sleep and sex.

- Eliminate blue lights, which can disrupt sleep. Maintain darkness by covering small indicator lights and using an eye mask, blackout blinds, or heavy curtains.
- Consider a food dispenser with an automatic timer to feed animals that might otherwise wake you in the night.
- A white-noise generator may be helpful.
- If environmental noise is an issue, use ear plugs.

GETTING HELP

- Apps featuring guided meditations or peaceful sounds help.
- Make an appointment with your GP to explore management of primary and secondary sleep deficiency. Treatment depends on the underlying cause(s). These can include conditions such as chronic pain, gastrointestinal issues, and upper respiratory infection; sleep disorders such as obstructive sleep apnoea, restless leg syndrome, circadian rhythm disorders, and insomnia; and mental health conditions, including bipolar disorder, depression, anxiety, attention-deficit/hyperactivity disorder, and post-traumatic stress disorder. Pregnancy can also interfere with sleep.
- Your GP can refer you to a sleep specialist.
- Allied health professionals such as physiotherapists can help treat musculoskeletal pain.

Getting a decent sleep makes a huge difference to how we feel. It can improve concentration, productivity, and mood. It helps aid memory retention, which helps us learn new information and skills, which allows us to better care for our patients. Adequate sleep (at least 8 hours per night) promotes healing, restoration, and homeostasis of the cardiovascular, musculoskeletal, central nervous, and endocrine systems. It increases our resilience and helps contribute to healthy energy levels to meet the demands of veterinary work. And healthy sleep fortifies the crucial communications between neurons comprising the brain's signalling network. The lapses in memory and problems concentrating due to chronic fatigue could result in self-injury, medical mistakes, and impairment overall in functioning in the world. Daytime drowsiness and microsleep episodes are less likely to occur … such as while you are driving home after a long shift.

REFERENCES

De Bruin, E. J. & Dewald-Kaufmann, J. F. (2021) What is 'chronic' in 'chronic sleep reduction' and what are its consequences? A systematic scoping review of the literature. *Current Sleep Medicine Reports* 7:129–154. doi: 10.1007/s40675-021-00214-1.

Ho, N. T. Z., Santoro, F., Palacious Jimenez, C. & Pelligand, L. (2023) Cross-sectional survey of sleep, fatigue and mental health in veterinary anaesthesia personnel. *Veterinary Anaesthesia and Analgesia* 50(4):315–324. doi: 10.1016/j.vaa.2023.03.003.

Lowrie, J. & Brownlow, H. (2020) The impact of sleep deprivation and alcohol on driving: a comparative study. *BMC Public Health* 20(1):980. doi: 10.1186/s12889-020-09095-5.

Nappier, M. T., Bartl-Wilson, L., Shoop, T. & Borowski, S. (2019) Sleep quality and sleepiness among veterinary medical students over an academic year. *Frontiers in Veterinary Science* 6:119. doi: 10.3389/fvets.2019.00119.

Royal, K. D., Hunt, S. A., Borst, L. B. & Gerard, M. (2018) Sleep hygiene among veterinary medical students. *Journal of Education and Health Promotion* 7:47. doi: 10.4103/jehp.jehp_114_17.

Scharf, V. F., McPhetridge, J. B. & Dickson, R. (2022) Sleep patterns, fatigue, and working hours among veterinary house officers: a cross-sectional survey study. *Journal of the American Veterinary Medical Association* 260(11):1377–1385. doi: 10.2460/javma.21.05.0234.

Page numbers in **bold** refer to discussion in the answers; those in Roman relate to the questions, where there is often a photograph.